Register Now for Online Access to Your Book!

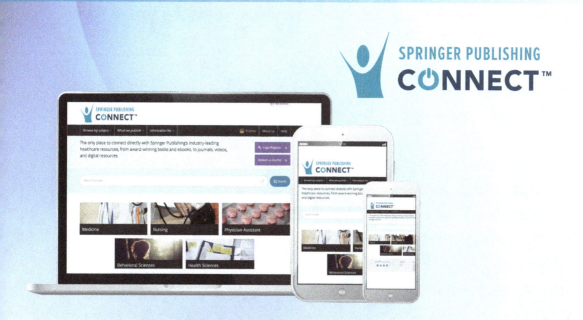

Your print purchase of *Symptom Management Guidelines for Oncology Nursing,* **includes online access to the contents of your book**—increasing accessibility, portability, and searchability!

Access today at:
http://connect.springerpub.com/content/reference-book/978-0-8261-8524-2
or scan the QR code at the right with your smartphone. Log in or register, then click "Redeem a voucher" and use the code below.

UEU8NGCJ

Scan here for quick access.

Having trouble redeeming a voucher code?
Go to https://connect.springerpub.com/redeeming-voucher-code
If you are experiencing problems accessing the digital component of this product, please contact our customer service department at cs@springerpub.com
The online access with your print purchase is available at the publisher's discretion and may be removed at any time without notice.
Publisher's Note: New and used products purchased from third-party sellers are not guaranteed for quality, authenticity, or access to any included digital components.

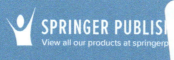

Symptom Management Guidelines for Oncology Nursing

Anne Katz, PhD, RN, FAAN, is a certified sexuality counselor at CancerCare Manitoba and a clinical nurse specialist at the Manitoba Prostate Centre. She has authored more than 15 books, including most recently *Woman Cancer Sex* (Second Edition) by Routledge, and numerous journal articles. She also served as the editor of the cancer research journal *Oncology Nursing Forum*. She has been an invited speaker at multiple international conferences and meetings in North America, Europe, and beyond where she has educated healthcare providers and cancer survivors about cancer, sexuality, and survivorship. She was inducted into the American Academy of Nursing in 2014.

Symptom Management Guidelines for Oncology Nursing

Anne Katz, PhD, RN, FAAN

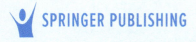

Copyright © 2025 Springer Publishing Company, LLC
All rights reserved.

No part of this publication may be reproduced, stored in a retrieval system, or transmitted in any form or by any means, electronic, mechanical, photocopying, recording, or otherwise, without the prior permission of Springer Publishing Company, LLC, or authorization through payment of the appropriate fees to the Copyright Clearance Center, Inc., 222 Rosewood Drive, Danvers, MA 01923, 978-750-8400, fax 978-646-8600, info@copyright.com or at www.copyright.com.

Springer Publishing Company, LLC
www.springerpub.com
connect.springerpub.com

Acquisitions Editor: John Zaphyr
Production Editor: Joseph Stubenrauch
Compositor: diacriTech

ISBN: 978-0-8261-8527-3
ebook ISBN: 978-0-8261-8528-0
DOI: 9780826185280

SUPPLEMENTS:

 A robust set of instructor resources designed to supplement this text is located at http://connect.springerpub.com/content/reference-book/978-0-8261-8524-2. Qualifying Instructors may request access by emailing **textbook@springerpub.com**.

Instructor PowerPoint Presentations ISBN: 978-0-8261-8529-7

Printed by LSI

The author and the publisher of this Work have made every effort to use sources believed to be reliable to provide information that is accurate and compatible with the standards generally accepted at the time of publication. Because medical science is continually advancing, our knowledge base continues to expand. Therefore, as new information becomes available, changes in procedures become necessary. We recommend that the reader always consult current research and specific institutional policies before performing any clinical procedure or delivering any medication. The author and publisher shall not be liable for any special, consequential, or exemplary damages resulting, in whole or in part, from the readers' use of, or reliance on, the information contained in this book. The publisher has no responsibility for the persistence or accuracy of URLs for external or third-party Internet websites referred to in this publication and does not guarantee that any content on such websites is, or will remain, accurate or appropriate.

Library of Congress Cataloging-in-Publication Data

Name: Katz, Anne (Anne Jennifer), 1958- author.
Title: Symptom management guidelines for oncology nursing / Anne Katz.
Description: New York, NY : Springer Publishing, [2024] | Includes index.
Identifiers: LCCN 2023053143 (print) | LCCN 2023053144 (ebook) | ISBN 9780826185273 (paperback) | ISBN 9780826185280 (ebook)
Subjects: MESH: Neoplasms–nursing | Oncology Nursing–methods | Symptom Assessment–nursing | Patient Care Management–methods
Classification: LCC RC266 (print) | LCC RC266 (ebook) | NLM WY 156 | DDC 616.99/40231–dc23/eng/20240105
LC record available at https://lccn.loc.gov/2023053143
LC ebook record available at https://lccn.loc.gov/2023053144

Contact sales@springerpub.com to receive discount rates on bulk purchases.

Publisher's Note: **New and used products purchased from third-party sellers are not guaranteed for quality, authenticity, or access to any included digital components.**

Eternal ISBN for reference work: 978-0-8261-8524-2

Printed in the United States of America.

This book is dedicated to oncology nurses who care for men and women using the experience accumulated through hours of direct patient care and the best evidence we can find.

Contents

Preface   ix
Acknowledgments   xi
Springer Publishing Resources   xiii

SECTION I: INTRODUCTION TO SYMPTOM MANAGEMENT

Chapter 1   Introduction   3
Chapter 2   Measuring Symptoms   5

SECTION II: GENERAL SYMPTOMS

Chapter 3   Cancer-Related Fatigue   15
Chapter 4   Cancer Pain   25
Chapter 5   Sleep Disturbances   43
Chapter 6   Lymphedema   55
Chapter 7   Alopecia   67
Chapter 8   Xerostomia and Oral Mucositis   75
Chapter 9   Fever   85
Chapter 10   Hot Flashes   89

SECTION III: GASTROINTESTINAL SYMPTOMS

Chapter 11   Constipation   101
Chapter 12   Diarrhea   107
Chapter 13   Nausea and Vomiting   115
Chapter 14   Anorexia and Cachexia   125
Chapter 15   Dysphagia   137

SECTION IV: GENITOURINARY SYMPTOMS

Chapter 16   Incontinence   145
Chapter 17   Sexual Dysfunction in Women   161

viii CONTENTS

Chapter 18	Sexual Dysfunction in Men	183

SECTION V: PULMONARY SYMPTOMS

Chapter 19	Dyspnea	197
Chapter 20	Hemoptysis	207

SECTION VI: NEUROLOGIC SYMPTOMS

Chapter 21	Hearing Loss	213
Chapter 22	Peripheral Neuropathy	219
Chapter 23	Cognitive Dysfunction	227

SECTION VII: CUTANEOUS SYMPTOMS

Chapter 24	Skin and Nail Changes	237

SECTION VIII: PSYCHOSOCIAL SYMPTOMS

Chapter 25	Anxiety	249
Chapter 26	Depression	257
Chapter 27	Distress	267
Chapter 28	Answers to Case Studies	275

Index   285

Preface

The oncology nurse provides comprehensive clinical care to patients with cancer and their families along the disease trajectory, from initial diagnosis to end of life. The care of these patients is often complex, with various and sometimes concurrent symptoms and side effects that nurses must manage. To provide optimum care for the best patient outcomes, clinicians need the latest evidence-based information. With 22 million people expected to be living with cancer by 2030, nurses working outside oncology settings must be prepared for the care of the individual with cancer. *Symptom Management Guidelines for Oncology Nursing* uses a systems-based approach addressing common symptoms experienced by patients with cancer during and after treatment. This new text provides evidence-based clinical guidelines for key pharmaceutical and supportive interventions in an easy-to-read format that clinicians can use in their daily practice.

Each section of the book offers a comprehensive examination of common cancer symptoms, offering clinical guidance on evidence-based management. Included are sections on general symptoms (fatigue, pain, alopecia), as well as gastrointestinal (nausea and vomiting, diarrhea, constipation), genitourinary (incontinence, sexuality), pulmonary (dyspnea, hemoptysis), neurologic (hearing loss, peripheral neuropathy), cutaneous (nail and skin disorders), and psychosocial (anxiety, depression, distress) symptoms. Each chapter explores issues such as prevalence, contributing factors, assessment, and management, and also includes a case study and questions. The text also addresses symptom assessment and measurement. *Symptom Management Guidelines for Oncology Nursing* is suitable for nurses specializing in oncology, as well as for clinicians who care for cancer patients in their practice.

Anne Katz, PhD, RN, FAAN

Acknowledgments

To two men who have encouraged and supported me through the years.

Dr. Alan Katz who has read every word of everything I have written and published.

John Zaphyr whose first word is almost always "yes" when I send him a book proposal.

My gratitude comes from the very last cell in my left ventricle.

Springer Publishing Resources

A robust set of instructor resources designed to supplement this text is located at http://connect.springerpub.com/content/reference-book/978-0-8261-8524-2. Qualifying Instructors may request access by emailing **textbook@springerpub.com**.

INSTRUCTOR RESOURCES

Available resources include:

- Instructor PowerPoint Presentations

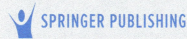

Visit https://connect.springerpub.com/ and look for the "**Show Supplementary**" button on the **book homepage**.

I

Introduction to Symptom Management

CHAPTER 1

INTRODUCTION

INTRODUCTION

The oncology nurse and most specifically the APRN provide comprehensive care for the person with cancer and their family. Cancer care has become increasingly complex with new treatment agents and protocols emerging constantly, all to the benefit of patients. However, treatments come with side effects and oncology nurses need to know how to both assess and manage symptoms in patients they care for. To do this, we need evidence-based interventions that are effective and provided in a timely manner.

The oncology nurse and APRN are immersed in the daily care of patients but nurses outside of specialized units and clinics will also see patients with symptoms related to their cancer and its treatment. This book will provide guidance in the management of symptoms, often from side effects of cancer treatments, that may not be top of mind when presented to the nononcology nurse.

The book is divided into eight sections.

Section I contains a chapter on measuring symptoms using patient-reported measures. These are useful in learning the patient's perspective of a wide variety of symptoms and their experience of these symptoms but also in designing studies that highlight the outcomes and patient experience of treatment.

Section II presents guidance on the management of general symptoms such as pain, fatigue, fever, and so on. Most patients with cancer will experience these symptoms as a result of treatment at some point in the cancer trajectory.

Section III contains information about gastrointestinal symptoms such as nausea and vomiting, alterations in bowel function, weight loss, and dysphagia.

Section IV addresses genitourinary symptoms including incontinence and problems with sexual function for both men and women.

Pulmonary symptoms (dyspnea and hemoptysis) are identified in Section V. Neurologic symptoms such as cognitive changes, hearing loss, and peripheral neuropathy are presented in Section VI.

Skin and nail changes are distressing to patients and these are described in Section VII.

Finally, in Section VIII psychosocial symptoms such as anxiety, depression, and distress are presented with guidance on interventions.

This book aims to provide evidence-based guidance in an easy to read format that addresses the most common symptoms we see in practice, both inpatient and outpatient, in hospital, clinic, and the community. "Need to know" information is presented in text boxes, and case studies and review questions are included to enhance learning and understanding.

 A robust set of instructor resources designed to supplement this text is located at http://connect.springerpub.com/content/reference-book/978-0-8261-8524-2. Qualifying Instructors may request access by emailing **textbook@springerpub.com**.

CHAPTER 2

MEASURING SYMPTOMS

INTRODUCTION

Clinical assessment can be enhanced by the use of patient-reported measures. The most well-known of these are patient-reported outcomes (PROs), using patient-reported outcome measures (PROMs); and patient-reportsed experience measures (PREMs), which provide the patient's perspective of their symptoms and care experience.

PATIENT-REPORTED OUTCOMES

PROs are important when trying to understand the voice of the patient. This is especially important in oncology because most patients experience physical and psychosocial symptoms as consequences of treatment and these may be underrecognized and undertreated (Howell et al., 2015). There is increasing evidence that measuring PROs in clinical care has many benefits (Chen et al., 2013), including but not limited to the clinician's understanding of the patient's experience of symptoms that require intervention during and between clinic visits (Basch et al., 2009). Other benefits include enhanced communication between healthcare clinicians and patients, managing symptoms between clinic visits, and improving patient outcomes (Watson et al., 2021).

Subjective patient-reported symptoms include health-related quality of life, mental health issues, adherence to medications, physical functioning, and bothersome symptoms. Historically used in clinical research where a core set of 12 symptoms were recommended to be measured (Reeve et al., 2014), it is now recognized that PROs should be included in routine clinical care (Ishaque et al., 2019), both in person at clinic visits as well as between visits using e-technology electronic patient-reported outcome measures (ePROMs).

PATIENT-REPORTED OUTCOME MEASURES

A large number of PROMs have been developed to measure a wide variety of symptoms in physical, emotional, and social health, as

6 SECTION I • INTRODUCTION TO SYMPTOM MANAGEMENT

well as the quality of life affected by cancer treatment (Howell et al., 2013). Those listed in Figure 2.1 represent a daunting number of tools. Clinicians should familiarize themselves with a few of these so that they can become comfortable with their use. These may be specific measures or more global measures of well-being.

1. Physical Health

a. Physical function
  i. Medical Outcomes Study-Physical Function Scale
  ii. ECOG Performance Status
  iii. Sickness Impact Profile
b. Symptom experience
  i. Overall Symptom Experience Measures
    1. Memorial symptom assessment scale
    2. MD Anderson symptom inventory
    3. ESAS
  ii. Pain
    1. Brief pain inventory
    2. McGill pain questionnaire
    3. Numeric rating scales
    4. Pain-O-meter
    5. Visual analog scale
  iii. Fatigue
    1. Cancer fatigue scale
    2. Revised piper fatigue scale
    3. Multidimensional fatigue symptom inventory
    4. FACT-fatigue
    5. Brief fatigue inventory
  iv. Nausea/Vomiting
    1. Functional living index emesis
    2. Index of nausea, vomiting, and retching
  v. Dyspnea
    1. Cancer dyspnea scale
  vi. Sleep/Wake Function Disturbance
    1. Pittsburgh sleep quality index
    2. Insomnia severity index
  vii. Sexual Function
    1. Derogatis interview for sexual functioning
    2. Sexual function questionnaire
    3. International index of erectile dysfunction

2. Emotional Health

a. Emotional distress/negative affect
  i. Anxiety
    1. HADS
    2. Profile of mood states—short form
    3. Spielberger state–trait anxiety scale
  ii. Depression
    1. HADS
    2. Center for epidemiological study (CES)-depression scale
    3. Profile of mood states-SF
b. Cognitive function
  i. FACT-cog
c. Psychological adjustment
  i. Overall Psychological Adjustment
    1. Mental adjustment to cancer (MAC) scale
    2. Mini MAC scale
  ii. Coping
    1. Cancer coping questionnaire
    2. Ways of coping questionnaire
    3. COPE-SF
  iii. Self-Concept/Body Image
    1. Body image scale
  iv. Subjective Well-Being
    1. Benefit finding scale
    2. Posttraumatic growth inventory

3. Social Health

a. Social health
  i. Social Function
    1. Psychosocial adjustment to illness
  ii. Social Support/Relationships
    1. Medical outcomes study social support survey
b. Quality of life
  i. Health-Related Quality of Life
    1. EORTC QLQ-C30
    2. FACT—general
    3. McGill QOL questionnaire
    4. Functional living index cancer
    5. Quick functional living index cancer
    6. Cancer care monitor

Figure 2.1 Patient-reported outcome domain framework and outcome measures.

PROMs are used in a variety of patient populations, including

- advanced cancer and palliative care (Kaufmann et al., 2022; Ratti et al., 2022; van Roij et al., 2018),

- skin cancer (Lee et al., 2013; Reinhardt et al., 2022),

- breast cancer (Salas et al., 2022; Srour et al., 2022; van Egdom et al., 2019),

- lung cancer (King-Kallimanis et al., 2018; Liao et al., 2022; Maguire et al., 2013),

- cancers in the pelvis and abdomen (Moss et al., 2021; Vistad, 2019),

- brain cancer (Romero et al., 2015),

- esophageal cancer (Straatman et al., 2016), and

- bladder cancer (Mason et al., 2018).

PROMs provide a patient-focused, reliable, and clinically relevant perspective on what the patient is experiencing (Bennett et al., 2012). When the data from PROMs are systematically collected, analysis of the data can be used to inform policies, planning of health services, performance measurement, and quality improvement (Canadian Institute for Health Information [CIHI, n.d.]).

Electronic Patient-Reported Outcome Measures

ePROMs are increasingly being used rather than pencil-and-paper questionnaires. Measures can be completed at home by patients, and symptoms or changes in symptoms are reported in real time. ePROMs allow for accurate reporting of symptoms and are available on a wide variety of devices (smartphones, tablets, personal computers, and wearable medical devices). When monitored by nurses, alerts for grades 3 or 4 side effects can be acted on promptly (Basch et al., 2016).

Barriers

Barriers to the use of PROMs have been identified by healthcare clinicians (Graupner et al., 2021). They include lack of time to read and interpret completed measures, lack of knowledge on how to use them, lack of IT (information technology) support, and administrative burden. Other concerns include challenges integrating PROMs and PROs into clinical workflows and not being able to act on the data obtained from these measures (Nguyen et al., 2021).

PATIENT-REPORTED EXPERIENCE MEASURES

PREMs are designed to capture the patient's perspective of the care they received during a clinical interaction (Bull et al., 2022). There are relational (provision of support, being treated with dignity and respect, being involved in treatment decisions) and functional (effective treatment, being treated in a timely manner, availability of physical support needs) aspects of the patient experience. PREMs are different from satisfaction measures in that they are subjective descriptions of experiences rather than comparisons with expectations (Kingsley & Patel, 2017). An example of a PREM is the Consultation and Relational Empathy (CARE) patient feedback measure (Mercer et al., 2004), a 10-item questionnaire that uses a Likert scale (from poor to excellent; Figure 2.2).

PREMs have been used in oncology settings, primarily to evaluate oncology services at a national level or to evaluate a specific intervention; however, data on the impact of their use are limited (Cook et al., 2020). PREMs also provide an opportunity for individual clinicians to receive patient feedback to support quality improvement.

Limitations with the use of PREMs have been identified (Manary et al., 2013) to include confounding factors not related to the quality of care and reflecting the patient's expectations of care rather than their actual experience.

How Was The Healthcare Provider At . . .

1. Making you feel at ease
2. Letting you tell your story
3. Really listening
4. Being interested in you as a whole person
5. Fully understanding your concerns
6. Showing care and compassion
7. Being positive
8. Explaining things clearly
9. Helping you to take control
10. Making a plan of action with you

Figure 2.2 Consultation and Relational Empathy patient feedback measure.

Source: From Mercer, S. W., Maxwell, M., Heaney, D., & Watt, G. C. M. (2004). The Consultation and Relational Empathy (CARE) measure: Development and preliminary validation and reliability of an empathy-based consultation process measure. *Family Practice, 21*(6), 699–705. https://doi.org/10.1093/fampra/cmh621.

RESOURCES

Examples of PROMs and PREMs are presented in the following:

Patient-Reported Outcome Measures

- www.cihi.ca/en/patient-reported-outcome-measures-proms
- www.patientreportedoutcomes.ca/what-are-pros/prom-examples/
- www.oecd.org/health/paris/OECD-PaRIS-PROMs-for-breast-cancer-care.pdf
- www.prom-select.eu/
- www.qportfolio.org/breast-q/breast-cancer/

Patient-Reported Experience Measures

- www.bqs.de/en/leistungen/picker-befragungen/patient-reported-experience-measures-prems.php

- www.cihi.ca/en/patient-experience/patient-reported-experience-measures-prems-frequently-asked-questions

A robust set of instructor resources designed to supplement this text is located at http://connect.springerpub.com/content/reference-book/978-0-8261-8524-2. Qualifying Instructors may request access by emailing **textbook@springerpub.com**.

REFERENCES

Basch, E., Deal, A. M., Kris, M. G., Scher, H. I., Hudis, C. A., Sabbatini, P., Rogak, L., Bennett, A. V., Dueck, A. C., Atkinson, T. M., Chou, J. F., Dulko, D., Sit, L., Barz, A., Novotny, P., Fruscione, M., Sloan, J. A., & Schrag, D. (2016). Symptom monitoring with patient-reported outcomes during routine cancer treatment: A randomized controlled trial. *Journal of Clinical Oncology, 34*(6), 557–565. https://doi.org/10.1200/jco.2015.63.0830

Basch, E., Jia, X., Heller, G., Barz, A., Sit, L., Fruscione, M., Appawu, M., Iasonos, A., Atkinson, T., Goldfarb, S., Culkin, A., Kris, M. G., & Schrag, D. (2009). Adverse symptom event reporting by patients vs clinicians: Relationships with clinical outcomes. *JNCI: Journal of the National Cancer Institute, 101*(23), 1624–1632. https://doi.org/10.1093/jnci/djp386

Bennett, A. V., Jensen, R. E., & Basch, E. (2012). Electronic patient-reported outcome systems in oncology clinical practice. *CA: A Cancer Journal for Clinicians, 62*(5), 336–347. https://doi.org/10.3322/caac.21150

Bull, C., Teede, H., Watson, D., & Callander, E. J. (2022). Selecting and implementing patient-reported outcome and experience measures to assess health system performance. *JAMA Health Forum, 3*(4), e220326. https://doi.org/10.1001/jamahealthforum.2022.0326

CIHI, Canadian Institute for Health Information. (n.d.). *Patient-reported outcome measures (PROMs)*. https://www.cihi.ca/en/patient-reported-outcome-measures-proms

Chen, J., Ou, L., & Hollis, S. J. (2013). A systematic review of the impact of routine collection of patient reported outcome measures on patients, providers and health organisations in an oncologic setting. *BMC Health Services Research, 13*(1), 211. https://doi.org/10.1186/1472-6963-13-211

Cook, O., Daiyan, Y., Yeganeh, L., Davies, A. G., Kwok, A., Webber, K., & Segelov, E. (2020). Exploration of the use and impact of patient-reported experience measures (PREMs) in oncology settings: A systematic review. *Journal of Clinical Oncology, 38*(29_suppl), 166–166. https://doi.org/10.1200/JCO.2020.38.29_suppl.166

Graupner, C., Breukink, S. O., Mul, S., Claessens, D., Slok, A. H. M., & Kimman, M. L. (2021). Patient-reported outcome measures in oncology: A qualitative study of the healthcare professional's perspective. *Supportive Care in Cancer*, 29(9), 5253–5261. https://doi.org/10.1007/s00520-021-06052-9

Howell, D., Fitch, M., Bakker, D., Green, E., Sussman, J., Mayo, S., Mohammed, S., Lee, C., & Doran, D. (2013). Core domains for a person-focused outcome measurement system in cancer (PROMS-Cancer Core) for routine care: A scoping review and Canadian Delphi consensus. *Value in Health*, 16(1), 76–87. https://doi.org/10.1016/j.jval.2012.10.017

Howell, D., Molloy, S., Wilkinson, K., Green, E., Orchard, K., Wang, K., & Liberty, J. (2015). Patient-reported outcomes in routine cancer clinical practice: A scoping review of use, impact on health outcomes, and implementation factors. *Annals of Oncology*, 26(9), 1846–1858. https://doi.org/10.1093/annonc/mdv181

Ishaque, S., Karnon, J., Chen, G., Nair, R., & Salter, A. B. (2019). A systematic review of randomised controlled trials evaluating the use of patient-reported outcome measures (PROMs). *Quality of Life Research*, 28(3), 567–592. https://doi.org/10.1007/s11136-018-2016-z

Kaufmann, T. L., Rocque, G. B., Kvale, E. A., Kamal, A., Pignone, M., Bennett, A. V., Saxton, J., Hernandez, R.-K., & Stover, A. M. (2022). Development of a patient-reported outcome measure (PROM) screening strategy for early palliative care needs in outpatients with advanced cancer. *Journal of Clinical Oncology*, 40(28_suppl), 203–203. https://doi.org/10.1200/JCO.2022.40.28_suppl.203

King-Kallimanis, B. L., Kanapuru, B., Blumenthal, G. M., Theoret, M. R., & Kluetz, P. G. (2018). Age-related differences in patient-reported outcomes in patients with advanced lung cancer receiving anti-PD-1/PD-L1 therapy. *Seminars in Oncology*, 45(4), 201–209. https://doi.org/10.1053/j.seminoncol.2018.06.003

Kingsley, C., & Patel, S. (2017). Patient-reported outcome measures and patient-reported experience measures. *BJA Education*, 17(4), 137–144. https://doi.org/10.1093/bjaed/mkw060

Lee, E. H., Klassen, A. F., Nehal, K. S., Cano, S. J., Waters, J., & Pusic, A. L. (2013). A systematic review of patient-reported outcome instruments of nonmelanoma skin cancer in the dermatologic population. *Journals of the American Academy of Dermatology*, 69(2), e59–e67. https://doi.org/10.1016/j.jaad.2012.09.017

Liao, K., Wang, T., Coomber-Moore, J., Wong, D. C., Gomes, F., Faivre-Finn, C., Sperrin, M., Yorke, J., & van der Veer, S. N. (2022). Prognostic value of patient-reported outcome measures (PROMs) in adults with non-small cell Lung Cancer: A scoping review. *BMC Cancer*, 22(1), 1076. https://doi.org/10.1186/s12885-022-10151-z

Maguire, R., Kotronoulas, G., Papadopoulou, C., Simpson, M. F., McPhelim, J., & Irvine, L. (2013). Patient-reported outcome measures for the identification of supportive care needs in people with lung cancer: Are we there yet? *Cancer Nursing*, 36(4), E1–E17. https://doi.org/10.1097/NCC.0b013e31826f3c8f

Manary, M. P., Boulding, W., Staelin, R., & Glickman, S. W. (2013). The patient experience and health outcomes. *The New England Journal of Medicine, 368*, 201–203. https://doi.org/10.1056/NEJMp1211775

Mason, S. J., Catto, J. W. F., Downing, A., Bottomley, S. E., Glaser, A. W., & Wright, P. (2018). Evaluating patient-reported outcome measures (PROMs) for bladder cancer: A systematic review using the COnsensus-based Standards for the selection of health Measurement INstruments (COSMIN) checklist. *BJU International, 122*(5), 760–773. https://doi.org/10.1111/bju.14368

Mercer, S. W., Maxwell, M., Heaney, D., & Watt, G. C. M. (2004). The consultation and relational empathy (CARE) measure: Development and preliminary validation and reliability of an empathy-based consultation process measure. *Family Practice, 21*(6), 699–705. https://doi.org/10.1093/fampra/cmh621

Moss, M. C. L., Aggarwal, A., Qureshi, A., Taylor, B., Guerrero-Urbano, T., & Van Hemelrijck, M. (2021). An assessment of the use of patient reported outcome measurements (PROMs) in cancers of the pelvic abdominal cavity: Identifying oncologic benefit and an evidence-practice gap in routine clinical practice. *Health and Quality of Life Outcomes, 19*(1), 20. https://doi.org/10.1186/s12955-020-01648-x

Nguyen, H., Butow, P., Dhillon, H., & Sundaresan, P. (2021). A review of the barriers to using Patient-Reported Outcomes (PROs) and Patient-Reported Outcome Measures (PROMs) in routine cancer care. *Journal of Medical Radiation Sciences, 68*(2), 186–195. https://doi.org/10.1002/jmrs.421

Ratti, M. M., Gandaglia, G., Sisca, E. S., Derevianko, A., Alleva, E., Beyer, K., Moss, C., Barletta, F., Scuderi, S., Omar, M. I., MacLennan, S., Williamson, P. R., Zong, J., MacLennan, S. J., Mottet, N., Cornford, P., Aiyegbusi, O. L., Van Hemelrijck, M., N'Dow, J., & Briganti, A. (2022). A systematic review to evaluate patient-reported outcome measures (PROMs) for metastatic prostate cancer according to the consensus-based standard for the selection of health measurement instruments (COSMIN) methodology. *Cancers, 14*, 5120. https://doi.org/10.3390/cancers14205120

Reeve, B. B., Mitchell, S. A., Dueck, A. C., Basch, E., Cella, D., Reilly, C. M., Minasian, L. M., Denicoff, A. M., O'Mara, A. M., Fisch, M. J., Chauhan, C., Aaronson, N. K., Coens, C., & Bruner, D. W. (2014). Recommended patient-reported core set of symptoms to measure in adult cancer treatment trials. *Journal of the National Cancer Institute, 106*(7), dju129. https://doi.org/10.1093/jnci/dju129

Reinhardt, M. E., Sun, T., Pan, C. X., Schmults, C. D., Lee, E. H., & Waldman, A. B. (2022). A systematic review of patient-reported outcome measures for advanced skin cancer patients. *Archives of Dermatological Research, 315*, 1473–1480. https://doi.org/10.1007/s00403-022-02479-0

Romero, M. M., Flood, L. S., Gasiewicz, N. K., Rovin, R., & Conklin, S. (2015). Validation of the national institutes of health patient-reported outcomes measurement information system survey as a quality-of-life instrument for patients with malignant brain tumors and their caregivers. *Nursing Clinics of North America, 50*(4), 679–690. https://doi.org/10.1016/j.cnur.2015.07.009

Salas, M., Mordin, M., Castro, C., Islam, Z., Tu, N., & Hackshaw, M. D. (2022). Health-related quality of life in women with breast cancer: A review of measures. *BMC Cancer, 22*(1), 66. https://doi.org/10.1186/s12885-021-09157-w

Srour, M. K., Tadros, A. B., Sevilimedu, V., Nelson, J. A., Cracchiolo, J. R., McCready, T. M., Silva, N., Moo, T.-A., & Morrow, M. (2022). Who are we missing: Does engagement in patient-reported outcome measures for breast cancer vary by age, race, or disease stage? *Annals of Surgical Oncology, 29*(13), 7964–7973. https://doi.org/10.1245/s10434-022-12477-1

Straatman, J., Joosten, P. J., Terwee, C. B., Cuesta, M. A., Jansma, E. P., & van der Peet, D. L. (2016). Systematic review of patient-reported outcome measures in the surgical treatment of patients with esophageal cancer. *Disease of the Esophagus, 29*(7), 760–772. https://doi.org/10.1111/dote.12405

van Egdom, L. S. E., Oemrawsingh, A., Verweij, L. M., Lingsma, H. F., Koppert, L. B., Verhoef, C., Klazinga, N. S., & Hazelzet, J. A. (2019). Implementing patient-reported outcome measures in clinical breast cancer care: A systematic review. *Value Health, 22*(10), 1197–1226. https://doi.org/10.1016/j.jval.2019.04.1927

van Roij, J., Fransen, H., van, de Poll-Franse., L, Zijlstra., M, & Raijmakers, N. (2018). Measuring health-related quality of life in patients with advanced cancer: A systematic review of self-administered measurement instruments. *Quality of Life Research, 27*(8), 1937–1955. https://doi.org/10.1007/s11136-018-1809-4

Vistad, I. (2019). Electronic patient-reported outcomes to monitor symptoms after gynecological cancer treatment. *Acta Obstetricia et Gynecologica Scandinavica, 98*(11), 1365–1366. https://doi.org/10.1111/aogs.13734

Watson, L., Delure, A., Qi, S., Link, C., Chmielewski, L., Photitai, É., & Smith, L. (2021). Utilizing Patient Reported Outcome Measures (PROMs) in ambulatory oncology in Alberta: Digital reporting at the micro, meso and macro level. *Journal of Patient-Reported Outcomes, 5*(2), 1–8. https://doi.org/10.1186/s41687-021-00373-3

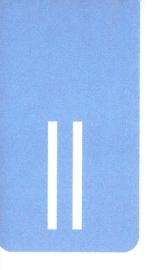

General Symptoms

CHAPTER 3

CANCER-RELATED FATIGUE

INTRODUCTION

Cancer-related fatigue (CRF) is a persistent and distressing subjective sense of tiredness or exhaustion related to cancer or cancer treatment that is disproportionate to activity and that interferes with daily functioning. The tiredness can be physical, emotional, or cognitive, and is not relieved by rest (Bower et al., 2014).

PREVALENCE

CRF is reported by up to 92% of patients, and 30% report feeling fatigued for months after the end of treatment (Lipsett et al., 2017). CRF is present during and after cancer treatment and tends to fluctuate over the course of treatment and may persist into the months and years of survivorship after active treatment (Al Maqbali, 2021). Chemotherapy causes fatigue in up to 80% of patients (Xian et al., 2021), and 25% of people on oral chemotherapy report fatigue (Poort et al., 2020). Radiation therapy causes an increase in CRF over the course of treatment and may persist for months after treatment is over (Dhruva et al., 2010). Newer treatments such as poly-ADP ribose polymerase (PARP) inhibitors (Poort et al., 2021) and tyrosine kinase inhibitors (Poort et al., 2019) are also associated with fatigue.

CRF is related to sleep disturbance and depression, and this forms a well-established symptom, the fatigue–depression–sleep disturbance symptom cluster (Charalambous et al., 2019). The other is the pain–fatigue–distress cluster (Bjerkeset et al., 2020).

CONTRIBUTING FACTORS

Multiple contributing factors to CRF have been identified; they are thought to be related to underlying mechanisms that are central (neural) and peripheral (muscular; O'Higgins et al., 2018). Sarcopenia contributes to fatigue due to the loss of muscle mass (Wang et al., 2020). Of importance is an understanding of the treatable factors that contribute to CRF (Figure 3.1).

Cardiac dysfunction	Arthritis
Endocrine dysfunction	Neuromuscular complications
Pulmonary dysfunction	Sleep disturbance
Renal dysfunction	Pain
Anemia	Distress

Figure 3.1 Treatable contributing factors.

Source: From Bower, J. E., Bak, K., Berger, A., Breitbart, W., Escalante, C. P., Ganz, P. A., Schnipper, H. H., Lacchetti, C., Ligibel, J. A., Lyman, G. H., Ogaily, M. S., Pirl, W. F., & Jacobsen, P. B. (2014). Screening, assessment, and management of fatigue in adult survivors of cancer: An American Society of Clinical oncology clinical practice guideline adaptation. *Journal of Clinical Oncology, 32*(17), 1840–1850. https://doi.org/10.1200/jco.2013.53.4495.

CASE STUDY

Your patient, a 47-year-old woman with ovarian cancer, has been treated with a total hysterectomy and debulking surgery. She is now having chemotherapy and appears thin and pale.

1. What questions do you want to ask her?

2. What objective measures could you use to further identify any problems?

Her daughter who is with her at the appointment states that her mother is exhausted all the time and is not able to do any of the things she usually likes to do.

3. What advice would you give your patient based on this?

4. What intervention has the most support for mitigating cancer-related fatigue (CRF)?

5. What medications would be appropriate for her?

ASSESSMENT

Screening for CRF should be done regularly, starting at diagnosis and continuing through active treatment and survivorship. The first step is to review and assess any factors that may be contributing to the experience of fatigue. There are a number of measures to assess CRF, both uni- and multidimensional, including emotional, behavioral, and cognitive domains (Amarsheda & Bhise, 2022; Figure 3.2).

- A brief tool, such as the one-item National Comprehensive Cancer Network (NCCN) screening question, is more efficient in the clinical setting.

- The Edmonton Symptom Assessment Scale Revised (ESAS-r) can also be utilized. This nine-item multidimensional instrument

How would you rate your fatigue on a scale of 0–10 over the past 7 days?
0 = no fatigue; 10 = worst fatigue imaginable

Mild = 0–3
Moderate = 4–6
Severe = 7–10

Figure 3.2 National Comprehensive Cancer Network fatigue screening question.

Source: From NCCN (2022). NCCN guidelines version 2.2024 cancer-related fatigue.

measures the severity of symptoms on a scale of 1 to 10 and includes single items for pain, activity, nausea, depression, anxiety, lack of appetite, well-being, and shortness of breath, in addition to tiredness (Gentile et al., 2022).

- There are a number of PROMIS (Patient-Reported Outcomes Measurement Information System) measures that assess fatigue, including short forms with four, six, seven, and eight items. The Functional Assessment of Chronic Illness Therapy-Fatigue Scale (FACIT-Fatigue) is a 13-item measure that is more comprehensive than the other short-form questionnaires. All are available on the HealthMeasures website (www.healthmeasures.net/index.php).

- The MD Anderson Symptom Inventory (MDASI) is a 13-item tool that has multiple language translations and also has additional modules for specific patient populations, including among others patients with leukemia, lung cancer, and ovarian cancer. The scale assesses symptom severity and interference with daily life (www.mdanderson.org/research/departments-labs-institutes/departments-divisions/symptom-research/symptom-assessment-tools/md-anderson-symptom-inventory.html).

Assessing muscle strength and nutritional markers may also serve as proxy measures for CRF (Schvartsman et al., 2017).

MANAGEMENT

All patients undergoing treatment for cancer should receive anticipatory guidance about the risk of fatigue, as well as advice on strategies to mitigate this symptom. Second, it is important to manage all contributing factors such as anemia, pain, and depression (Bower et al., 2014), as well as control physical symptoms such as pain, dyspnea, and nausea. Sleep disturbances should also be addressed with emphasis on sleep hygiene.

Patients may not always report fatigue to their healthcare clinicians (Smith et al., 2019) despite one study reporting that 78% were interested in learning skills to manage their fatigue (Krueger et al., 2021).

Identifying the goals of the individual patient in reducing fatigue may help target interventions that are specific and meet the needs of the individual, whether they are social or physical, in an effective manner (Hagan et al., 2017).

Pharmaceutical Interventions

The use of pharmacologic agents is not recommended in the management of fatigue, except for short-term use of dexamethasone or methylprednisolone in patients with metastatic cancer (Fabi et al., 2020), although these agents have significant side effects (Hagmann et al., 2018). Methylphenidate has not been shown to be more effective than placebo (Centeno et al., 2022). The efficacy of modafinil has also not been shown (Henson et al., 2020).

Nonpharmaceutical Interventions

- *Exercise:* Exercise is supported by evidence to manage CRF (Pearson et al., 2018) and may promote long-term survival (Palesh et al., 2018). It is recommended that anyone with cancer do 150 minutes of moderate-intensity aerobic exercise per week, in addition to 20 to 30 minutes of resistance exercise 2 days per week (Schmitz et al., 2010). Patients at higher risk for injury, for example, those with peripheral neuropathy, are advised to consult with a physical therapist or an exercise specialist before starting any exercise program (Bower et al., 2014). However, the recommendation for exercise may seem antithetical to the patient who is fatigued and therefore encouragement and a clear explanation are needed.

- *Yoga:* Yoga may also be helpful in reducing fatigue (Bower et al., 2005; Zetzl et al., 2021), and there is preliminary evidence on the use of acupuncture in CRF in women with breast cancer (Molassiotis et al., 2012).

- *Supplements and vitamins:* There is limited evidence to support the use of supplements and vitamins in the management of CRF (Aapro et al., 2017). A small study of *Panax ginseng* did not show benefit over placebo (Yennurajalingam et al., 2017). Guarana has also not shown to be of benefit (de Araujo et al., 2021).

- *Diet:* It is suggested that a diet rich in whole foods, fruits, vegetables, and omega-3 fatty acids may be helpful in managing CRF (Zick et al., 2017), especially if it is associated with other symptoms such as nausea, loss of appetite, stomatitis, and so on (David et al., 2021).

Psychosocial Interventions

Cognitive behavioral therapy (CBT) may be helpful during active treatment, whereas mindfulness-based cognitive therapy can be useful in the posttreatment scenario (Arring et al., 2019). Encouraging patients to conserve energy, when possible, by planning, pacing, and prioritizing activity may also be helpful (Chapman et al., 2022). Conserving energy is not the opposite of exercising; it means not doing activities that deplete energy and that may not be necessary. The benefits of these interventions are also useful to those experiencing symptom clusters, such as the pain–fatigue–sleep disturbance cluster (So et al., 2020).

Self-Management

Providing tailored information about CRF and how to manage it can support patients as they try a variety of interventions described above (Agbejule et al., 2022). Mobile health (mHealth) or electronic health (eHealth) interventions are a promising method for encouraging efforts to mitigate CRF; however, they may not be appropriate to those without access to the technology required (Seiler et al., 2017).

GUIDELINES

- **European Society for Medical Oncology (ESMO)**

    ESMO Clinical Practice Guidelines for Diagnosis and Treatment (Fabi et al., 2020)

- **National Comprehensive Cancer Network (NCCN)**

    NCCN Cancer-Related Fatigue Version 2.2022—February 9, 2022

    www.nccn.org/professionals/physician_gls/pdf/fatigue.pdf

- Oncology Nursing Society (ONS)

    Fatigue Guidelines

    www.ons.org/pep/fatigue?display=pepnavigator&sort_by=created&items_per_page=50

    Putting Evidence Into Practice: An update of Evidence-Based Interventions for CRF during and following treatment

    www.ons.org/cjon/18/6/supplement/putting-evidence-practice-update-evidence-based-interventions-cancer-related

SUMMARY

CRF is a distressing symptom that affects many individuals with cancer during and after treatment. There are limited pharmaceutical interventions for treatment, but exercise has been shown to be effective in mitigating this symptom. A number of psychosocial interventions show promise with few, if any, side effects.

A robust set of instructor resources designed to supplement this text is located at http://connect.springerpub.com/content/reference-book/978-0-8261-8524-2. Qualifying Instructors may request access by emailing **textbook@springerpub.com**.

REFERENCES

Aapro, M., Scotte, F., Bouillet, T., Currow, D., & Vigano, A. (2017). A practical approach to fatigue management in colorectal cancer. *Clinical Colorectal Cancer, 16*(4), 275–285. https://doi.org/10.1016/j.clcc.2016.04.010

Agbejule, O. A., Hart, N. H., Ekberg, S., Crichton, M., & Chan, R. J. (2022). Self-management support for cancer-related fatigue: A systematic review. *International Journal of Nursing Studies, 129,* 104206. https://doi.org/10.1016/j.ijnurstu.2022.104206

Al Maqbali, M. (2021). Cancer-related fatigue: An overview. *British Journal of Nursing, 30*(4), S36–S43. https://doi.org/10.12968/bjon.2021.30.4.S36

Amarsheda, S., & Bhise, A. R. (2022). Systematic review of cancer-related fatigue instruments in breast cancer patients. *Palliative & Supportive Care, 20*(1), 122–128. https://doi.org/10.1017/s1478951521000444

Arring, N. M., Barton, D. L., Brooks, T., & Zick, S. M. (2019). Integrative therapies for cancer-related fatigue. *The Cancer Journal, 25*(5), 349–356. https://doi.org/10.1097/ppo.0000000000000396

Bjerkeset, E., Röhrl, K., & Schou-Bredal, I. (2020). Symptom cluster of pain, fatigue, and psychological distress in breast cancer survivors: Prevalence and characteristics. *Breast Cancer Research and Treatment, 180*(1), 63–71. https://doi.org/10.1007/s10549-020-05522-8

Bower, J. E., Bak, K., Berger, A., Breitbart, W., Escalante, C. P., Ganz, P. A., Schnipper, H. H., Lacchetti, C., Ligibel, J. A., Lyman, G. H., Ogaily, M. S., Pirl, W. F., & Jacobsen, P. B. (2014). Screening, assessment, and management of fatigue in adult survivors of cancer: An American Society of Clinical oncology clinical practice guideline adaptation. *Journal of Clinical Oncology, 32*(17), 1840–1850. https://doi.org/10.1200/jco.2013.53.4495

Bower, J. E., Woolery, A., Sternlieb, B., & Garet, D. (2005). Yoga for cancer patients and survivors : Meta-analyses. *Cancer Control, 12*(3), 165–171. https://doi.org/10.1177/107327480501200304

Centeno, C., Rojí, R., Portela, M. A., De Santiago, A., Cuervo, M. A., Ramos, D., Gandara, A., Salgado, E., Gagnon, B., & Sanz, A. (2022). Improved cancer-related fatigue in a randomised clinical trial: Methylphenidate no better than placebo. *BMJ Support Palliat Care, 12*(2), 226–234. https://doi.org/10.1136/bmjspcare-2020-002454

Chapman, E. J., Martino, E. D., Edwards, Z., Black, K., Maddocks, M., & Bennett, M. I. (2022). Practice review: Evidence-based and effective management of fatigue in patients with advanced cancer. *Palliative Medicine, 36*(1), 7–14. https://doi.org/10.1177/02692163211046754

Charalambous, A., Berger, A. M., Matthews, E., Balachandran, D. D., Papastavrou, E., & Palesh, O. (2019). Cancer-related fatigue and sleep deficiency in cancer care continuum: Concepts, assessment, clusters, and management. *Supportive Care in Cancer, 27*(7), 2747–2753. https://doi.org/10.1007/s00520-019-04746-9

David, A., Hausner, D., & Frenkel, M. (2021). Cancer-related fatigue-is there a role for complementary and integrative medicine? *Current Oncology Reports, 23*(12), 145. https://doi.org/10.1007/s11912-021-01135-6

de Araujo, D. P., Pereira, P., Fontes, A. J. C., Marques, K. D. S., de, Moraes., É, B., Guerra, R. N. M., & Garcia, J. B. S. (2021). The use of guarana (Paullinia cupana) as a dietary supplement for fatigue in cancer patients: A systematic review with a meta-analysis. *Supportive Care in Cancer, 29*(12), 7171–7182. https://doi.org/10.1007/s00520-021-06242-5

Dhruva, A., Dodd, M., Paul, S. M., Cooper, B. A., Lee, K., West, C., Aouizerat, B. E., Swift, P. S., Wara, W., & Miaskowski, C. (2010). Trajectories of fatigue in patients with breast cancer before, during, and after radiation therapy. *Cancer Nursing, 33*(3), 201–212. https://doi.org/10.1097/NCC.0b013e3181c 75f2a

Fabi, A., Bhargava, R., Fatigoni, S., Guglielmo, M., Horneber, M., Roila, F., Weis, J., Jordan, K., & Ripamonti, C. I. (2020). Cancer-related fatigue: ESMO Clinical Practice Guidelines for diagnosis and treatment. *Annals of Oncology, 31*(6), 713–723. https://doi.org/10.1016/j.annonc.2020.02.016

Gentile, D., Beeler, D., Wang, X. S., Ben-Ayre, E., Zick, S. M., Bao, T., Carlson, L. E., Ghelman, R., Master, V. A., Tripathy, D., & Zhi, W. I. (2022). Cancer-related fatigue outcome measures in integrative oncology: Evidence for practice and research recommendations. *Oncology (Williston Park), 36*(5), 276–287. https://doi.org/10.46883/2022.25920958

Hagan, T. L., Arida, J. A., Hughes, S. H., & Donovan, H. S. (2017). Creating individualized symptom management goals and strategies for cancer-related fatigue for patients with recurrent ovarian cancer. *Cancer Nursing, 40*(4), 305–313. https://doi.org/10.1097/ncc.0000000000000407

Hagmann, C., Cramer, A., Kestenbaum, A., Durazo, C., Downey, A., Russell, M., Geluz, J., Ma, J. D., & Roeland, E. J. (2018). Evidence-based palliative care approaches to non-pain physical symptom management in cancer patients. *Seminars in Oncology Nursing, 34*(3), 227–240. https://doi.org/10.1016/j.son cn.2018.06.004

Henson, L. A., Maddocks, M., Evans, C., Davidson, M., Hicks, S., & Higginson, I. J. (2020). Palliative care and the management of common distressing symptoms in advanced cancer: Pain, breathlessness, nausea and vomiting, and fatigue. *Journal of Clinical Oncology, 38*(9), 905–914. https://doi.org/10.1200/jco.19.00470

Krueger, E., Secinti, E., Mosher, C. E., Stutz, P. V., Cohee, A. A., & Johns, S. A. (2021). Symptom treatment preferences of cancer survivors: Does fatigue level make a difference? *Cancer Nursing, 44*(6), E540–e546. https://doi.org/10.1097/ncc.0000000000000941

Lipsett, A., Barrett, S., Haruna, F., Mustian, K., & O'Donovan, A. (2017). The impact of exercise during adjuvant radiotherapy for breast cancer on fatigue and quality of life: A systematic review and meta-analysis. *The Breast, 32*, 144–155. https://doi.org/10.1016/j.breast.2017.02.002

Molassiotis, A., Bardy, J., Finnegan-John, J., Mackereth, P., Ryder, D. W., Filshie, J., Ream, E., & Richardson, A. (2012). Acupuncture for cancer-related fatigue in patients with breast cancer: A pragmatic randomized controlled trial. *Journal of Clinical Oncology, 30*(36), 4470–4476. https://doi.org/10.1200/jco.2012.41.6222

O'Higgins, C. M., Brady, B., O'Connor, B., Walsh, D., & Reilly, R. B. (2018). The pathophysiology of cancer-related fatigue: Current controversies. *Supportive Care in Cancer, 26*(10), 3353–3364. https://doi.org/10.1007/s00520-018-4318-7

Palesh, O., Scheiber, C., Kesler, S., Mustian, K., Koopman, C., & Schapira, L. (2018). Management of side effects during and post-treatment in breast cancer survivors. *The Breast Journal, 24*(2), 167–175. https://doi.org/10.1111/tbj.12862

Pearson, E. J. M., Morris, M. E., di Stefano, M., & McKinstry, C. E. (2018). Interventions for cancer-related fatigue: A scoping review. *European Journal of Cancer Care (England), 27*(1), e12516. https://doi.org/10.1111/ecc.12516

Poort, H., Fenton, A., Thompson, E., Dinardo, M. M., Liu, J. F., Arch, J. J., & Wright, A. A. (2021). Lived experiences of women reporting fatigue during PARP inhibitor maintenance treatment for advanced ovarian cancer: A qualitative study. *Gynecologic Oncology, 160*(1), 227–233. https://doi.org/10.1016/j.ygyno.2020.10.034

Poort, H., Jacobs, J. M., Pirl, W. F., Temel, J. S., & Greer, J. A. (2020). Fatigue in patients on oral targeted or chemotherapy for cancer and associations with anxiety, depression, and quality of life. *Palliat Support Care, 18*(2), 141–147. https://doi.org/10.1017/s147895151900066x

Poort, H., Onghena, P., Abrahams, H. J. G., Jim, H. S. L., Jacobsen, P. B., Blijlevens, N. M. A., & Knoop, H. (2019). Cognitive behavioral therapy for treatment-related fatigue in chronic myeloid leukemia patients on tyrosine kinase inhibitors: A mixed-method study. *Journal of Clinical Psychology in Medical Settings, 26*(4), 440–448. https://doi.org/10.1007/s10880-019-09607-5

Schmitz, K., Courneya, K., Matthews, C., Demark-Wahnefried, W., Galvão, D., Pinto, B., Irwin, M., Wolin, K., Segal, R., Lucia, A., Schneider, C., von Gruenigen, V., & Schwartz, A. (2010). American College of Sports Medicine roundtable on exercise guidelines for cancer survivors. *Medicine & Science in Sports and Exercise, 42*(7), 1409–1426. https://doi.org/10.1249/MSS.0b013e3181e0c112

Schvartsman, G., Park, M., Liu, D. D., Yennu, S., Bruera, E., & Hui, D. (2017). Could objective tests be used to measure fatigue in patients with advanced cancer? *Journal of Pain and Symptom Management, 54*(2), 237–244. https://doi.org/10.1016/j.jpainsymman.2016.12.343

Seiler, A., Klaas, V., Tröster, G., & Fagundes, C. P. (2017). eHealth and mHealth interventions in the treatment of fatigued cancer survivors: A systematic review and meta-analysis. *Psychooncology, 26*(9), 1239–1253. https://doi.org/10.1002/pon.4489

Smith, T. G., Troeschel, A. N., Castro, K. M., Arora, N. K., Stein, K., Lipscomb, J., Brawley, O. W., McCabe, R. M., Clauser, S. B., & Ward, E. (2019). Perceptions of patients with breast and colon cancer of the management of cancer-related pain, fatigue, and emotional distress in community oncology. *Journal of Clinical Oncology, 37*(19), 1666–1676. https://doi.org/10.1200/jco.18.01579

So, W. K. W., Law, B. M. H., Chan, D. N. S., Xing, W., Chan, C. W. H., & McCarthy, A. L. (2020). The Effect of nonpharmacological interventions on managing symptom clusters among cancer patients: A systematic review. *Cancer Nursing, 43*(6), E304–e327. https://doi.org/10.1097/ncc.0000000000000730

Wang, B., Thapa, S., Zhou, T., Liu, H., Li, L., Peng, G., & Yu, S. (2020). Cancer-related fatigue and biochemical parameters among cancer patients with different stages of sarcopenia. *Supportive Care in Cancer, 28*(2), 581–588. https://doi.org/10.1007/s00520-019-04717-0

Xian, X., Zhu, C., Chen, Y., Huang, B., & Xu, D. (2021). A longitudinal analysis of fatigue in colorectal cancer patients during chemotherapy. *Supportive Care in Cancer, 29*(9), 5245–5252. https://doi.org/10.1007/s00520-021-06097-w

Yennurajalingam, S., Tannir, N. M., Williams, J. L., Lu, Z., Hess, K. R., Frisbee-Hume, S., House, H. L., Lim, Z. D., Lim, K.-H., Lopez, G., Reddy, A., Azhar, A., Wong, A., Patel, S. M., Kuban, D. A., Kaseb, A. O., Cohen, L., & Bruera, E. (2017). A double-blind, randomized, placebo-controlled trial of panax ginseng for cancer-related fatigue in patients with advanced cancer. *Journal of the National Comprehensive Cancer Network, 15*(9), 1111–1120. https://doi.org/10.6004/jnccn.2017.0149

Zetzl, T., Renner, A., Pittig, A., Jentschke, E., Roch, C., & van Oorschot, B. (2021). Yoga effectively reduces fatigue and symptoms of depression in patients with different types of cancer. *Supportive Care in Cancer, 29*(6), 2973–2982. https://doi.org/10.1007/s00520-020-05794-2

Zick, S. M., Colacino, J., Cornellier, M., Khabir, T., Surnow, K., & Djuric, Z. (2017). Fatigue reduction diet in breast cancer survivors: A pilot randomized clinical trial. *Breast Cancer Research and Treatment, 161*(2), 299–310. https://doi.org/10.1007/s10549-016-4070-y

CHAPTER 4

CANCER PAIN

INTRODUCTION

Pain is a complex phenomenon that may persist both during and after treatment for cancer. *Pain* is defined as "an unpleasant sensory and emotional experience associated with or resembling that associated with actual or potential tissue damage" (Raja et al., 2020). Pain may be acute or chronic and causes suffering for both the person with cancer and their caregivers. Unrelieved severe pain has been associated with suicide in older men with cancer (Aboumrad et al., 2018). Culture can affect the experience of pain, as well as the person's beliefs about pain and their behavior (Crombez et al., 2019). Cancer pain is also different from other kinds of acute and chronic pain (Khatooni, 2021). Cancer pain may be nociceptive (skin, musculoskeletal, or visceral) or neuropathic (damage to the nervous system), but can also be a combination of both (Yoong & Poon, 2018). It is important to individualize the management of pain, which requires a comprehensive knowledge of pain medications and alternative interventions. The involvement of the patient's caregivers is important as they play an integral role in administering medications to a family member with cancer.

PREVALENCE

A recent systematic review and meta-analysis found the prevalence of pain was 40% in those on active treatment, lasting up to 3 months after treatment (Evenepoel et al., 2022). Despite advances in assessment and management, pain remains a problem with consequences in all aspects of quality of life. The prevalence of pain is higher in those with advanced cancer. In the last weeks of life, almost 70% of people report moderate to severe pain (Seow et al., 2021).

CONTRIBUTING FACTORS

Multiple factors contribute to the experience of pain, including the type of cancer, treatment modalities, psychological factors, and preexisting

26 SECTION II • GENERAL SYMPTOMS

conditions (Gulati, 2021). Treatment-related pain is caused by surgery, chemotherapy, and radiation therapy. Structural changes in the body (Gress et al., 2020) and inflammation at the cellular level also contribute to pain (Kwekkeboom et al., 2018). Depression (Azizoddin et al., 2021), anxiety, fatigue, sleep disturbance, and cognitive dysfunction also contribute to acute (Shin et al., 2022a) and persistent pain (Sipilä et al., 2020). A history of opioid and/or alcohol use is associated with chronic pain (Berger et al., 2020).

ASSESSMENT

Guidelines on the management of pain in people with cancer recommend that cancer pain be assessed at every visit. Assessment should include the intensity and quality of pain, location, variation and duration, if the pain radiates or is referred, chronicity, and any alleviating or exacerbating factors (Webb & LeBlanc, 2018). Nociceptive pain is described as aching, throbbing, or a sense of pressure in the skin, muscle, or bone. Visceral pain is described as aching, cramping, gnawing, or sharp. Neuropathic pain is shooting, sharp, stabbing, or tingling, and is often described as a feeling of electric shocks (Fallon et al., 2018; Figure 4.1).

Patients may not recall their pain or may overestimate their level of pain; patient-reported experience measures (PREMs) may improve their subjective assessment of pain and increase the frequency of pain discussions with healthcare clinicians (Adam et al., 2017). For those who are nonverbal or have cognitive impairment, observing pain-related behavior (facial expression, body movements, vocalization) can measure the presence of pain but not its intensity (Fallon et al., 2018). A bidirectional association of pain and distress should be considered in all patients, and assessing the role of pain is warranted in those who report distress (see Chapter 27 for distress).

Numeric Rating Scale

A simple screening question using a numerical rating scale is the first step in the assessment.

The Numeric Rating Scale (NRS) is a commonly used brief pain assessment tool that asks the question "What number describes your pain from 0 (no pain) to 10 (worst pain you can imagine)?" No pain = 0; mild pain = 1 to 3; moderate pain = 4 to 6; and severe pain = 7 to 10.

- Ask about breakthrough pain.
- Ask about any pharmaceutical and nonpharmaceutical treatment and their effectiveness.
- Ask whether they are satisfied with their pain relief.
- Ask whether pain interferes with their daily life.
- Ask caregivers for additional information where necessary.
- Consider psychological, cultural, spiritual, and social aspects of the pain experience.

Figure 4.1 Additional questions related to pain.

Assessing current pain, average pain, and least pain in the past 24 hours provides additional information.

Additional qualifiers can be used, for example, pain in the past week, pain at rest, or pain with movement (NCCN Clinical Practice Guidelines in Oncology: Adult Cancer Pain Version 1.2022).

Visual Analog Scale

The Visual Analog Scale (VAS) asks the patient to indicate on a 100-mm scale which level best represents their pain. The score is determined by measuring the distance from 0 to 100, with a higher score indicating more severe pain (Hawker et al., 2011). The VAS has been rated lowest for those with advanced cancer (Jeter et al., 2018; Kim & Jung, 2020) and so should be used with caution in this population. If the pain is rated at 3 or above, or if the person is distressed by the pain, a more detailed assessment is warranted.

Faces Pain Rating Scale

The Faces Pain Rating Scale (Revised) is used for children with cancer or individuals with low or absent literacy. This scale depicts six faces expressing the intensity of pain, ranging from no pain to a lot of pain, and is rated on a scale from 0 to 10. Validated tools to assess pain are available and these are shown in Figure 4.2.

Referral to a pain specialist has been shown to be helpful in managing pain (Patton et al., 2021). *Early palliative care*—defined as family-centered care that optimizes the quality of life by anticipating, preventing, and treating suffering (Ferrell et al., 2017)—addresses pain and suffering (Haun et al., 2017). This care is described as "symptom management" in some institutions or cancer centers. Referral to palliative care is especially important when advanced care nurses are not able to prescribe certain classes of pain medication.

- Visual Analog Scale for Pain (VAS)
- Numeric Rating Scale for Pain (NRS)
- The Brief Pain Inventory (BPI)
- McGill Pain Questionnaire (MPQ)
- Short-Form McGill Pain Questionnaire (SF-MPQ)
- Edmonton Symptom Assessment System-Revised (ESAS-r)

Figure 4.2 Pain measures.

Sources: From Hawker, G. A., Mian, S., Kendzerska, T., & French, M. (2011). Measures of adult pain: Visual Analog Scale for Pain (VAS Pain), Numeric Rating Scale for Pain (NRS Pain), McGill Pain Questionnaire (MPQ), Short-Form McGill Pain Questionnaire (SF-MPQ), Chronic Pain Grade Scale (CPGS), Short Form-36 Bodily Pain Scale (SF-36 BPS), and Measure of Intermittent and Constant Osteoarthritis Pain (ICOAP). *Arthritis Care & Research, 63*(S11), S240–S252. https://doi.org/10.1002/acr.20543; Lopes-Júnior, L. C., Rosa, G. S., Pessanha, R. M., Schuab, S., Nunes, K. Z., & Amorim, M. H. C. (2020). Efficacy of the complementary therapies in the management of cancer pain in palliative care: A systematic review. *Revista Latino-Americana de Enfermagem, 28*, e3377. https://doi.org/10.1590/1518-8345.4213.3377.

MANAGEMENT

Determining the source of pain is essential in the management of this symptom. The type of pain (nociceptive, visceral, or neuropathic) may indicate the cause, which then suggests the most effective treatment.

Pharmaceutical Management of Cancer Pain

The National Comprehensive Cancer Network (NCCN; www.nccn.org/professionals/physician_gls/pdf/pain.pdf) has clear guidelines on the management of cancer pain in both opioid-naïve and opioid-tolerant individuals. In addition, the NCCN offers advice on the management of patients in severe pain or in pain crisis. Prevention of drug side effects, for example, constipation, is very important, and acute or severe pain may require admission to hospital or hospice. Regular analgesia with long-acting medications and short-acting analgesia for breakthrough pain lies at the core of pain management (Figure 4.3).

The European Society for Medical Oncology (ESMO) guideline (Fallon et al., 2018a) refers to the World Health Organization's Analgesic Ladder, which has three levels of pain management:

- *Step 1:* nonsteroidal anti-inflammatories (NSAIDs) for treatment of mild pain

- *Step 2:* tramadol, dihydrocodeine, and codeine for mild to moderate pain

- *Step 3:* strong opioids (morphine, oxycodone, hydromorphone) for treatment of moderate to severe pain; may also consider methadone, fentanyl, and buprenorphine

The fourth step to the Analgesic Ladder is the use of nerve blocks, epidural, spinal stimulators, and other nonopioid methods to manage severe (Scarborough & Smith, 2018) or intractable pain (Dziedzic & Albert, 2021; Hao et al., 2021).

Ketamine may also be helpful in refractory pain (Cheung et al., 2020). Antidepressants and anticonvulsants may be useful in chemotherapy-induced peripheral neuropathy. Gabapentin and pregabalin have increasingly been used off-label for the management of

- Analgesia (optimize pain relief)
- Activities (optimize activities of daily living)
- Adverse effects (minimize side effects)
- Aberrant drug taking (avoid misuse of pain medications)
- Affect (assess relationship between pain and mood)

Figure 4.3 The five As of pain management.

Source: From NCCN guidelines version 1.2023 survivorship: Pain

neuropathic pain despite the lack of evidence on their effectiveness (Fauer et al., 2020). **When used at the same time as opioids, occurring in 49% of patients with advanced cancer, the addition of these medications has potentially lethal side effects (Madden et al., 2021).**

Metastatic bone pain is also treated in a stepwise manner, starting with NSAIDs, then opioids, followed by bisphosphonates, tricyclic antidepressants, corticosteroids, growth factors, and signaling molecules. Radiation therapy is helpful in this context; radioactive isotopes can also be used (Ahmad et al., 2018).

The American Society of Clinical Oncology (ASCO) states that opioids should be offered at the lowest possible dose to achieve pain control and patient goals. For patients with a history of substance abuse, consultation with a specialist in this area is recommended. Education of the patient and their family caregivers on the risks and benefits of long-term opioid use should be provided, as well as education on safe storage and disposal information. For a full discussion, see the ASCO guidelines (Paice et al., 2022).

Opioid use has declined in the 5 years from 2013 to 2018 (Chen et al., 2022), from 40.2% to 34.5%, due in part to concerns about overuse of these drugs, despite the exclusion of people with cancer from the guidelines (www.cdc.gov/mmwr/volumes/65/rr/rr6501e1.htm).

Barriers to Pain Management

Concerns about tolerance and addiction as well as negative attitudes toward cancer pain persist among healthcare clinicians and family caregivers (Makhlouf et al., 2020). Additional barriers include lack of knowledge about pharmacologic pain management and lack of psychological interventions for pain control (Darawad et al., 2019).

Systematic pain assessment and management protocols have been shown to improve pain outcomes for hospitalized patients (Marie Fallon et al., 2018b).

Nonpharmaceutical Management of Cancer Pain

There is limited evidence on the effectiveness of nonpharmaceutical interventions for the management of cancer pain, but some interventions do appear to offer relief to some patients (Ruano et al., 2022) and may be worth suggesting as there is little to no harm associated with them. Mindfulness-based cognitive therapy, guided imagery, and progressive muscle relaxation are three interventions suggested as the most effective. Other integrative therapies with evidence of effectiveness are presented in Figure 4.4.

CANNABIS

The use of cannabis to manage pain is widespread among people with cancer (Nugent et al., 2020). A national study reported that 8% of cancer survivors used cannabis in the previous year (Do et al., 2021);

SECTION II • GENERAL SYMPTOMS

Therapeutic Exercise

- Hydrotherapy
- Cold or heat
- TENS

Mind–Body Therapies

- Relaxation therapy
- Imagery (guided)
- Hypnosis
- Biofeedback
- Meditation

- Creative arts
- Biofield therapies (Reiki, therapeutic or healing touch)
- Reflexology

Manual Interventions

- Massage
- Acupuncture, acupoint stimulation, electroacupuncture

Figure 4.4 Integrative therapies for pain.

TENS, transcutaneous electrical nerve stimulation.

Source: From Anderson, K. D., & Downey, M. (2021). Foot reflexology: An intervention for pain and nausea among inpatients with cancer. *Clinical Journal of Oncology Nursing, 25*(5), 539–545. https://doi.org/10.1188/21.Cjon.539-545; Cadet, T., Davis, C., Wilson, P., & Elks, J. (2022). The experiences of touch therapies in symptom management of rural and regional cancer patients in Australia. *International Journal of Therapeutic Massage & Bodywork, 15*(1), 66–71. https://doi.org/10.3822/ijtmb.v15i1.687; Lopes-Júnior, L. C., Rosa, G. S., Pessanha, R. M., Schuab, S., Nunes, K. Z., & Amorim, M. H. C. (2020). Efficacy of the complementary therapies in the management of cancer pain in palliative care: A systematic review. *Revista Latino-Americana de Enfermagem, 28*, e3377. https://doi.org/10.1590/1518-8345.4213.3377; Mantoudi, A., Parpa, E., Tsilika, E., Batistaki, C., Nikoloudi, M., Kouloulias, V., Kostopoulou, S., Galanos, A., & Mystakidou, K. (2020). Complementary therapies for patients with cancer: Reflexology and relaxation in integrative palliative care. A randomized controlled comparative study. *Journal of Alternative and Complementary Medicine, 26*(9), 792–798. https://doi.org/10.1089/acm.2019.0402; Sikorskii, A., Niyogi, P. G., Victorson, D., Tamkus, D., & Wyatt, G. (2020). Symptom response analysis of a randomized controlled trial of reflexology for symptom management among women with advanced breast cancer. *Supportive Care in Cancer, 28*(3), 1395–1404. https://doi.org/10.1007/s00520-019-04959-y; Sine, H., Achbani, A., & Filali, K. (2022). The effect of hypnosis on the intensity of pain and anxiety in cancer patients: A systematic review of controlled experimental trials. *Cancer Investigation, 40*(3), 235–253. https://doi.org/10.1080/07357907.2021.1998520; Yang, J., Wahner-Roedler, D. L., Zhou, X., Johnson, L. A., Do, A., Pachman, D. R., Chon, T. Y., Salinas, M., Millstine, D., & Bauer, B. A. (2021). Acupuncture for palliative cancer pain management: Systematic review. *BMJ Support Palliat Care, 11*(3), 264–270. https://doi.org/10.1136/bmjspcare-2020-002638.

however, in another study, 42.5% of patients were using cannabis (Potts et al., 2022). Use of cannabis for pain has been reported by 77% (Bar-Lev Schleider et al., 2018) to 89% of patients (Zolotov et al., 2021). In one study, 30% of young adults tested positive for tetrahydrocannabinol (THC) in their urine (Donovan et al., 2020; Figure 4.5).

Cannabis appears to be most useful in neuropathic pain (Abu-Amna et al., 2021) and may work synergistically with opioids to improve pain control (Abrams, 2022). The side effects of cannabis are mild and include dizziness, nausea, vomiting, somnolence, and fatigue (Boland et al., 2020). Of concern is the belief by some that cannabis can cure cancer (Buchwald et al., 2020).

Tetrahydrocannabinoid (THC)
• Has psychoactive properties—euphoria, relaxation, time distortion
Cannabidiol (CBD)
• No psychoactive properties • Causes drowsiness
Cannabis sativa
• Greater THC concentration
Cannabis indica
• Higher CBD concentration

Figure 4.5 Types of cannabinoids.

Sources: From Clark, C. S. (2018). Medical cannabis: The oncology nurse's role in patient education about the effects of marijuana on cancer palliation. *Clinical Journal of Oncology Nursing, 22*(1), E1–E6. https://doi.org/10.1188/18.Cjon.E1-e6; Kleckner, A. S., Kleckner, I. R., Kamen, C. S., Tejani, M. A., Janelsins, M. C., Morrow, G. R., & Peppone, L. J. (2019). Opportunities for cannabis in supportive care in cancer. *Therapeutic Advances in Medical Oncology, 11*, 1758835919866362. https://doi.org/10.1177/1758835919866362.

Approved products include dronabinol oral solution (Syndros) and capsules (Marinol), as well as nabilone capsules (Cesamet; Vinette et al., 2022). Oromucosal spray (Sativex) is not yet approved in the United States (Worster et al., 2022). Smoking cannabis is common but can cause respiratory problems; vaporization may be safer. Both of these methods of inhalation have a rapid onset (Worster et al., 2022).

Drug–drug interactions are concerning and cannabis has shown to cause decreased response rate with nivolumab as well as increased side effects from tamoxifen (Bouquié et al., 2018). Advising patients to "start low and go slow" and on the development of tolerance is important, and if the side effects of THC are bothersome, the addition of cannabidiol (CBD) can be helpful (Clark, 2018).

Some patients regard cannabis as more natural than opioids, and cannabis has reduced the overall number of prescription medications that they needed (McTaggart-Cowan et al., 2021). Concerns about the legality and access to cannabis products may be a barrier to use, especially in areas where restrictive laws exist (Singh et al., 2019). Lack of knowledge on the part of oncology care clinicians is also a barrier when patients ask for their advice about cannabis use (Abrams, 2022). However, attitudes are changing among primary care clinicians, with more than 50% believing that, for people with cancer, cannabis can be helpful in managing symptoms, especially intractable pain (Philpot et al., 2019). Patients may access cannabis through informal social networks or illicit sources, but some may obtain a medical marijuana certificate from a clinician who is not part of their oncology team (Braun et al., 2021). These clinicians do not know the person's cancer history and interactions are usually brief and superficial.

SECTION II • GENERAL SYMPTOMS

CASE STUDY

Your patient is a 22-year-old man with lymphoma. He had a successful stem cell transplant 6 months ago, but he frequently misses appointments. He calls the clinic a few times a month, requesting repeat prescriptions for oxycodone. He is frequently not available on his cell phone when you try to respond to his messages.

1. What is most concerning to you at this time?

2. What do you need to assess before addressing his requests for repeat prescriptions?

He finally comes to see the oncology team. He is disheveled and falls asleep in the examination room while waiting to see the oncologist.

3. What might be the reason for this behavior?

4. What questions do you want to ask him about his apparent fatigue?

SELF-MANAGEMENT

Outside of the inpatient setting, patients and/or their caregivers are responsible for managing pain. Up to 80% of patients in the community experience ongoing pain that is associated with high levels of stress (Shin et al., 2022a, b). Patients may put themselves at risk in attempting to reduce their opioid use. These actions include cutting pills, mixing nonopioid medications with prescribed opioids, using illicit drugs instead of prescription pain medications, and self-tapering off opioids (Meghani et al., 2020).

Family caregivers must carefully monitor for signs of pain and act accordingly, adjusting pain medication where necessary (Ullgren et al., 2018). Family caregivers who are distressed may not be able to assess the patient's pain level, resulting in less pain relief (Smyth et al., 2018). Support from nurses (Han et al., 2018) and skills training (Check et al., 2021) may help reduce the risk of both the patient and their family caregivers undertreating pain.

GUIDELINES

■ **American College of Chest Physicians (ACCP)**

Complementary Therapies and Integrative Oncology in Lung Cancer: ACCP Evidence-Based Clinical Practice Guidelines (Second Edition; Cassileth et al., 2007)

- **American Society of Clinical Oncology (ASCO)**

  Use of Opioids for Adults With Pain From Cancer or Cancer Treatment: ASCO Guideline (Paice et al., 2022)

- **American Society of Pain and Neuroscience (ASPN)**

  Best Practices and Guidelines for the Interventional Management of Cancer-Associated Pain (Aman et al., 2021)

- **European Society for Medical Oncology (ESMO)**

  Clinical Practice Guidelines: Management of Cancer Pain in Adult Patients (Fallon et al., 2018)

- **National Cancer Institute (NCI)**

  Cancer Pain. Health Professional Version (2021)

  www.cancer.gov/about-cancer/treatment/side-effects/pain/pain-hp-pdq

- **National Comprehensive Cancer Network (NCCN)**

  Clinical Practice Guidelines in Oncology

  Adult Cancer Pain Version 1.2022

  www.nccn.org/professionals/physician_gls/pdf/pain.pdf

- **Oncology Nursing Society (ONS)**

  Position Statement on Cancer Pain Management (Revised 2022)

  www.ons.org/make-difference/ons-center-advocacy-and-health-policy/position-statements/cancer-pain-management

  Position Statement on Refractory/Intractable Pain (2009)

  www.ons.org/pep/refractoryintractable-pain?display=pepnavigator&sort_by=created&items_per_page=50

  Position Statement on Chronic Pain (2019)

  www.ons.org/pep/chronic-pain?display=pepnavigator&sort_by=created&items_per_page=50

  Position Statement on Breakthrough Pain (2019)

  www.ons.org/pep/breakthrough-pain?display=pepnavigator&sort_by=created&items_per_page=50

- **Society for Integrative Oncology**

  ASCO Guideline Summary and Q&A (Mao et al., 2023)

  Use of Cannabinoids in Cancer Patients: A Society of Gynecologic Oncology (SGO) Clinical Practice Statement (Whitcomb et al., 2020)

- **World Health Organization (WHO)**

    WHO Guidelines for the Pharmacological and Radiotherapeutic Management of Cancer Pain in Adults and Adolescents

    www.who.int/publications/i/item/9789241550390

SUMMARY

Analgesics are an important part of patient care because both acute and chronic cancer pain impact on quality of life, including sleep disturbance, activities of daily living, and social functioning. The role of pain and palliative care specialists cannot be underestimated in pain control for patients at all stages of disease.

A robust set of instructor resources designed to supplement this text is located at http://connect.springerpub.com/content/reference-book/978-0-8261-8524-2. Qualifying Instructors may request access by emailing **textbook@springerpub.com**.

REFERENCES

Aboumrad, M., Shiner, B., Riblet, N., Mills, P. D., & Watts, B. V. (2018). Factors contributing to cancer-related suicide: A study of root-cause analysis reports. *Psychooncology*, 27(9), 2237–2244. https://doi.org/10.1002/pon.4815

Abrams, D. I. (2022). Cannabis, cannabinoids and cannabis-based medicines in cancer care. *Integrative Cancer Therapies*, 21, 15347354221081772. https://doi.org/10.1177/15347354221081772

Abu-Amna, M., Salti, T., Khoury, M., Cohen, I., & Bar-Sela, G. (2021). Medical cannabis in oncology: A valuable unappreciated remedy or an undesirable risk? *Current Treatment Options in Oncology*, 22(2), 16. https://doi.org/10.1007/s11864-020-00811-2

Adam, R., Burton, C. D., Bond, C. M., de Bruin, M., & Murchie, P. (2017). Can patient-reported measurements of pain be used to improve cancer pain management? A systematic review and meta-analysis. *BMJ Supportive & Palliative Care*, 7(4), 00. https://doi.org/10.1136/bmjspcare-2016-001137

Ahmad, I., Ahmed, M. M., Ahsraf, M. F., Naeem, A., Tasleem, A., Ahmed, M., & Farooqi, M. S. (2018). Pain management in metastatic bone disease: A literature review. *Cureus*, 10(9), e3286. https://doi.org/10.7759/cureus.3286

Aman, M. M., Mahmoud, A., Deer, T., Sayed, D., Hagedorn, J. M., Brogan, S. E., Singh, V., Gulati, A., Strand, N., Weisbein, J., Goree, J. H., Xing, F., Valimahomed, A., Pak, D. J., El Helou, A., Ghosh, P., Shah, K., Patel, V., Escobar, A., ... Narang, S. (2021). The American Society of Pain and Neuroscience (ASPN) Best practices and guidelines for the interventional management of cancer-associated pain. *Journal of Pain Research*, 14, 2139–2164. https://doi.org/10.2147/JPR.S315585

Anderson, K. D., & Downey, M. (2021). Foot reflexology: An intervention for pain and nausea among inpatients with cancer. *Clinical Journal of Oncology Nursing*, *25*(5), 539–545. https://doi.org/10.1188/21.Cjon.539-545

Azizoddin, D. R., Schreiber, K., Beck, M. R., Enzinger, A. C., Hruschak, V., Darnall, B. D., Edwards, R. R., Allsop, M. J., Tulsky, J. A., Boyer, E., & Mackey, S. (2021). Chronic pain severity, impact, and opioid use among patients with cancer: An analysis of biopsychosocial factors using the CHOIR learning health care system. *Cancer*, *127*(17), 3254–3263. https://doi.org/10.1002/cncr.33645

Bar-Lev Schleider, L., Mechoulam, R., Lederman, V., Hilou, M., Lencovsky, O., Betzalel, O., Shbiro, L., & Novack, V. (2018). Prospective analysis of safety and efficacy of medical cannabis in large unselected population of patients with cancer. *European Journal of Internal Medicine*, *49*, 37–43. https://doi.org/10.1016/j.ejim.2018.01.023

Berger, J. M., Longhitano, Y., Zanza, C., & Sener, S. F. (2020). Factors affecting the incidence of chronic pain following breast cancer surgery: Preoperative history, anesthetic management, and surgical technique. *Journal of Surgical Oncology*, *122*(7), 1307–1314. https://doi.org/10.1002/jso.26176

Boland, E. G., Bennett, M. I., Allgar, V., & Boland, J. W. (2020). Cannabinoids for adult cancer-related pain: Systematic review and meta-analysis. *BMJ Support Palliat Care*, *10*(1), 14–24. https://doi.org/10.1136/bmjspcare-2019-002032

Bouquié, R., Deslandes, G., Mazaré, H., Cogné, M., Mahé, J., Grégoire, M., & Jolliet, P. (2018). Cannabis and anticancer drugs: Societal usage and expected pharmacological interactions—A review. *Fundamental & Clinical Pharmacology*, *32*(5), 462–484. https://doi.org/10.1111/fcp.12373

Braun, I. M., Nayak, M. M., Revette, A., Wright, A. A., Chai, P. R., Yusufov, M., Pirl, W. F., & Tulsky, J. A. (2021). Cancer patients' experiences with medicinal cannabis—related care. *Cancer*, *127*(1), 67–73. https://doi.org/10.1002/cncr.33202

Buchwald, D., Brønnum, D., Melgaard, D., & Leutscher, P. D. C. (2020). Living with a hope of survival is challenged by a lack of clinical evidence: An interview study among cancer patients using cannabis-based medicine. *Journal of Palliative Medicine*, *23*(8), 1090–1093. https://doi.org/10.1089/jpm.2019.0298

Cadet, T., Davis, C., Wilson, P., & Elks, J. (2022). The experiences of touch therapies in symptom management of rural and regional cancer patients in Australia. *International Journal of Therapeutic Massage & Bodywork*, *15*(1), 66–71. https://doi.org/10.3822/ijtmb.v15i1.687

Cassileth, B. R., Deng, G. E., Gomez, J. E., Johnstone, P. A. S., Kumar, N., & Vickers, A. J. (2007). Complementary therapies and integrative oncology in lung cancer: ACCP evidence-based clinical practice guidelines (2nd edition). *Chest*, *132*(3 Suppl), 340S-354S. https://doi.org/10.1378/chest.07-1389

Check, D. K., Winger, J. G., Jones, K. A., & Somers, T. J. (2021). Predictors of response to an evidence-based behavioral cancer pain management intervention: An exploratory analysis from a clinical trial. *Journal of Pain and Symptom Management*, 62(2), 391–399. https://doi.org/10.1016/j.jpainsymman.2020.12.020

Chen, Y., Spillane, S., Shiels, M. S., Young, L., Quach, D., Berrington de González, A., & Freedman, N. D. (2022). Trends in opioid use among cancer patients in the United States: 2013–2018. *JNCI Cancer Spectrum*, 6(1), pkab095. https://doi.org/10.1093/jncics/pkab095

Cheung, K. W. A., Chan, P. C., & Lo, S. H. (2020). The use of ketamine in the management of refractory cancer pain in a palliative care unit. *Annals of Palliative Medicine*, 9(6), 4478–4489. https://doi.org/10.21037/apm.2019.09.09

Clark, C. S. (2018). Medical cannabis: The oncology nurse's role in patient education about the effects of marijuana on cancer palliation. *Clinical Journal of Oncology Nursing*, 22(1), E1–E6. https://doi.org/10.1188/18.Cjon.E1-e6

Crombez, P., Bron, D., & Michiels, S. (2019). Multicultural approaches of cancer pain. *Current Opinion in Oncology*, 31(4), 268–274. https://doi.org/10.1097/cco.0000000000000547

Darawad, M., Alnajar, M. K., Abdalrahim, M. S., & El-Aqoul, A. M. (2019). Cancer pain management at oncology units: Comparing knowledge, attitudes and perceived barriers between physicians and nurses. *Journal of Cancer Education*, 34(2), 366–374. https://doi.org/10.1007/s13187-017-1314-4

Do, E. K., Ksinan, A. J., Kim, S. J., Del Fabbro, E. G., & Fuemmeler, B. F. (2021). Cannabis use among cancer survivors in the United States: Analysis of a nationally representative sample. *Cancer*, 127(21), 4040–4049. https://doi.org/10.1002/cncr.33794

Donovan, K. A., Oberoi-Jassal, R., Chang, Y. D., Rajasekhara, S., Haas, M. F., Randich, A. L., & Portman, D. G. (2020). Cannabis use in young adult cancer patients. *Journal of Adolescent and Young Adult Oncology*, 9(1), 30–35. https://doi.org/10.1089/jayao.2019.0039

Dziedzic, K. L., & Albert, R. H. (2021). Management of intractable symptoms in oncologic care. *Current Oncology Reports*, 23(8), 93. https://doi.org/10.1007/s11912-021-01082-2

Evenepoel, M., Haenen, V., De Baerdemaecker, T., Meeus, M., Devoogdt, N., Dams, L., Van Dijck, S., Van der Gucht, E., & De Groef, A. (2022). Pain prevalence during cancer treatment: a systematic review and meta-analysis. *Journal of Pain and Symptom Management*, 63(3), e317–e335. https://doi.org/10.1016/j.jpainsymman.2021.09.011

Fallon, M., Giusti, R., Aielli, F., Hoskin, P., Rolke, R., Sharma, M., & Ripamonti, C. I. (2018a). Management of cancer pain in adult patients: ESMO clinical practice guidelines. *Annals of Oncology*, 29(Suppl 4), iv166–iv191. https://doi.org/10.1093/annonc/mdy152

Fallon, M., Walker, J., Colvin, L., Rodriguez, A., Murray, G., Sharpe, M., & Group, M. T. S. (2018b). Pain management in cancer center inpatients: A cluster randomized trial to evaluate a systematic integrated approach— The Edinburgh pain assessment and management tool. *Journal of Clinical Oncology, 36*(13), 1284–1290. https://doi.org/10.1200/jco.2017.76.1825

Fauer, A. J., Davis, M. A., Choi, S. W., Wallner, L. P., & Friese, C. R. (2020). Use of gabapentinoid medications among US adults with cancer, 2005–2015. *Supportive Care in Cancer, 28*(1), 5–8. https://doi.org/10.1007/s00520-019-05100-9

Ferrell, B. R., Temel, J. S., Temin, S., Alesi, E. R., Balboni, T. A., Basch, E. M., Firn, J. I., Paice, J. A., Peppercorn, J. M., Phillips, T., Stovall, E. L., Zimmermann, C., & Smith, T. J. (2017). Integration of palliative care into standard oncology care: American Society of Clinical Oncology Clinical Practice Guideline update. *Journal of Clinical Oncology, 35*(1), 96–112. https://doi.org/10.1200/jco.2016.70.1474

Gress, K. L., Charipova, K., Kaye, A. D., Viswanath, O., & Urits, I. (2020). An overview of current recommendations and options for the management of cancer pain: A comprehensive review. *Oncology and Therapy, 8*(2), 251–259. https://doi.org/10.1007/s40487-020-00128-y

Gulati, R. R. (2021). The challenge of cancer pain assessment. *Ulster Medical Journal, 90*(1), 37–40.

Han, C. J., Chi, N. C., Han, S., Demiris, G., Parker-Oliver, D., Washington, K., Clayton, . M. F., Reblin, M., & Ellington, L. (2018). Communicating caregivers' challenges with cancer pain management: An analysis of home hospice visits. *Journal of Pain and Symptom Management, 55*(5), 1296–1303. https://doi.org/10.1016/j.jpainsymman.2018.01.004

Hao, D., Sidharthan, S., Cotte, J., Decker, M., Salisu-Orhurhu, M., Olatoye, D., Karri, J., Hagedorn, J. M., Adekoya, P., Odonkor, C., Gulati, A., & Orhurhu, V. (2021). Interventional therapies for pain in cancer patients: A narrative review. *Current Pain and Headache Reports, 25*(7), 44. https://doi.org/10.1007/s11916-021-00963-2

Haun, M. W., Estel, S., Rücker, G., Friederich, H. C., Villalobos, M., Thomas, M., & Hartmann, M. (2017). Early palliative care for adults with advanced cancer. *Cochrane Database of Systematic Reviews, 6*. https://doi.org/10.1002/14651858.CD011129.pub2

Hawker, G. A., Mian, S., Kendzerska, T., & French, M. (2011). Measures of adult pain: Visual analog scale for pain (VAS Pain), numeric rating scale for pain (NRS Pain), McGill Pain Questionnaire (MPQ), short-form McGill Pain Questionnaire (SF-MPQ), chronic pain grade scale (CPGS), short form-36 bodily pain scale (SF-36 BPS), and measure of intermittent and constant osteoarthritis pain (ICOAP). *Arthritis Care & Research, 63*(S11), S240–S252. https://doi.org/10.1002/acr.20543

Jeter, K., Blackwell, S., Burke, L., Joyce, D., Moran, C., Conway, E. V., Cremen, I., O'Connor, B., Ui Dhuibhir, P., & Walsh, D. (2018). Cancer symptom scale preferences: Does one size fit all? *BMJ Support Palliat Care, 8*(2), 198–203. https://doi.org/10.1136/bmjspcare-2015-001018

Khatooni, M. (2021). Cancer pain: An evolutionary concept analysis. *Professional Case Management, 26*(6), 275–285. https://doi.org/10.1097/ncm.0000000000 000509

Kim, H. J., & Jung, S. O. (2020). Comparative evaluations of single-item pain-intensity measures in cancer patients: Numeric rating scale vs. verbal rating scale. *Journal of Clinical Nursing, 29*(15–16), 2945–2952. https://doi.org/10.1111/jocn.15341

Kleckner, A. S., Kleckner, I. R., Kamen, C. S., Tejani, M. A., Janelsins, M. C., Morrow, G. R., & Peppone, L. J. (2019). Opportunities for cannabis in supportive care in cancer. *Therapeutic Advances in Medical Oncology, 11*, 1758835919866362. https://doi.org/10.1177/1758835919866362

Kwekkeboom, K. L., Tostrud, L., Costanzo, E., Coe, C. L., Serlin, R. C., Ward, S. E., & Zhang, Y. (2018). The Role of Inflammation in the pain, fatigue, and sleep disturbance symptom cluster in advanced cancer. *Journal of Pain and Symptom Management, 55*(5), 1286–1295. https://doi.org/10.1016/j.jpainsy mman.2018.01.008

Lopes-Júnior, L. C., Rosa, G. S., Pessanha, R. M., Schuab, S., Nunes, K. Z., & Amorim, M. H. C. (2020). Efficacy of the complementary therapies in the management of cancer pain in palliative care: A systematic review. *Revista Latino-Americana de Enfermagem, 28*, e3377. https://doi.org/10.1590/1518-8 345.4213.3377

Madden, K., Haider, A., Rozman De Moraes, A., Naqvi, S. M., Enriquez, P. A., Wu, J., Williams, J., Liu, D., & Bruera, E. (2021). Frequency of concomitant use of gabapentinoids and opioids among patients with cancer-related pain at an outpatient palliative care clinic. *Journal of Palliative Medicine, 24*(1), 91–96. https://doi.org/10.1089/jpm.2019.0614

Makhlouf, S. M., Pini, S., Ahmed, S., & Bennett, M. I. (2020). Managing pain in people with cancer-a systematic review of the attitudes and knowledge of professionals, patients, caregivers and public. *Journal of Cancer Education, 35*(2), 214–240. https://doi.org/10.1007/s13187-019-01548-9

Mantoudi, A., Parpa, E., Tsilika, E., Batistaki, C., Nikoloudi, M., Kouloulias, V., Kostopoulou, S., Galanos, A., & Mystakidou, K. (2020). Complementary therapies for patients with cancer: Reflexology and relaxation in integrative palliative care. A randomized controlled comparative study. *Journal of Alternative and Complementary Medicine, 26*(9), 792–798. https://doi.org/10.1089/acm.2019.0402

Mao, J. J., Greenlee, H., Bao, T., Ismaila, N., Bruera, E., & on behalf of the SIO-ASCO Expert Panel. (2023). Integrative medicine for pain management in oncology: Society for integrative oncology-ASCO guideline summary and Q&A. *JCO Oncology Practice, 19*, 45–48. https://doi.org/10.1200/op.22.00622

McTaggart-Cowan, H., Bentley, C., Raymakers, A., Metcalfe, R., Hawley, P., & Peacock, S. (2021). Understanding cancer survivors' reasons to medicate with cannabis: A qualitative study based on the theory of planned behavior. *Cancer Medicine, 10*(1), 396–404. https://doi.org/10.1002/cam4.3536

Meghani, S. H., Wool, J., Davis, J., Yeager, K. A., Mao, J. J., & Barg, F. K. (2020). When patients take charge of opioids: Self-management concerns and practices among cancer outpatients in the context of opioid crisis. *Journal of Pain and Symptom Management, 59*(3), 618–625. https://doi.org/10.1016/j.jpainsymman.2019.10.029

Nugent, S. M., Meghani, S. H., Rogal, S. S., & Merlin, J. S. (2020). Medical cannabis use among individuals with cancer: An unresolved and timely issue. *Cancer, 126*(9), 1832–1836. https://doi.org/10.1002/cncr.32732

Paice, J. A., Bohlke, K., Barton, D., Craig, D. S., El-Jawahri, A., Hershman, D. L., Kong, L. R., Kurita, G. P., LeBlanc, T. W., Mercadante, S., Novick, K. L. M., Sedhom, R., Seigel, C., Stimmel, J., & Bruera, E. (2022). Use of opioids for adults with pain from cancer or cancer treatment: ASCO guideline. *Journal of Clinical Oncology, 41*, 914–930. https://doi.org/10.1200/JCO.22.02198

Patton, L., Avsar, P., Nugent, D. L., O'Connor, T., Patton, D., & Moore, Z. (2021). What is the impact of specialist palliative care outpatient consultations on pain in adult patients with cancer? A systematic review. *European Journal of Oncology Nursing, 55*, 102034. https://doi.org/10.1016/j.ejon.2021.102034

Philpot, L. M., Ebbert, J. O., & Hurt, R. T. (2019). A survey of the attitudes, beliefs and knowledge about medical cannabis among primary care providers. *BMC Family Practice, 20*(1), 17. https://doi.org/10.1186/s12875-019-0906-y

Potts, J. M., Getachew, B., Vu, M., Nehl, E., Yeager, K. A., Leach, C. R., & Berg, C. J. (2022). Use and perceptions of opioids versus marijuana among cancer survivors. *Journal of Cancer Education, 37*(1), 91–101. https://doi.org/10.1007/s13187-020-01791-5

Raja, S. N., Carr, D. B., Cohen, M., Finnerup, N. B., Flor, H., Gibson, S., Keefe, F. J., Mogil, J. S., Ringkamp, M., Sluka, K. A., Song, X.-J., Stevens, B., Sullivan, M. D., Tutelman, P. R., Ushida, T., & Vader, K. (2020). The revised International Association for the Study of Pain definition of pain: concepts, challenges, and compromises. *Pain, 161*(9), 1976–1982. https://doi.org/10.1097/j.pain.0000000000001939

Ruano, A., García-Torres, F., Gálvez-Lara, M., & Moriana, J. A. (2022). Psychological and non-pharmacologic treatments for pain in cancer patients: A systematic review and meta-analysis. *Journal of Pain and Symptom Management, 63*(5), e505–e520. https://doi.org/10.1016/j.jpainsymman.2021.12.021

Scarborough, B. M., & Smith, C. B. (2018). Optimal pain management for patients with cancer in the modern era. *CA: A Cancer Journal for Clinicians, 68*(3), 182–196. https://doi.org/10.3322/caac.21453

Seow, H., Guthrie, D. M., Stevens, T., Barbera, L. C., Burge, F., McGrail, K., Chan, K. K. W., Peacock, S. J., & Sutradhar, R. (2021). Trajectory of end-of-life pain and other physical symptoms among cancer patients receiving home care. *Current Oncology, 28*(3), 1641–1651. https://doi.org/10.3390/curronco l28030153

Shin, J., Harris, C., Oppegaard, K., Kober, K. M., Paul, S. M., Cooper, B. A., Hammer, M., Conley, Y., Levine, J. D., & Miaskowski, C. (2022a). Worst pain severity profiles of oncology patients are associated with significant stress and multiple co-occurring symptoms. *The Journal of Pain, 23*(1), 74–88. https://doi.org/10.1016/j.jpain.2021.07.001

Shin, J., Oppegaard, K., Calvo-Schimmel, A., Harris, C., Cooper, B. A., Paul, S. M., Conley, Y. P., Hammer, M. J., Cartwright, F., Kober, K. M., Levine, J., & Miaskowski, C. (2022b). Distinct worst pain profiles in oncology outpatients undergoing chemotherapy. *Cancer Nursing, 46,* 176–188. https://doi.org/ 10.1097/ncc.0000000000001095

Sine, H., Achbani, A., & Filali, K. (2022). The effect of hypnosis on the intensity of pain and anxiety in cancer patients: A systematic review of controlled experimental trials. *Cancer Investigation, 40*(3), 235–253. https://doi.org/10. 1080/07357907.2021.1998520

Singh, V., Zarrabi, A. J., Curseen, K. A., Sniecinski, R., Welsh, J. W., McKenzie-Brown, A. M., Baer, W., & Gillespie, T. W. (2019). Concerns of patients with cancer on accessing cannabis products in a state with restrictive medical marijuana laws: a survey study. *JCO Oncology Practice, 15*(10), 531–538. https:// doi.org/10.1200/jop.19.00184

Sipilä, R., Kalso, E., & Lötsch, J. (2020). Machine-learned identification of psychological subgroups with relation to pain interference in patients after breast cancer treatments. *Breast, 50,* 71–80. https://doi.org/10.1016/j.breas t.2020.01.042

Smyth, J. A., Dempster, M., Warwick, I., Wilkinson, P., & McCorry, N. K. (2018). A systematic review of the patient- and carer-related factors affecting the experience of pain for advanced cancer patients cared for at home. *Journal of Pain and Symptom Management, 55*(2), 496–507. https://doi.org/10.1016/j.jp ainsymman.2017.08.012

Ullgren, H., Tsitsi, T., Papastavrou, E., & Charalambous, A. (2018). How family caregivers of cancer patients manage symptoms at home: A systematic review. *International Journal of Nursing Studies, 85,* 68–79. https://doi.org/ 10.1016/j.ijnurstu.2018.05.004

Vinette, B., Côté, J., El-Akhras, A., Mrad, H., Chicoine, G., & Bilodeau, K. (2022). Routes of administration, reasons for use, and approved indications of medical cannabis in oncology: A scoping review. *BMC Cancer, 22*(1), 319. https://doi.org/10.1186/s12885-022-09378-7

Webb, J. A., & LeBlanc, T. W. (2018). Evidence-based management of cancer pain. *Seminars in Oncology Nursing, 34*(3), 215–226. https://doi.org/10.1016 /j.soncn.2018.06.003

Whitcomb, B., Lutman, C., Pearl, M., Medlin, E., Prendergast, E., Robison, K., & Burke, W. (2020). Use of cannabinoids in cancer patients: A Society of Gynecologic Oncology (SGO) clinical practice statement. *Gynecologic Oncology, 157*(2), 307–311. https://doi.org/10.1016/j.ygyno.2019.12.013

Worster, B., Hajjar, E. R., & Handley, N. (2022). Cannabis use in patients with cancer: A clinical review. *JCO Oncology Practice, 18*, Op2200080. https://doi.org/10.1200/op.22.00080

Yang, J., Wahner-Roedler, D. L., Zhou, X., Johnson, L. A., Do, A., Pachman, D. R., Chon, T. Y., Salinas, M., Millstine, D., & Bauer, B. A. (2021). Acupuncture for palliative cancer pain management: Systematic review. *BMJ Support Palliat Care, 11*(3), 264–270. https://doi.org/10.1136/bmjspcare-2020-002638

Yoong, J., & Poon, P. (2018). Principles of cancer pain management: An overview and focus on pharmacological and interventional strategies. *Australian Journal of General Practice, 47*(11), 758–762. https://doi.org/10.31128/ajgp-07-18-4629

Zolotov, Y., Eshet, L., & Morag, O. (2021). Preliminary assessment of medical cannabis consumption by cancer survivors. *Complementary Therapies in Medicine, 56*, 102592. https://doi.org/10.1016/j.ctim.2020.102592

CHAPTER 5

SLEEP DISTURBANCES

INTRODUCTION

Sleep is important for quality of life, and sleep disturbance leads to adverse outcomes, especially for people with cancer (Matthews et al., 2018a). Poor sleep is associated with pain and depression (Zdanys & Steffens, 2015), both of which are common problems during and after cancer treatment. Sleep worsens pain and depression, and pain and depression impact sleep. Sleep disorders include insomnia, hypersomnia, and circadian rhythm disorders (López et al., 2016). Sleep disturbances, including both short and long sleep duration, are also associated with cancer-specific and all-cause mortality (Stone et al., 2019). Poor sleep may worsen pain intensity; it also plays a role in posttraumatic stress disorder (Lillis et al., 2018) and higher symptom burden (Calvo-Schimmel et al., 2022). While there appears to be a bidirectional association between sleep and the development of cancer (Mogavero et al., 2021), this chapter will focus on sleep disturbance as a symptom of cancer, rather than a contributing cause.

PREVALENCE

Much of the research on sleep disturbance has been conducted in women with breast cancer. In one systematic review in this population, 40% of women experienced this symptom (Leysen et al., 2019). In men with prostate cancer, 39% experienced sleep disturbance across the disease trajectory (Zenger et al., 2010). Of those with lung cancer, 40% report sleep problems (Rades et al., 2021). As a comparison, 30% of the general population report some form of sleep disorder.

CONTRIBUTING FACTORS

Both physical and psychological factors contribute to problems with sleep; psychological factors appear to be a larger contributor to sleep disturbance than physical factors (Schulte et al., 2021).

- In women with breast cancer, depression, distress, hot flashes, and anxiety, as well as poor physical function, contribute to sleep disturbance (Kreutz et al., 2019). Younger age is also a contributing factor in this population (Berger et al., 2019). Being treated with radiation and/or chemotherapy also contributes to the development of sleep disorders (Grayson et al., 2022). Pain and fatigue are also involved (Leysen et al., 2019). While anxiety contributes to poor sleep in the early phase of treatment, fatigue and perceived stress appear to be involved later (Yang et al., 2022).

- In men with prostate cancer, urinary symptoms and hot flashes are also contributing factors for those on androgen deprivation (Robbins et al., 2022). Sleep disturbance is linked to depression, which may make treatment decision-making more challenging (Sharpley et al., 2021).

- Alterations in body image and the need to urinate contribute to sleep disturbance in women with gynecologic cancer (Aquil et al., 2021).

- Depression and anxiety, as well as physical problems (dyspnea, pain, and fatigue), impact sleep of lung cancer survivors (Rades et al., 2021).

- Fear of recurrence, cancer-related distress, and intrusive thoughts contribute to poor sleep in people treated with autologous stem cell transplant (Nelson et al., 2018).

- Higher body mass and previous sleep problems are also risk factors for poor sleep in those treated with chemotherapy (Mark et al., 2017).

- The sleep quality of the partner also impacts the sleep quality of the person with cancer (Otto et al., 2019).

- Among hospitalized patients, multiple factors impact sleep; few institutions employ sleep-friendly initiatives, such as decreasing overhead announcements and decreasing ambient lighting in the hallways, among other actions that improve sleep quality (Affini et al., 2022).

ASSESSMENT

A formal assessment of sleep quality and quantity is rarely conducted in people with cancer (Khater et al., 2019); however, there are a number of tools that can be used to identify sleep disturbance that if corrected can improve the quality of life of this population. A *sleep history* or a *sleep diary* can help identify factors that disturb sleep, but it does rely on subjective recall and may not be accurate enough to make a diagnosis.

Pittsburgh Sleep Quality Index

The most commonly cited measure is the Pittsburgh Sleep Quality Index (PSQI). This 19-item self-report measure assesses sleep quality and duration, sleep efficiency, sleep latency (the time it takes to fall asleep), sleep disturbances, daytime function, and the use of sleep medication over the previous month (Buysse et al., 1989).

Patient-Reported Outcomes Measurement Information System Sleep Disturbance Short Form

The PROMIS (Patient-Reported Outcomes Measurement Information System) Sleep Disturbance Short Form contains eight questions about sleep over the past 7 days, including questions about sleep quality and satisfaction, as well as problems falling asleep, restlessness, and worry (file:///C:/Users/akatz2/Downloads/PROMIS_Short_Form_v1.0_-_Sleep_Disturbance_-_8a_16Mar2020.pdf).

Insomnia Severity Index

The Insomnia Severity Index (ISI; Morin et al., 2011) is a seven-item self-report questionnaire that measures sleep latency, staying asleep, early awakening, sleep interference, worry, sleep satisfaction, and how noticeable sleep problems are to others.

Jenkins Sleep Scale

The four-item Jenkins Sleep Scale (JSS) was developed to measure sleep problems in clinical research (Jenkins et al., 1988). This self-report questionnaire measures trouble falling asleep and staying asleep, as well as waking during the night and feeling tired on waking.

A single item on the European Organisation for Research and Treatment of Cancer Quality of Life Questionnaire (EORTC QLQ-sC30)—"Have you had trouble sleeping?"—is comparable with the JSS, but a single item should not be used as stand-alone to assess sleep (Hofmeister et al., 2020).

It is suggested that adding a sleep item assessing insomnia to the Edmonton Symptom Assessment Scale-Revised (ESAS-r) is valuable. A score of 2 or higher on a 0 to 10 scale has high sensitivity in identifying those with sleep disturbance (Savard & Ivers, 2019).

Dysfunctional Beliefs and Attitudes About Sleep Scale for Cancer Patients

The Dysfunctional Beliefs and Attitudes About Sleep Scale for Cancer Patients (C-DBAS-14) is a newly developed 14-item questionnaire (Youn et al., 2020) that measures four factors, namely sleep expectation and consequences of insomnia, worry about sleep, medication use, and cancer concerns. It may be useful in educating patients and dispelling inaccurate beliefs about sleep as part of a comprehensive assessment.

See Figure 5.1 for screening questions from the National Comprehensive Cancer Network (NCCN).

Objective measures of sleep include polysomnography, which requires specialized equipment; and actigraphy, which uses a device on the wrist (Chen & Fang, 2018).

See Figure 5.1.

Are you having problems falling asleep, staying asleep, waking up too early, or with poor sleep quality?

Are you experiencing excessive sleepiness (sleepiness or falling asleep in inappropriate situations or sleeping more during a 24-hour period than in the past)?

Have you been told that you snore frequently or stop breathing during sleep?

Figure 5.1 National Comprehensive Cancer Network screening questions.

Source: From NCCN (2023). NCCN guidelines version 1.2023 survivorship: Sleep disorders.

MANAGEMENT

Assessment and treatment of modifiable contributing factors is the first step in managing sleep disorders. Contributing factors include alcohol or substance abuse, caffeine intake, anemia, medications, pain, fatigue, distress, depression, anxiety, chemotherapy-induced peripheral neuropathy, and so on.

Nonpharmaceutical Interventions

Cancer survivors will often attempt to manage sleep disturbances by themselves using a variety of methods, including herbal supplements and going to bed early (Reynolds-Cowie & Fleming, 2021); these are generally not effective and may increase the frustration and worry that the person experiences.

Cognitive Behavioral Interventions

Cognitive behavioral interventions are recommended for the management of sleep–wake disturbances in adults with cancer (Edinger et al., 2021; Matthews et al., 2018a). These include sleep restrictions during the day, stimulus control, education about sleep hygiene, and cognitive behavioral therapy with or without relaxation exercises (Morin & Benca, 2012). These interventions have been shown to be effective in patients undergoing chemotherapy (Palesh et al., 2018), and can be done at home (Barton et al., 2020) or as part of a group facilitated by sleep experts (Zhou et al., 2020).

Exercise

Exercise has been shown to be effective in improving the sleep quality of women with cancer (Armbruster et al., 2018); physical activity needs to be moderate to vigorous to be effective as well as aerobic to improve sleep (Matthews et al., 2018b). See Figure 5.2 for a listing of mind–body interventions that improve sleep.

Sleep Hygiene

Educating patients about sleep hygiene may be enough to improve both sleep quality and insomnia (Figure 5.3).

- Yoga has been shown to improve sleep quality for some (Lin et al., 2019; Selvan et al., 2022); however, this has not been shown to be effective in reducing insomnia (Wang et al., 2020).
- Tai Chi Chih, a form of mindful movement when accompanied by traditional cognitive behavioral therapy for insomnia, also results in improvement in sleep quality (Irwin et al., 2017).
- Acupuncture has also been shown to be effective in improving sleep quality in breast cancer survivors (Zhang et al., 2022).
- The use of bright light in the morning (Wu et al., 2018) may be useful but to date there has been imited evidence, although it has been used successfully to treat seasonal affective disorder (Bean et al., 2020).

Figure 5.2 Mind–body interventions.

- Keep to a regular bedtime and waketime every day.
- Perform regular exercise in the morning.
- Increase exposure to bright light during the day.
- Reduce exposure to bright light (computers, phone screens) within a few hours of bedtime and during the night.
- Avoid heavy meals before bedtime.
- Limit fluids within 3 hours of bedtime.
- Limit caffeine during the day and avoid within 4 hours of bedtime.
- Sleep in a dark, quiet room that is at a comfortable temperature.
- Try not to look at the clock if waking up during the night.
- Limit daytime naps to once a day, no longer than 30 minutes.
- Turn off light-emitting sources at bedtime.
- If unable to sleep within 45 minutes or upon waking in the night, get up and go to a different location that is dark and avoid any stimulating activity. Instead read a book or watch a relaxing TV program and then return to bed when feeling sleepy.

Figure 5.3 Sleep hygiene.

Source: NCCN Guidelines Version 1.2022 Survivorship: Sleep Disorders. https://www.nccn.org/professionals/physician_gls/pdf/survivorship.pdf.

Pharmaceutical Sleep Agents

Pharmaceutical sleep agents should only be used if other methods have not been successful. There is a risk of dependence, abuse, and withdrawal with many hypnotics, and regular assessment for the continued need of these medications is necessary.

See Figure 5.4.

Second-line use of hypnotics may be used if the patient has difficulty falling or staying asleep. The following medications help with both sleep initiation and maintenance: zolpidem CR, eszopiclone, temazepam, suvorexant, and lemborexant (www.nccn.org/professionals/physician_gls/pdf/survivorship.pdf). Melatonin, valerian, or tryptophan should not be used for sleep initiation or maintenance (Sateia et al., 2017).

The **Choosing Wisely** initiative states that hypnotics should not be used as the sole initial treatment for chronic insomnia for adults; rather use cognitive behavioral therapy methods including stimulus control and sleep restriction.

https://www.choosingwisely.org/clinician-lists/aasm-hypnotics-for-chronic-insomnia/

Figure 5.4 The Choosing Wisely initiative.

48 SECTION II • GENERAL SYMPTOMS

CASE STUDY

Your patient is a 54-year-old nurses' aid who does shift work. She was treated with brachytherapy for endometrial cancer 1 year ago. At her follow-up appointment, she says that she is still fatigued and wonders what might help her.

1. What further questions should you ask her?

She says she has seen a naturopath who sold her some pills but they have not helped.

2. What suggestions can you make that might be effective in managing her sleep disturbance?

She says she has heard that there are sleeping pills that can help and she wants to try those.

3. What is your response to this request?

GUIDELINES

- **American Academy of Sleep Medicine**

  Behavioral and Psychological Treatments for Chronic Insomnia Disorder in Adults: An American Academy of Sleep Medicine Clinical Practice Guideline (Edinger et al., 2021)

  Establishes clinical practice recommendations on the use of behavioral and psychological treatments for chronic insomnia disorder in adults (2016)

  https://jcsm.aasm.org/doi/10.5664/jcsm.8986

- **American Academy of Sleep Medicine**

  Clinical Practice Guideline for the Pharmacologic Treatment of Chronic Insomnia in Adults: An American Academy of Sleep Medicine Clinical Practice Guideline (Sateia et al., 2017)

  Establishes clinical practice recommendations for the pharmacologic treatment of chronic insomnia in adults; contains information about Food and Drug Administration (FDA)-approved medications for the treatment of insomnia in adults (2017)

  https://jcsm.aasm.org/doi/10.5664/jcsm.6470

- **American College of Physicians**

  Management of Chronic Insomnia Disorder in Adults: A Clinical Practice Guideline From the American College of Physicians (2016)

Provides the evidence in support of clinical management of insomnia in adults

https://www.acpjournals.org/doi/10.7326/m15-2175

- **National Comprehensive Cancer Network**

    NCCN Guidelines Version 1.2022 Survivorship: Sleep Disorders

    Provides comprehensive guidance on the assessment and management of sleep disorders in people with cancer

    www.nccn.org/professionals/physician_gls/pdf/survivorship.pdf

SUMMARY

Sleep disturbance is common along the disease trajectory and is associated with other symptoms such as anxiety and depression. Pharmaceutical agents should only be used if first-line interventions, such as education about sleep hygiene and mind–body interventions, have not been helpful.

A robust set of instructor resources designed to supplement this text is located at http://connect.springerpub.com/content/reference-book/978-0-8261-8524-2. Qualifying Instructors may request access by emailing **textbook@springerpub.com**.

REFERENCES

Affini, M. I., Arora, V. M., Gulati, J., Mason, N., Klein, A., Cho, H. J., Clarke, K., Lee, V., McDaniel, L. M., & Orlov, N. M. (2022). Defining existing practices to support the sleep of hospitalized patients: A mixed-methods study of top-ranked hospitals. *Journal of Hospital Medicine*, 17(8), 633–638. https://doi.org/10.1002/jhm.12917

Aquil, A., El Kherchi, O., El Azmaoui, N., Mouallif, M., Guerroumi, M., Chokri, A., Jayakumar, A. R., Benider, A., & Elgot, A. (2021). Body image dissatisfaction and lower self-esteem as major predictors of poor sleep quality in gynecological cancer patients after surgery: Cross-sectional study. *BMC Womens Health*, 21(1), 229. https://doi.org/10.1186/s12905-021-01375-5

Armbruster, S. D., Song, J., Gatus, L., Lu, K. H., & Basen-Engquist, K. M. (2018). Endometrial cancer survivors' sleep patterns before and after a physical activity intervention: A retrospective cohort analysis. *Gynecologic Oncology*, 149(1), 133–139. https://doi.org/10.1016/j.ygyno.2018.01.028

Barton, D. L., Atherton, P. J., Satele, D. V., Qin, R., Dakhil, S., Pipe, T., Hobday, T., Fee-Schroeder, K., & Loprinzi, C. L. (2020). A randomized phase II trial evaluating two non-pharmacologic interventions in cancer survivors for the treatment of sleep-wake disturbances: NCCTG N07C4 (Alliance).

Supportive Care in Cancer, 28(12), 6085–6094. https://doi.org/10.1007/s005 20-020-05461-6

Berger, A. M., Kupzyk, K. A., Djalilova, D. M., & Cowan, K. H. (2019). Breast Cancer Collaborative Registry informs understanding of factors predicting sleep quality. *Supportive Care in Cancer, 27*(4), 1365–1373. https://doi.org/10.1007/s00520-018-4417-5

Buysse, D. J., Reynolds, C. F., Monk, T. H., Berman, S. R., & Kupfer, D. J. (1989). The Pittsburgh sleep quality index: A new instrument for psychiatric practice and research. *Psychiatry Research, 28*(2), 193–213. https://doi.org/10.1016/0165-1781(89)90047-4

Calvo-Schimmel, A., Paul, S. M., Cooper, B. A., Harris, C., Shin, J., Oppegaard, K., Hammer, M. J., Dunn, L. B., Conley, Y. P., Kober, K. M., Levine, J. D., & Miaskowski, C. (2022). Oncology outpatients with worse depression and sleep disturbance profiles are at increased risk for a higher symptom burden and poorer quality of life outcomes. *Sleep Medicine, 95*, 91–104. https://doi.org/10.1016/j.sleep.2022.04.023

Chen, D. Y. Z., & Fang, B. (2018). Measurements and status of sleep quality in patients with cancers. *Supportive Care in Cancer, 26*(2), 405–414. https://doi.org/10.1007/s00520-017-3927-x

Edinger, J. D., Arned., J. T., Bertisch, S. M., Carney, C. E., Harrington, J. J., Lichstein, K. L., Sateia, M. J., Troxel, W. M., Zhou, E. S., Kazmi, U., Heald, J. L., & Martin, J. L. (2021). Behavioral and psychological treatments for chronic insomnia disorder in adults: An American Academy of Sleep Medicine clinical practice guideline. *Journal of Clinical Sleep Medicine, 17*(2), 255–262. https://doi.org/10.5664/jcsm.8986

Grayson, S., Sereika, S., Harpel, C., Diego, E., Steiman, J. G., McAuliffe, P. F., & Wesmiller, S. (2022). Factors associated with sleep disturbances in women undergoing treatment for early-stage breast cancer. *Supportive Care in Cancer, 30*(1), 157–166. https://doi.org/10.1007/s00520-021-06373-9

Hofmeister, D., Schulte, T., & Hinz, A. (2020). Sleep problems in cancer patients: A comparison between the Jenkins Sleep Scale and the single-item sleep scale of the EORTC QLQ-C30. *Sleep Medicine, 71*, 59–65. https://doi.org/10.1016/j.sleep.2019.12.033

Jenkins, C. D., Stanton, B.-A., Niemcryk, S. J., & Rose, R. M. (1988). A scale for the estimation of sleep problems in clinical research. *Journal of Clinical Epidemiology, 41*(4), 313–321. https://doi.org/10.1016/0895-4356(88)90138-2

Khater, W., Masha'al, D., & Al-Sayaheen, A. (2019). Sleep assessment and interventions for patients living with cancer from the patients' and nurses' perspective. *International Journal of Palliative Nursing, 25*(7), 316–324. https://doi.org/10.12968/ijpn.2019.25.7.316

Kreutz, C., Schmidt, M. E., & Steindorf, K. (2019). Effects of physical and mind-body exercise on sleep problems during and after breast cancer treatment: A systematic review and meta-analysis. *Breast Cancer Research and Treatment, 176*(1), 1–15. https://doi.org/10.1007/s10549-019-05217-9

Leysen, L., Lahousse, A., Nijs, J., Adriaenssens, N., Mairesse, O., Ivakhnov, S., Bilterys, T., Van Looveren, E., Pas, R., & Beckwée, D. (2019). Prevalence and risk factors of sleep disturbances in breast cancer survivors: Systematic review and meta-analyses. *Supportive Care in Cancer, 27*(12), 4401–4433. https://doi.org/10.1007/s00520-019-04936-5

Lillis, T. A., Gerhart, J., Bouchard, L. C., Cvengros, J., O'Mahony, S., Kopkash, K., Kabaker, K. B., & Burns, J. (2018). Sleep disturbance mediates the association of post-traumatic stress disorder symptoms and pain in patients with cancer. *American Journal of Hospice and Palliative Medicine, 35*(5), 788–793. https://doi.org/10.1177/1049909117739299

López, E., de, la Torre-Luque., A, Lazo., A, Álvarez., J, & Buela-Casal, G. (2016). Assessment of sleep disturbances in patients with cancer: Cross-sectional study in a radiotherapy department. *European Journal of Oncology Nursing, 20*, 71–76. https://doi.org/10.1016/j.ejon.2014.12.008

Mark, S., Cataldo, J., Dhruva, A., Paul, S. M., Chen, L. M., Hammer, M. J., Levine, J. D., Wright, F., Melisko, M., Lee, K., Conley, Y. P., & Miaskowski, C. (2017). Modifiable and non-modifiable characteristics associated with sleep disturbance in oncology outpatients during chemotherapy. *Supportive Care in Cancer, 25*(8), 2485–2494. https://doi.org/10.1007/s00520-017-3655-2

Matthews, E. E., Carter, P., Page, M., Dean, G., & Berger, A. (2018a). Sleep-wake disturbance: A systematic review of evidence-based interventions for management in patients with cancer. *Clinical Journal of Oncology Nursing, 22*(1), 37–52. https://doi.org/10.1188/18.Cjon.37-52

Matthews, E. E., Janssen, D. W., Djalilova, D. M., & Berger, A. M. (2018b). Effects of exercise on sleep in women with breast cancer: A systematic review. *Sleep Medicine Clinics, 13*(3), 395–417. https://doi.org/10.1016/j.jsmc.2018.04.007

Mogavero, M. P., DelRosso, L. M., Fanfulla, F., Bruni, O., & Ferri, R. (2021). Sleep disorders and cancer: State of the art and future perspectives. *Sleep Medicine Reviews, 56*, 101409. https://doi.org/10.1016/j.smrv.2020.101409

Morin, C. M., Belleville, G., Bélanger, L., & Ivers, H. (2011). The insomnia severity index: Psychometric indicators to detect insomnia cases and evaluate treatment response. *Sleep, 34*(5), 601–608. https://doi.org/10.1093/sleep/34.5.601

Morin, C. M., & Benca, R. (2012). Chronic insomnia. *The Lancet, 379*(9821), 1129–1141. https://doi.org/10.1016/S0140-6736(11)60750-2

Nelson, A. M., Jim, H. S. L., Small, B. J., Nishihori, T., Gonzalez, B. D., Cessna, J. M., Hyland, K. A., Rumble, M. E., & Jacobsen, P. B. (2018). Sleep disruption among cancer patients following autologous hematopoietic cell transplantation. *Bone Marrow Transplant, 53*(3), 307–314. https://doi.org/10.1038/s41409-017-0022-3

Otto, A. K., Gonzalez, B. D., Heyman, R. E., Vadaparampil, S. T., Ellington, L., & Reblin, M. (2019). Dyadic effects of distress on sleep duration in advanced cancer patients and spouse caregivers. *Psychooncology*, *28*(12), 2358–2364. https://doi.org/10.1002/pon.5229

Palesh, O., Scheiber, C., Kesler, S., Janelsins, M. C., Guido, J. J., Heckler, C., Cases, M. G., Miller, J., Chrysson, N. G., & Mustian, K. M. (2018). Feasibility and acceptability of brief behavioral therapy for cancer-related insomnia: Effects on insomnia and circadian rhythm during chemotherapy: a phase II randomised multicentre controlled trial. *British Journal of Cancer*, *119*(3), 274–281. https://doi.org/10.1038/s41416-018-0154-2

Rades, D., Kopelke, S., Tvilsted, S., Kjaer, T. W., Schild, S. E., & Bartscht, T. (2021). Sleep disturbances in lung cancer patients assigned to definitive or adjuvant irradiation. *In Vivo*, *35*(6), 3333–3337. https://doi.org/10.21873/invivo.12630

Reynolds-Cowie, P., & Fleming, L. (2021). Living with persistent insomnia after cancer: A qualitative analysis of impact and management. *British Journal of Health Psychology*, *26*(1), 33–49. https://doi.org/10.1111/bjhp.12446

Robbins, R., Cole, R., Ejikeme, C., Orstad, S. L., Porten, S., Salter, C. A., Nolasco, T. S., Vieira, D., & Loeb, S. (2022). Systematic review of sleep and sleep disorders among prostate cancer patients and caregivers: A call to action for using validated sleep assessments during prostate cancer care. *Sleep Medicine*, *94*, 38–53. https://doi.org/10.1016/j.sleep.2022.03.020

Sateia, M. J., Buysse, D. J., Krystal, A. D., Neubauer, D. N., & Heald, J. L. (2017). Clinical practice guideline for the pharmacologic treatment of chronic insomnia in adults: An American academy of sleep medicine clinical practice guideline. *Journal of Clinical Sleep Medicine*, *13*(02), 307–349. https://doi.org/10.5664/jcsm.6470

Savard, J., & Ivers, H. (2019). Screening for clinical insomnia in cancer patients with the Edmonton Symptom Assessment System-Revised: A specific sleep item is needed. *Supportive Care in Cancer*, *27*(10), 3777–3783. https://doi.org/10.1007/s00520-019-4662-2

Schulte, T., Hofmeister, D., Mehnert-Theuerkauf, A., Hartung, T., & Hinz, A. (2021). Assessment of sleep problems with the Insomnia Severity Index (ISI) and the sleep item of the Patient Health Questionnaire (PHQ-9) in cancer patients. *Supportive Care in Cancer*, *29*(12), 7377–7384. https://doi.org/10.1007/s00520-021-06282-x

Sharpley, C. F., Christie, D. R. H., & Bitsika, V. (2021). Deterioration in sleep quality affects cognitive depression in prostate cancer patients. *American Journal of Men's Health*, *15*(2), 15579883211001201. https://doi.org/10.1177/15579883211001201

Stone, C. R., Haig, T. R., Fiest, K. M., McNeil, J., Brenner, D. R., & Friedenreich, C. M. (2019). The association between sleep duration and cancer-specific mortality: A systematic review and meta-analysis. *Cancer Causes Control*, *30*(5), 501–525. https://doi.org/10.1007/s10552-019-01156-4

Yang, G. S., Starkweather, A. R., Lynch Kelly, D., Meegan, T., Byon, H. D., & Lyon, D. E. (2022). Longitudinal analysis of sleep disturbance in breast cancer survivors. *Nursing Research*, *71*(3), 177–188. https://doi.org/10.1097/nnr.0000000000000578

Youn, S., Kim, C., Lee, J., Yeo, S., Suh, S., & Chung, S. (2020). Development of dysfunctional beliefs and attitude about sleep scale for cancer patients. *Behavioral Sleep Medicine*, *18*(3), 287–297. https://doi.org/10.1080/15402002.2019.1578773

Zdanys, K. S., & Steffens, D. (2015). Sleep disturbances in the elderly. *Psychiatric Clinics of North America*, *38*(4), 723–741.

Zenger, M., Lehmann-Laue, A., Stolzenburg, J. U., Schwalenberg, T., Ried, A., & Hinz, A. (2010). The relationship of quality of life and distress in prostate cancer patients compared to the general population. *Psychosocial Medicine*, *7*, Doc02. https://doi.org/10.3205/psm000064

CHAPTER 6

LYMPHEDEMA

INTRODUCTION

Lymphedema is one of the most dreaded side effects of treatment for breast, gynecologic, and head and neck cancer. The swelling of the affected limb or body part is caused by an excess of interstitial fluid in the tissues (Abouelazayem et al., 2021). The underlying cause of lymphedema is interference with lymph drainage, but the exact mechanisms are not well-understood (DiSipio et al., 2013). Lymphedema is associated with distress and has an impact on quality of life, including difficulty finding clothing that fits. In turn, this may impact the willingness of the individual to engage in social activities. Lymphedema also has an economic impact on patients and society as a whole (De Vrieze et al., 2020).

PREVALENCE

Studies suggest that up to 21% of women with breast cancer will develop lymphedema. However, this statistic is based on studies with different methods of diagnosing and measuring the phenomenon (DiSipio et al., 2013). For women with gynecologic cancer, the estimated prevalence of lower limb lymphedema ranges from 0% to 69% (Bona et al., 2020). For patients treated for head and neck cancer, 75% have some form of lymphedema that may be present internally, externally, or both (Deng et al., 2012a).

CONTRIBUTING FACTORS

Axillary lymph node dissection is a major contributing factor for women treated for breast cancer, and the number of lymph nodes removed, mastectomy, and high body mass are additional risk factors (McLaughlin et al., 2020). Axillary radiation therapy is a significant risk factor for lymphedema in this population (Chaput et al., 2020; Lin et al., 2021). Women who receive taxane-based chemotherapy are also at increased risk (Michelotti et al., 2019).

56 SECTION II • GENERAL SYMPTOMS

Contributing factors for women with gynecologic cancer include the number of lymph nodes removed, adjuvant radiation therapy, higher body mass index, and little physical activity (Bona et al., 2020), as well as younger age (Guliyeva et al., 2020). Open surgery (laparotomy) for cervical cancer also contributes to the development of lymphedema (Li et al., 2021). Multimodal treatment (concurrent chemotherapy and radiation therapy) for head and neck cancer increases the risk of lymphedema. High body mass is another risk factor (Tribius et al., 2020).

In the past, caution was advised for certain activities that were thought to increase the risk of lymphedema. Newer research has changed the recommendations to avoid these activities as follows: There is not sufficient evidence to support the use of compression garments for air travel as prevention; avoidance of blood pressure measurement and avoidance of skin puncture on the affected side are also not warranted (Ahn & Port, 2016). Exercise and progressive weight training under supervision do not increase the risk or progression of lymphedema (www.issuu.com/lymphnet/docs/exercise).

ASSESSMENT

There are a number of measures that can be used in the diagnosis of lymphedema secondary to treatment for *breast cancer*; these range from measuring the circumference of the arm, to displacement of water to measure the volume of the affected limb, to more sophisticated technology (Table 6.1).

TABLE 6.1 Measuring the Affected Limb in Breast Cancer Survivors

Limb circumference	Measures several points on the affected arm	Simple, low-cost Reliable but with questionable sensitivity due to shape of arm
Water displacement	Immersion of arm in water Displacement of 200 mL or 10% of volume = lymphedema	Concerns about infection Time-consuming Imprecise
Perometry	Optical scanner that calculates arm volume	Expensive Not portable
Ultrasonography	Compares thickness of skin and subcutaneous tissue	Safe, cheap, accessible, noninvasive

(continued)

TABLE 6.1 Measuring the Affected Limb in Breast Cancer Survivors (*continued*)

MRI	Visualizes skin and subcutaneous tissue	Expensive Not portable
3D laser scanner	Emerging technique Accurate volume measurement	Noninvasive Reliable
BIS	Measures tissue resistance to electrical current	Noninvasive Expensive
Lymphoscintigraphy	Allows for visualization of lymphatic function	Accurate Expensive Uses radiotracer

BIS, bioimpedance spectroscopy.

Sources: From Michelotti, A., Invernizzi, M., Lopez, G., Lorenzini, D., Nesa, F., De Sire, A., & Fusco, N. (2019). Tackling the diversity of breast cancer related lymphedema: Perspectives on diagnosis, risk assessment, and clinical management. *Breast, 44,* 15–23. https://doi.org/10.1016/j.breast.2018.12.009; McLaughlin, S. A., Brunelle, C. L., & Taghian, A. (2020). Breast cancer-related lymphedema: Risk factors, screening, management, and the impact of locoregional treatment. *Journal of Clinical Oncology, 38*(20), 2341–2350. https://doi.org/10.1200/jco.19.02896.

According to the National Comprehensive Cancer Network (NCCN) guideline (www.nccn.org/professionals/physician_gls/pdf/survivorship.pdf), asking about swelling of the affected limb, a feeling of heaviness or fullness, pain, range of motion, strength, and fatigue should be done at each visit to promote early identification of developing lymphedema.

The most commonly reported subjective symptoms are swelling and heaviness in the affected limb (Gursen et al., 2021). Patient-reported measures are important in the diagnosis of lymphedema. A baseline measure of the limb on both the affected and unaffected sides should be taken.

A systematic review of patient-reported outcome measures for lymphedema and health-related quality of life concluded that, of the 35 measures reviewed, none could be recommended because they do not measure the totality of the experience of those with the condition (Beelen et al., 2021).

In an earlier systematic review, Pusic et al. (2013) found that only one of the measures reviewed was valid; the Upper Limb Lymphedema 27 (Launois et al., 2002) measures physical function and psychological and social domains.

For measurement of *lower limb lymphedema* after treatment for gynecologic cancer, circumference measures conducted in a consistent

58 SECTION II • GENERAL SYMPTOMS

manner are frequently used and both limbs should be measured. Perometry may also be used, but it is expensive and many clinicians are not able to use this method. Water displacement remains the gold standard, but it is not frequently used (Figure 6.1).

The Lymphedema Symptom Intensity and Distress Survey-Lower Limb (LSIDS-L) contains 31 items (Ridner, 2018).

Self-report Lower Extremity Lymphedema Screening Questionnaire contains 13 items (Yost, Cheville, Weaver, Al Hilli, & Dowdy, 2013).

The Gynecologic Cancer Lymphedema Questionnaire (SCLQ) has 20 items (Carter et al., 2010).

A single item (lymphedema) on the European Organisation for Research Treatment of Cancer (EORTC) Quality-of-Life Questionnaire cervical cancer module (QLQ-CX24) measures the quality of life of women with cervical cancer (Greimel et al., 2006).

Figure 6.1 Patient-reported measures for lower extremity lymphedema.

Assessment of *head and neck edema* is conducted using a variety of methods, including patient-reported outcomes (Lymphedema Symptom Intensity and Distress Survey [LSIDS-H&N]; Deng et al., 2012b). Clinician-reported measures are fraught with difficulties due to the challenges with the characteristics of head and neck lymphedema, which is often both internal and external (Deng et al., 2015). However, clinical examination remains important in the assessment of external lymphedema (Deng et al., 2012a). Imaging may be used, and digital photography can be useful to measure external changes over time. CT, MRI, and ultrasound are additional techniques that can be considered (Deng et al., 2015). A referral to a lymphedema specialist who can accurately measure the affected body part is warranted for anyone at risk of lymphedema; these professionals can also make recommendations for treatment (Figure 6.2).

• Stage 0 (latent/subclinical)—subtle symptoms without swelling; feeling of heaviness or fatigue in the limb
• Stage 1 (spontaneous reversible)—fluid causing swelling; pitting edema possible; increased girth, heaviness, stiffness; relieved with elevation of the limb
• Stage 2 (irreversible)—spongy tissue with pitting edema; tissue fibrosis causing hardness and increase in size; swelling not relieved with elevation of limb
• Stage 3 (lymphostatic elephantiasis)—dry, thickened, scaly skin; increased girth and swelling; fluid leakage and blisters on limbs; no pitting due to deposition of fat and fibrosis

Figure 6.2 Stages of lymphedema.

Source: From NCCN Guidelines Version 1.2000 Survivorship: Lymphedema. https://www.nccn.org/professionals/physician_gls/pdf/survivorship.pdf.

MANAGEMENT

Prevention

Prevention of lymphedema by limiting axillary surgery and radiation in women with breast cancer, as well as early detection of subclinical and latent stages, is important to limit progression. Surveillance, comprising at least three assessments and early treatment of lymphedema, is effective in preventing chronic lymphedema (Rafn et al., 2022).

Prehabilitation using some combination of physical therapy, progressive resistance training, compression garments, and manual lymphatic drainage (MLD) may be helpful (Heller et al., 2019).

Patient education is also key (Michelotti et al., 2019). This includes awareness of when the patient can contact their healthcare clinician/lymphedema specialist should they feel any heaviness, swelling, or tightness in the limb of the affected side. Some women report a feeling of numbness in the affected limb as one of the first signs of a developing lymphedema (Armer et al., 2003).

A healthy diet and exercise as well as skin hygiene and avoidance of injury and trauma to the affected side are additional components of patient education. Losing weight has been shown to decrease the volume of both the affected and unaffected limbs, but not with decreased severity of lymphedema when the volume of both limbs is compared (Tsai et al., 2020). Self-management with exercise, massage, and prevention has been shown to be effective at preventing the development of this condition after breast cancer treatment (Temur & Kapucu, 2019).

Lymphatic Therapy

Decongestive or complex lymphatic therapy (DLT or CDT) is the gold standard for management of upper arm lymphedema after breast cancer treatment (Chaput et al., 2020). These therapies comprise intensive MLD and application of compression bandages by a lymphedema specialist daily and maintenance use of compression garments thereafter. These therapies have been shown to be somewhat effective in women with breast cancer who presented with lymphedema within 12 months of developing symptoms (Jeffs et al., 2018). There is limited evidence on the effectiveness of MLD in the early stages after breast cancer treatment to avoid progression to more severe symptoms, but it may help reduce the volume of mild lymphedema (Marchica et al., 2021; Thompson et al., 2021).

Exercise

Resistance exercise, once thought to cause or accelerate upper arm lymphedema, has been shown to decrease it (Hasenoehrl et al., 2020a, 2020b; Olsson Möller et al., 2019). While strength/resistance training is the form of exercise most often recommended, other forms of physical activity, including yoga, Pilates, and aerobic exercise, may also be effective in reducing swelling and improving quality of life (Panchik et al., 2019). Swimming and aquatic exercises may also be helpful (Baumann et al., 2018), although the evidence on their effectiveness is inconclusive (Mur-Gimeno et al., 2022).

- *Kinesio taping* is as effective as other manual methods in women after mastectomy and is noninvasive (Kasawara et al., 2018).

- *Acupuncture* may be of benefit in the management of upper arm lymphedema, with some evidence of improvement (Chien et al., 2019; Hou et al., 2019; Yu et al., 2020). The addition of moxibustion (heat generated by lighting a moxa stick) may provide additional benefit to acupuncture (Gao et al., 2021).

- *Photobiomodulation therapy* (low-level laser therapy) may be of potential benefit in the management of lymphedema; however, the evidence is limited (Baxter et al., 2017; Chen et al., 2019).

Surgery

Microsurgical techniques that either resect fibrous tissue or reconnect lymphatic vessels to blood vessels may have a role to play in the prevention or management of upper arm lymphedema (McLaughlin et al., 2020; Michelotti et al., 2019). Similar methods to treat *lower limb lymphedema* are used (Liao et al., 2012). *Manual lymph drainage, liposuction, and surgical treatments* may be factors in reducing lymphedema in head and neck cancer (Tyker et al., 2019).

CASE STUDY

Your patient is a 48-year-old woman who is scheduled for a unilateral mastectomy next week. She is very tearful at her presurgery appointment with you. She tells you that her older sister had the same surgery 5 years ago and now has "bad swelling" in her right arm. She is terrified that the same thing will happen to her.

1. What advice would you give her?

2. What is the most important thing she should do before the surgery?

She comes to see you 2 weeks after her surgery. She is feeling well and is a little embarrassed that she "made such a fuss" before the surgery.

3. What should you do regarding her arm on the affected side at this visit?

4. What other instructions should you provide her with?

GUIDELINES

- A Systematic Review of Guidelines for Lymphedema and the Need for Contemporary Intersocietal Guidelines for the Management of Lymphedema(O'Donnell et al., 2020)

    Provides a systematic review of clinical practice guidelines not specific to cancer-related lymphedema

- **American Society of Clinical Oncology (ASCO)**

    ASCO Guideline on Integrative Therapies During and After Breast Cancer Treatment 2018

    Contains recommendations for a variety of symptoms, including lymphedema

    Suggests that low-level laser therapy, MLD, and compression bandages may help

    www.asco.org/practice-patients/guidelines/supportive-care-and-treatment-related-issues#/31666

- Best Practice Guidelines in Assessment, Risk Reduction, Management, and Surveillance for Post-breast Cancer Lymphedema(Armer et al., 2013)

    Provides guidance on the surveillance, assessment, risk reduction, and management of lymphedema after treatment for breast cancer

- **National Comprehensive Cancer Network (NCCN)**

    Provides a comprehensive overview of the principles, assessment, diagnosis, and treatment of lymphedema

    NCCN Guidelines Version 1.2022 Survivorship: Lymphedema

    www.nccn.org/professionals/physician_gls/pdf/survivorship.pdf

- **National Lymphedema Network**

    Position papers of the National Lymphedema Network

    Has a number of position statements on lymphedema, including risk reduction, diagnosis and treatment, screening and measurement, exercise, and healthy habits

    www.lymphnet.org/position-papers

SUMMARY

Lymphedema is a distressing side effect of surgery and radiation therapy for some cancers. While potentially reversible when recognized early, later stages of the condition are not reversible and the consequences have a negative impact on quality of life. Patient education and consistent surveillance are vital to early identification, and the role of the lymphedema specialist is invaluable for both assessment and treatment.

 A robust set of instructor resources designed to supplement this text is located at http://connect.springerpub.com/content/reference-book/978-0-8261-8524-2. Qualifying Instructors may request access by emailing textbook@springerpub.com.

REFERENCES

Abouelazayem, M., Elkorety, M., & Monib, S. (2021). Breast lymphedema after conservative breast surgery: An up-to-date systematic review. *Clinical Breast Cancer, 21*(3), 156–161. https://doi.org/10.1016/j.clbc.2020.11.017

Ahn, S., & Port, E. R. (2016). Lymphedema precautions: Time to abandon old practices? *Journal of Clinical Oncology, 34*(7), 655–658. https://doi.org/10.1200/jco.2015.64.9574

Armer, J. M., Hulett, J. M., Bernas, M., Ostby, P., Stewart, B. R., & Cormier, J. N. (2013). Best practice guidelines in assessment, risk reduction, management, and surveillance for post-breast cancer lymphedema. *Current Breast Cancer Reports, 5*(2), 134–144. https://doi.org/10.1007/s12609-013-0105-0

Armer, J. M., Radina, M. E., Porock, D., & Culbertson, S. D. (2003). Predicting breast cancer-related lymphedema using self-reported symptoms. *Nursing Research, 52*(6), 370–379. https://doi.org/10.1097/00006199-200311000-00004

Baumann, F. T., Reike, A., Reimer, V., Schumann, M., Hallek, M., Taaffe, D. R., Newton, R. U., & Galvao, D. A. (2018). Effects of physical exercise on breast cancer-related secondary lymphedema: A systematic review. *Breast Cancer Research and Treatment, 170*(1), 1–13. https://doi.org/10.1007/s10549-018-4725-y

Baxter, G. D., Liu, L., Petrich, S., Gisselman, A. S., Chapple, C., Anders, J. J., & Tumilty, S. (2017). Low level laser therapy (Photobiomodulation therapy) for breast cancer-related lymphedema: A systematic review. *BMC Cancer, 17*(1), 833. https://doi.org/10.1186/s12885-017-3852-x

Beelen, L. M., van Dishoeck, A.-M., Tsangaris, E., Coriddi, M., Dayan, J. H., Pusic, A. L., Klassen, A., & Vasilic, D. (2021). Patient-reported outcome measures in lymphedema: A systematic review and COSMIN analysis. *Annals of Surgical Oncology, 28*(3), 1656–1668. https://doi.org/10.1245/s10434-020-09346-0

Bona, A. F., Ferreira, K. R., Carvalho, R. B. M., Thuler, L. C. S., & Bergmann, A. (2020). Incidence, prevalence, and factors associated with lymphedema after treatment for cervical cancer: A systematic review. *International Journal of Gynecological Cancer, 30*(11), 1697–1704. https://doi.org/10.1136/ijgc-2020-001682

Carter, J., Raviv, L., Appollo, K., Baser, R. E., Iasonos, A., & Barakat, R. R. (2010). A pilot study using the Gynecologic Cancer Lymphedema Questionnaire (GCLQ) as a clinical care tool to identify lower extremity lymphedema in gynecologic cancer survivors. *Gynecologic Oncology, 117*(2), 317–323. https://doi.org/10.1016/j.ygyno.2010.01.022

Chaput, G., Ibrahim, M., & Towers, A. (2020). Cancer-related lymphedema: Clinical pearls for providers. *Current Oncology, 27*(6), 336–340. https://doi.org/10.3747/co.27.7225

Chen, H. Y., Tsai, H. H., Tam, K. W., & Huang, T. W. (2019). Effects of photobiomodulation therapy on breast cancer-related lymphoedema: A systematic review and meta-analysis of randomised controlled trials. *Complementary Therapies in Medicine, 47*, 102200. https://doi.org/10.1016/j.ctim.2019.102200

Chien, T. J., Liu, C. Y., & Fang, C. J. (2019). The effect of acupuncture in breast cancer-related lymphoedema (BCRL): A systematic review and meta-analysis. *Integrative Cancer Therapies, 18*, 1534735419866910. https://doi.org/10.1177/1534735419866910

De Vrieze, T., Nevelsteen, I., Thomis, S., De Groef, A., Tjalma, W. A. A., Gebruers, N., & Devoogdt, N. (2020). What are the economic burden and costs associated with the treatment of breast cancer-related lymphoedema? A systematic review. *Supportive Care in Cancer, 28*(2), 439–449. https://doi.org/10.1007/s00520-019-05101-8

Deng, J., Ridner, S. H., Aulino, J. M., & Murphy, B. A. (2015). Assessment and measurement of head and neck lymphedema: State-of-the-science and future directions. *Oral Oncology, 51*(5), 431–437. https://doi.org/10.1016/j.oraloncology.2015.01.005

Deng, J., Ridner, S. H., Dietrich, M. S., Wells, N., Wallston, K. A., Sinard, R. J., Cmelak, A. J., & Murphy, B. A. (2012a). Prevalence of secondary lymphedema in patients with head and neck cancer. *Journal of Pain and Symptom Management, 43*(2), 244–252. https://doi.org/10.1016/j.jpainsymman.2011.03.019

Deng, J., Ridner, S. H., Murphy, B. A., & Dietrich, M. S. (2012b). Preliminary development of a lymphedema symptom assessment scale for patients with head and neck cancer. *Supportive Care in Cancer, 20*(8), 1911–1918. https://doi.org/10.1007/s00520-011-1294-6

DiSipio, T., Rye, S., Newman, B., & Hayes, S. (2013). Incidence of unilateral arm lymphoedema after breast cancer: A systematic review and meta-analysis. *The Lancet Oncology, 14*(6), 500–515. http://dx.doi.org/10.1016/S1470-2045(13)70076-7

Gao, Y., Ma, T., Han, M., Yu, M., Wang, X., Lv, Y., & Wang, X. (2021). Effects of acupuncture and moxibustion on breast cancer-related lymphedema: A systematic review and meta-analysis of randomized controlled trials. *Integrative Cancer Therapies, 20*, 15347354211044107. https://doi.org/10.1177/15347354211044107

Greimel, E. R., Kuljanic Vlasic, K., Waldenstrom, A.-C., Duric, V. M., Jensen, P. T., Singer, S., Chie, W., Nordin, A., Radisic, V. B., Wydra, D., & European Organization for Research and Treatment of Cancer Quality-of-Life Group. (2006). The European organization for research and treatment of cancer (EORTC) quality-of-life questionnaire cervical cancer module. *Cancer*, *107*(8), 1812–1822. https://doi.org/10.1002/cncr.22217

Guliyeva, G., Huayllani, M. T., Avila, F. R., Boczar, D., Lu, X., & Forte, A. J. (2020). Younger age as a risk factor for gynecologic cancer-related lymphedema: A systematic review. *Anticancer Research*, *40*(12), 6609–6612. https://doi.org/10.21873/anticanres.14685

Gursen, C., Dylke, E. S., Moloney, N., Meeus, M., De Vrieze, T., Devoogdt, N., & De Groef, A. (2021). Self-reported signs and symptoms of secondary upper limb lymphoedema related to breast cancer treatment: Systematic review. *European Journal of Cancer Care (England)*, *30*(5), e13440. https://doi.org/10.1111/ecc.13440

Hasenoehrl, T., Keilani, M., Palma, S., & Crevenna, R. (2020a). Resistance exercise and breast cancer related lymphedema—A systematic review update. *Disability and Rehabilitation*, *42*(1), 26–35. https://doi.org/10.1080/09638288.2018.1514663

Hasenoehrl, T., Palma, S., Ramazanova, D., Kölbl, H., Dorner, T. E., Keilani, M., & Crevenna, R. (2020b). Resistance exercise and breast cancer-related lymphedema—A systematic review update and meta-analysis. *Supportive Care in Cancer*, *28*(8), 3593–3603. https://doi.org/10.1007/s00520-020-05521-x

Heller, D. R., Killelea, B. K., & Sanft, T. (2019). Prevention is key: Importance of early recognition and referral in combating breast cancer-related lymphedema. *JCO Oncology Practice*, *15*(5), 263–264. https://doi.org/10.1200/jop.19.00148

Hou, W., Pei, L., Song, Y., Wu, J., Geng, H., Chen, L., Wang, Y., Hu, Y., Zhou, J., & Sun, J. (2019). Acupuncture therapy for breast cancer-related lymphedema: A systematic review and meta-analysis. *Journal of Obstetrics and Gynaecology Research*, *45*(12), 2307–2317. https://doi.org/10.1111/jog.14122

Jeffs, E., Ream, E., Taylor, C., & Bick, D. (2018). Clinical effectiveness of decongestive treatments on excess arm volume and patient-centered outcomes in women with early breast cancer-related arm lymphedema: A systematic review. *JBI Database of Systematic Reviews and Implementation Reports*, *16*(2), 453–506. https://doi.org/10.11124/jbisrir-2016-003185

Kasawara, K. T., Mapa, J. M. R., Ferreira, V., Added, M. A. N., Shiwa, S. R., Carvas, N., Jr., & Batista, P. A. (2018). Effects of Kinesio taping on breast cancer-related lymphedema: A meta-analysis in clinical trials. *Physiotherapy Theory and Practice*, *34*(5), 337–345. https://doi.org/10.1080/09593985.2017.1419522

Launois, R., Megnigbeto, A., Pocquet, K., Alliot, F., Campisi, C., & Witte, M. (2002). A specific quality of life scale in upper limb lymphedema: The ULL-27 questionnaire. *Lymphology*, *35*(1–760), 181–187.

Li, Y., Kong, Q., Wei, H., & Wang, Y. (2021). Comparison of the complications between minimally invasive surgery and open surgical treatments for early-stage cervical cancer: A systematic review and meta-analysis. *PLOS ONE, 16*(7), e0253143. https://doi.org/10.1371/journal.pone.0253143

Liao, S. F., Li, S. H., & Huang, H. Y. (2012). The efficacy of complex decongestive physiotherapy (CDP) and predictive factors of response to CDP in lower limb lymphedema (LLL) after pelvic cancer treatment. *Gynecologic Oncology, 125*(3), 712–715. https://doi.org/10.1016/j.ygyno.2012.03.017

Lin, Y., Xu, Y., Wang, C., Song, Y., Huang, X., Zhang, X., Cao, X., & Sun, Q. (2021). Loco-regional therapy and the risk of breast cancer-related lymphedema: A systematic review and meta-analysis. *Breast Cancer, 28*(6), 1261–1272. https://doi.org/10.1007/s12282-021-01263-8

Marchica, P., D'Arpa, S., Magno, S., Rossi, C., Forcina, L., Capizzi, V., Oieni, S., Amato, C., Piazza, D., & Gebbia, V. (2021). Integrated treatment of breast cancer-related lymphedema: A descriptive review of the state of the art. *Anticancer Research, 41*(7), 3233–3246. https://doi.org/10.21873/anticanres.15109

McLaughlin, S. A., Brunelle, C. L., & Taghian, A. (2020). Breast cancer-related lymphedema: Risk factors, screening, management, and the impact of locoregional treatment. *Journal of Clinical Oncology, 38*(20), 2341–2350. https://doi.org/10.1200/jco.19.02896

Michelotti, A., Invernizzi, M., Lopez, G., Lorenzini, D., Nesa, F., De Sire, A., & Fusco, N. (2019). Tackling the diversity of breast cancer related lymphedema: Perspectives on diagnosis, risk assessment, and clinical management. *Breast, 44*, 15–23. https://doi.org/10.1016/j.breast.2018.12.009

Mur-Gimeno, E., Postigo-Martin, P., Cantarero-Villanueva, I., & Sebio-Garcia, R. (2022). Systematic review of the effect of aquatic therapeutic exercise in breast cancer survivors. *European Journal of Cancer Care (England), 31*(1), e13535. https://doi.org/10.1111/ecc.13535

O'Donnell, T. F., Jr., Allison, G. M., & Iafrati, M. D. (2020). A systematic review of guidelines for lymphedema and the need for contemporary intersocietal guidelines for the management of lymphedema. *Journal of Vascular Surgery: Venous and Lymphatic Disorders, 8*(4), 676–684. https://doi.org/10.1016/j.jvsv.2020.03.006

Olsson Möller, U., Beck, I., Rydén, L., & Malmström, M. (2019). A comprehensive approach to rehabilitation interventions following breast cancer treatment—A systematic review of systematic reviews. *BMC Cancer, 19*(1). https://doi.org/10.1186/s12885-019-5648-7

Panchik, D., Masco, S., Zinnikas, P., Hillriegel, B., Lauder, T., Suttmann, E., Chinchilli, V., McBeth, M., & Hermann, W. (2019). Effect of exercise on breast cancer-related lymphedema: What the lymphatic surgeon needs to know. *Journal of Reconstructive Microsurgery, 35*(1), 37–45. https://doi.org/10.1055/s-0038-1660832

Pusic, A. L., Cemal, Y., Albornoz, C., Klassen, A., Cano, S., Sulimanoff, I., Hernandez, M., Massey, M., Cordeiro, P., Morrow, M., & Mehrara, B. (2013). Quality of life among breast cancer patients with lymphedema: A systematic review of patient-reported outcome instruments and outcomes. *Journal of Cancer Survivorship, 7*(1), 83–92. https://doi.org/10.1007/s11764-012-0247-5

Rafn, B. S., Christensen, J., Larsen, A., & Bloomquist, K. (2022). Prospective surveillance for breast cancer-related arm lymphedema: A systematic review and meta-analysis. *Journal of Clinical Oncology, 40*(9), 1009–1026. https://doi.org/10.1200/jco.21.01681

Ridner, S., Doersam, J., Stolldorf, D., & Dietrich, M. (2018). Development and validation of the lymphedema symptom intensity and distress survey-lower limb. *Lymphatic Research and Biology, 16*(6), 538–546. https://doi.org/10.1089/lrb.2017.0069

Temur, K., & Kapucu, S. (2019). The effectiveness of lymphedema self-management in the prevention of breast cancer-related lymphedema and quality of life: A randomized controlled trial. *European Journal of Oncology Nursing, 40*, 22–35. https://doi.org/10.1016/j.ejon.2019.02.006

Thompson, B., Gaitatzis, K., Janse de Jonge, X., Blackwell, R., & Koelmeyer, L. A. (2021). Manual lymphatic drainage treatment for lymphedema: A systematic review of the literature. *Journal Cancer Survivorship, 15*(2), 244–258. https://doi.org/10.1007/s11764-020-00928-1

Tribius, S., Pazdyka, H., Tennstedt, P., Busch, C.-J., Hanken, H., Krüll, A., & Petersen, C. (2020). Prognostic factors for lymphedema in patients with locally advanced head and neck cancer after combined radio(chemo)therapy—results of a longitudinal study. *Oral Oncology, 109*, 104856. https://doi.org/10.1016/j.oraloncology.2020.104856

Tsai, C. L., Chih-Yang, H., Chang, W. W., & Yen-Nung, L. (2020). Effects of weight reduction on the breast cancer-related lymphedema: A systematic review and meta-analysis. *Breast, 52*, 116–121. https://doi.org/10.1016/j.breast.2020.05.007

Tyker, A., Franco, J., Massa, S. T., Desai, S. C., & Walen, S. G. (2019). Treatment for lymphedema following head and neck cancer therapy: A systematic review. *American Journal of Otolaryngology, 40*(5), 761–769. https://doi.org/10.1016/j.amjoto.2019.05.024

Yost, K. J., Cheville, A. L., Weaver, A. L., Al Hilli, M., & Dowdy, S. C. (2013). Development and validation of a self-report lower-extremity lymphedema screening questionnaire in women. *Physical Therapy, 93*(5), 694–703. https://doi.org/10.2522/ptj.20120088

Yu, S., Zhu, L., Xie, P., Jiang, S., Yang, Z., He, J., & Ren, Y. (2020). Effects of acupuncture on breast cancer-related lymphoedema: A systematic review and meta-analysis. *Explore (NY), 16*(2), 97–102. https://doi.org/10.1016/j.explore.2019.06.002

CHAPTER 7

ALOPECIA

INTRODUCTION

Hair loss is one of the most distressing side effects of cancer treatment and one that is dreaded, especially by women. It is a public and private sign of cancer and one that many associate with stigma (Paterson et al., 2021), and for women a loss of femininity and attractiveness (Boland et al., 2020). Both men and women are equally affected by the impact on body image (Can et al., 2013). Hair loss is reported not just on the head; loss of eyelashes and eyebrows as well as pubic hair also occurs (Jayde et al., 2013). Alopecia is associated with depression and impacts on emotional, social, and role functioning (Choi et al., 2014). Hair loss may be permanent, but is also reversible, with regrowth often occurring within 3 to 6 months; 65% of people experience a change in color or texture of the new hair (Yun & Kim, 2007).

PREVALENCE

It is estimated that 65% of people who receive chemotherapy will experience some degree of alopecia (Rossi et al., 2020). Estimates for specific agents are as follows: more than 80% for antimicrotubule agents, 60% to 100% for topoisomerase inhibitors, 10% to 50% for antimetabolites, and more than 60% for alkylating agents (Rossi et al., 2017). Given that chemotherapy is commonly prescribed for treatment of both solid and hematologic cancers, the number of people affected and the impact cannot be overestimated.

CONTRIBUTING FACTORS

The most important risk factor is the type of chemotherapy and, increasingly, immunotherapy received (Paus et al., 2013). The amount of alopecia depends on the specific agent, the dose received, the route of administration, and the schedule of treatment. Chemotherapy agents that are given at lower doses, via oral route, and once weekly are less likely to cause alopecia. Patients who develop graft-versus-host disease are also at greater risk. However, multiple factors contribute to hair loss from cancer treatment, including age, nutritional and hormonal status, and comorbidities (Figure 7.1).

- Alkylating agents (cyclophosphamide; ifosfamide)
- Anti-estrogen therapy (tamoxifen; aromatase inhibitors)
- Checkpoint inhibitors (pembrolizumab; nivolumab; cemiplimab; ipilimumab)
- Cytotoxics (doxorubicin; daunorubicin)
- Epidermal growth factor receptor therapy (vismodegib; gefitinib)
- Taxanes (docetaxel; paclitaxel)
- Topoisomerase inhibitors (etoposide)
- Tyrosine kinase inhibitors (ripretinib most likely)

Figure 7.1 Agents causing alopecia.

Sources: From Belum, V. R., Marulanda, K., Ensslin, C., Gorcey, L., Parikh, T., Wu, S., Wu, S., Busam, K. J., Gerber, P. A., & Lacouture, M. E. (2015). Alopecia in patients treated with molecularly targeted anticancer therapies. *Annals of Oncology*, 26(12), 2496–2502. https://doi.org/10.1093/annonc/mdv390; Donovan, J. C., Ghazarian, D. M., & Shaw, J. C. (2008). Scarring alopecia associated with use of the epidermal growth factor receptor inhibitor gefitinib. *Archives of Dermatology*, 144(11), 1524–1525. https://doi.org/10.1001/archderm.144.11.1524; Paus, R., Haslam, I. S., Sharov, A. A., & Botchkarev, V. A. (2013). Pathobiology of chemotherapy-induced hair loss. *The Lancet Oncology*, 14(2), e50–e59. https://doi.org/10.1016/S1470-2045(12)70553-3.

ASSESSMENT

Alopecia is graded by the National Cancer Institute (NCI) Common Terminology Criteria for Adverse Events (CTCAE; cancer.gov).

- *Grade 1:* hair loss of less than 50% of normal for the person that is not visible from a distance but may be noticed on close inspection; does not require a wig or head covering

- *Grade 2:* hair loss of greater than 50% of normal for the person and is easily seen by others; may require a wig or head covering

Patient-Reported Outcomes-Common Terminology Criteria for Adverse Events Scale

The Patient-Reported Outcomes (PRO)-CTCAE scale (Kluetz et al., 2016) asks about hair loss in the past 7 days (not at all; a little bit; somewhat; quite a bit; very much).

Dean Scale

The Dean Scale has a more accurate grading scale but one that may be challenging to use due to the need to estimate the percentage of hair loss (Figure 7.2).

Chemotherapy-Induced Alopecia Distress Scale

Designed for use in women with breast cancer, the Chemotherapy-Induced Alopecia Distress Scale (CADS; Cho et al., 2014) is a validated

Grade 0	No hair loss
Grade 1	>0 to ≤25% hair loss
Grade 2	>25% to ≤50% hair loss
Grade 3	>50% to ≤75% hair loss
Grade 4	>75% hair loss

Figure 7.2 The Dean Scale.

Source: From Dean, J. C., Salmon, S. E., & Griffith, K. S. (1979). Prevention of doxorubicin-induced hair loss with scalp hypothermia. *New England Journal of Medicine, 301*(26), 1427–1429. https://doi.org/10.1056/nejm197912273012605.

17-item scale that measures physical, emotional, activity, and relationship factors related to distress.

CASE STUDY

Your patient is a 72-year-old man who is receiving docetaxel for advanced prostate cancer. His spouse tells you that he is depressed, and while they expected that with the treatment he has started to dress and undress in the bathroom and refuses to go to the beach with his son's family. She is confused about why this is happening.

1. What factors might be contributing to this behavior?

2. Is this a common complaint for men on treatment for advanced prostate cancer?

On questioning, he admits that he is embarrassed that he has lost almost all his chest hair. He tells you that he is "a proud man and this makes him feel like a little boy."

3. What advice can you offer him?

4. How would you treat this?

MANAGEMENT

While educating the patient and providing support, as well as providing advice about head coverings and wigs, a more recent focus has been on preventing hair loss. It is important to warn patients that loss of body hair (not hair on the head) cannot be hidden, and that loss of pubic hair in particular can have a significant impact on sexual self-image.

Scalp Cooling

Scalp cooling has been proposed as an effective method to reduce the risk of alopecia; however, a recent meta-analysis including 2,022 participants suggests the efficacy and effectiveness were just 61% (Wang et al., 2021). Side effects include headache, scalp and/or neck pain, dizziness, nausea, feeling cold, and a feeling of heaviness of the head. An earlier meta-analysis of 654 participants found that scalp cooling reduced the risk of alopecia by 43% in those with solid tumors (Rugo & Voigt, 2018). Another systematic review reported that, while two of the four studies included in the review found that scalp cooling was effective depending on the chemotherapy used, the quality of life was not improved in the population of women with breast cancer (Marks et al., 2019).

Currently, there are two Food and Drug Administration (FDA)-approved devices for scalp cooling—the DigniCap (www.dignicap.com) and the Paxman system (www.paxmanscalpcooling.com). Other devices that are not FDA-approved include Penguin, Elastogel, Polar, Arctic, and Chemo cold caps. These caps need to be frozen before use and changed every 30 minutes, as opposed to the DigniCap and Paxman systems, which maintain a preset temperature. Scalp cooling devices are more effective in patients who are receiving taxane-based chemotherapy compared with anthracycline-based regimens (Kruse & Abraham, 2018).

The cooling device needs to be used at least 30 minutes prior to the start of the chemotherapy infusion and kept on for a variable amount of time, including after the end of the infusion. In one study using the Paxman system, 20 minutes of postinfusion cooling time was more effective than 45 minutes (Lugtenberg et al., 2022). Extending the use of the same cooling system from 90 minutes to 150 minutes of postinfusion cooling did not have any additional benefit (Komen et al., 2019). A small study showed that scalp cooling improved regrowth of hair (Bajpai et al., 2020).

The extended chair time needed for use of these scalp cooling devices has an impact on patient flow in chemotherapy units (Kruse & Abraham, 2018), and the costs associated with their use range from $1,500 to $3,000 per patient, depending on the number of chemotherapy treatments, and these are not always covered by insurance.

There have been concerns raised about the risk of scalp metastases, although a meta-analysis of 1,959 patients did not show evidence of increased risk (Rugo et al., 2017). The manufacturer of DigniCap suggests that the device should not be used in those with hematologic cancers, in those undergoing bone marrow or stem cell transplantation, or in those with skin cancers as well as other cancers (www.dignicap.com).

Scalp cooling may not be effective in Black patients due to hair thickness and volume and the design of the cooling cap (Araoye et al., 2020; Dilawari et al., 2021).

Botanical and Herbal Supplements

Botanical and herbal supplements have shown some preliminary effectiveness in protecting against permanent hair loss (Dell'Acqua et al., 2020; Kang et al., 2020; Yu et al., 2019). However, these are not in widespread use.

Pharmaceutical Agents

Pharmaceutical agents show limited evidence in the management of chemotherapy-induced alopecia.

Minoxidil and bimatoprost should not be used during the duration of chemotherapy treatment but can be used after discontinuation of chemotherapy. Thus, these agents are not preventive but rather encourages hair regrowth (Rossi et al., 2020; Figure 7.3).

Minoxidil	Does not prevent alopecia	(Duvic et al., 1996; Rodriguez et al., 1994)
Finasteride	Not recommended	(Rozner et al., 2019)
Spironolactone	May increase levels of estrogen	(Rozner et al., 2019)
Topical calcitriol	Not recommended	(Hidalgo et al., 1999)
Bimatoprost	May be used for loss of eyelashes	(Glaser et al., 2015)

Figure 7.3 Pharmaceutical agents.

GUIDELINES

There are no formal guidelines for managing chemotherapy-induced alopecia. A clinical review from the American Society of Clinical Oncology (Kruse & Abraham, 2018) provides a comprehensive overview and suggestions.

SUMMARY

Despite alopecia being one of the most traumatic and distressing side effects of chemotherapy, few options for management are available. Anticipatory guidance based on the risks from specific chemotherapy agents and supportive counseling are essential, as well as advice about head coverings, wigs, and information about the timeline for regrowth.

A robust set of instructor resources designed to supplement this text is located at http://connect.springerpub.com/content/reference-book/978-0-8261-8524-2. Qualifying Instructors may request access by emailing **textbook@springerpub.com**.

REFERENCES

Araoye, E. F., Stearns, V., & Aguh, C. (2020). Considerations for the use of scalp cooling devices in black patients. *Journal of Clinical Oncology, 38*(30), 3575–3576. https://doi.org/10.1200/jco.20.02130

Bajpai, J., Kagwade, S., Chandrasekharan, A., Dandekar, S., Kanan, S., Kembhavi, Y., Ghosh, J., Banavali, S. D., & Gupta, S. (2020). Randomised controlled trial of scalp cooling for the prevention of chemotherapy induced alopecia. *Breast, 49*, 187–193. https://doi.org/10.1016/j.breast.2019.12.004

Belum, V. R., Marulanda, K., Ensslin, C., Gorcey, L., Parikh, T., Wu, S., Wu, S., Busam, K. J., Gerber, P. A., & Lacouture, M. E. (2015). Alopecia in patients treated with molecularly targeted anticancer therapies. *Annals of Oncology, 26*(12), 2496–2502. https://doi.org/10.1093/annonc/mdv390

Boland, V., Brady, A.-M., & Drury, A. (2020). The physical, psychological and social experiences of alopecia among women receiving chemotherapy: An integrative literature review. *European Journal of Oncology Nursing, 49,* 101840. https://doi.org/10.1016/j.ejon.2020.101840

Can, G., Demir, M., Erol, O., & Aydiner, A. (2013). A comparison of men and women's experiences of chemotherapy-induced alopecia. *European Journal of Oncology Nursing, 17*(3), 255–260. https://doi.org/10.1016/j.ejon.2012.06.003

Cho, J., Choi, E. K., Kim, I. R., Im, Y. H., Park, Y. H., Lee, S., Lee, J. E., Yang, J H., & Nam, S. J. (2014). Development and validation of Chemotherapy-induced Alopecia Distress Scale (CADS) for breast cancer patients. *Annals of Oncology, 25*(2), 346–351. https://doi.org/10.1093/annonc/mdt476

Choi, E. K., Kim, I.-R., Chang, O., Kang, D., Nam, S.-J., Lee, J. E., Lee, S. K., Im, Y.-H., Park, Y. H., Yang, J.-H., & Cho, J. (2014). Impact of chemotherapy-induced alopecia distress on body image, psychosocial well-being, and depression in breast cancer patients. *Psycho-Oncology, 23*(10), 1103–1110. https://doi.org/10.1002/pon.3531

Dean, J. C., Salmon, S. E., & Griffith, K. S. (1979). Prevention of doxorubicin-induced hair loss with scalp hypothermia. *New England Journal of Medicine, 301*(26), 1427–1429. https://doi.org/10.1056/nejm197912273012605

Dell'Acqua, G., Richards, A., & Thornton, M. J. (2020). The potential role of nutraceuticals as an adjuvant in breast cancer patients to prevent hair loss induced by endocrine therapy. *Nutrients, 12*(11), 3537. https://doi.org/10.3390/nu12113537

Dilawari, A., Gallagher, C., Alintah, P., Chitalia, A., Tiwari, S., Paxman, R., Adams-Campbell, L., & Dash, C. (2021). Does scalp cooling have the same efficacy in black patients receiving chemotherapy for breast cancer? *Oncologist, 26*(4), 292–e548. https://doi.org/10.1002/onco.13690

Donovan, J. C., Ghazarian, D. M., & Shaw, J. C. (2008). Scarring alopecia associated with use of the epidermal growth factor receptor inhibitor gefitinib. *Archives of Dermatology, 144*(11), 1524–1525. https://doi.org/10.1001/archderm.144.11.1524

Duvic, M., Lemak, N. A., Valero, V., Hymes, S. R., Farmer, K. L., Hortobagyi, G. N., Trancik, R. J., Bandstra, B. A., & Compton, L. D. (1996). A randomized trial of minoxidil in chemotherapy-induced alopecia. *Journal of the America n Academy of Dermatology, 35*(1), 74–78. https://doi.org/10.1016/s0190-9622(96)90500-9

Glaser, D. A., Hossain, P., Perkins, W., Griffiths, T., Ahluwalia, G., Weng, E., & Beddingfield, F. C. (2015). Long-term safety and efficacy of bimatoprost solution 0·03% application to the eyelid margin for the treatment of idiopathic and chemotherapy-induced eyelash hypotrichosis: A randomized controlled trial. *British Journal of Dermatology, 172*(5), 1384–1394. https://doi.org/10.1111/bjd.13443

Hidalgo, M., Rinaldi, D., Medina, G., Griffin, T., Turner, J., & Von Hoff, D. D. (1999). A phase I trial of topical topitriol (calcitriol, 1,25-dihydroxyvitamin D3) to prevent chemotherapy-induced alopecia. *Anticancer Drugs, 10*(4), 393–395. https://doi.org/10.1097/00001813-199904000-00007

Jayde, V., Boughton, M., & Blomfield, P. (2013). The experience of chemotherapy-induced alopecia for Australian women with ovarian cancer. *European Journal of Cancer Care, 22*(4), 503–512. https://doi.org/10.1111/ecc.12056

Kang, D., Kim, I. R., Park, Y. H., Im, Y. H., Zhao, D., Guallar, E., Ahn, J. S., & Cho, J. (2020). Impact of a topical lotion, CG428, on permanent chemotherapy-induced alopecia in breast cancer survivors: A pilot randomized double-blind controlled clinical trial (VOLUME RCT). *Supportive Care in Cancer, 28*(4), 1829–1837. https://doi.org/10.1007/s00520-019-04982-z

Kluetz, P. G., Chingos, D. T., Basch, E. M., & Mitchell, S. A. (2016). Patient-reported outcomes in cancer clinical trials: Measuring symptomatic adverse events with the national cancer institute's patient-reported outcomes version of the common terminology criteria for adverse events (PRO-CTCAE). *American Society of Clinical Oncology Educational Book, 35*, 67–73. https://doi.org/10.1200/edbk_159514

Komen, M. M. C., van den Hurk, C. J. G., Nortier, J. W. R., van der Ploeg, T., Nieboer, P., van der Hoeven, J. J. M., & Smorenburg, C. H. (2019). Prolonging the duration of post-infusion scalp cooling in the prevention of anthracycline-induced alopecia: A randomised trial in patients with breast cancer treated with adjuvant chemotherapy. *Supportive Care in Cancer, 27*(5), 1919–1925. https://doi.org/10.1007/s00520-018-4432-6

Kruse, M., & Abraham, J. (2018). Management of chemotherapy-induced alopecia with scalp cooling. *Journal of Oncology Practice, 14*(3), 149–154. https://doi.org/10.1200/jop.17.00038

Lugtenberg, R. T., van den Hurk, C. J. G., Smorenburg, C. H., Mosch, L., Houtsma, D., Deursen, M., Kaptein, A., Gelderblom, H., & Kroep, J. R. (2022). Comparable effectiveness of 45- and 20-min post-infusion scalp cooling time in preventing paclitaxel-induced alopecia—A randomized controlled trial. *Supportive Care in Cancer, 30*(8), 6641–6648. https://doi.org/10.1007/s00520-022-07090-7

Marks, D. H., Okhovat, J. P., Hagigeorges, D., Manatis-Lornell, A. J., Isakoff, S. J., Lacouture, M. E., & Senna, M. M. (2019). The effect of scalp cooling on CIA-related quality of life in breast cancer patients: A systematic review. *Breast Cancer Research and Treatment, 175*(2), 267–276. https://doi.org/10.1007/s10549-019-05169-0

Paterson, C., Kozlovskaia, M., Turner, M., Strickland, K., Roberts, C., Ogilvie, R., Pranavan, G., & Craft, P. (2021). Identifying the supportive care needs of men and women affected by chemotherapy-induced alopecia? A systematic review. *Journal of Cancer Survivorship, 15*(1), 14–28. https://doi.org/10.1007/s11764-020-00907-6

Paus, R., Haslam, I. S., Sharov, A. A., & Botchkarev, V. A. (2013). Pathobiology of chemotherapy-induced hair loss. *The Lancet Oncology, 14*(2), e50–e59. https://doi.org/10.1016/S1470-2045(12)70553-3

Rodriguez, R., Machiavelli, M., Leone, B., Romero, A., Cuevas, M. A., Langhi, M., Romero Acuna, L., Romero Acuna, J., Amato, S., Barbieri, M., Vallejo, C., Rabinovich, M., Perez, J., Sabatini, C., Ortiz, E., Salvadori, M., & Lacava, J. (1994). Minoxidil (Mx) as a prophylaxis of doxorubicin—induced alopecia. *Annals of Oncology, 5*(8), 769–770. https://doi.org/10.1093/oxfordjournals.annonc.a058986

Rossi, A., Caro, G., Fortuna, M. C., Pigliacelli, F., D'Arino, A., & Carlesimo, M. (2020). Prevention and treatment of chemotherapy-induced alopecia. *Dermatolgy Practical & Conceptual, 10*(3), e2020074. https://doi.org/10.5826/dpc.1003a74

Rossi, A., Fortuna, M. C., Caro, G., Pranteda, G., Garelli, V., Pompili, U., & Carlesimo, M. (2017). Chemotherapy-induced alopecia management: Clinical experience and practical advice. *Journal of Cosmetic Dermatology, 16*(4), 537–541. https://doi.org/10.1111/jocd.12308

Rozner, R. N., Freites-Martinez, A., Shapiro, J., Geer, E. B., Goldfarb, S., & Lacouture, M. E. (2019). Safety of 5α-reductase inhibitors and spironolactone in breast cancer patients receiving endocrine therapies. *Breast Cancer Research and Treatment, 174*(1), 15–26. https://doi.org/10.1007/s10549-018-4996-3

Rugo, H. S., Melin, S. A., & Voigt, J. (2017). Scalp cooling with adjuvant/neoadjuvant chemotherapy for breast cancer and the risk of scalp metastases: Systematic review and meta-analysis. *Breast Cancer Research and Treatment, 163*(2), 199–205. https://doi.org/10.1007/s10549-017-4185-9

Rugo, H. S., & Voigt, J. (2018). Scalp hypothermia for preventing alopecia during chemotherapy. A systematic review and meta-analysis of randomized controlled trials. *Clinical Breast Cancer, 18*(1), 19–28. https://doi.org/10.1016/j.clbc.2017.07.012

Wang, S., Yang, T., Shen, A., Qiang, W., Zhao, Z., & Zhang, F. (2021). The scalp cooling therapy for hair loss in breast cancer patients undergoing chemotherapy: A systematic review and meta-analysis. *Supportive Care in Cancer, 29*(11), 6943–6956. https://doi.org/10.1007/s00520-021-06188-8

Yu, F., Li, Y., Zou, J., Jiang, L., Wang, C., Tang, Y., Gao, B., Luo, D., & Jiang, X. (2019). The Chinese herb Xiaoaiping protects against breast cancer chemotherapy-induced alopecia and other side effects: a randomized controlled trial. *Journal of International Medical Research, 47*(6), 2607–2614. https://doi.org/10.1177/0300060519842781

Yun, S. J., & Kim, S. J. (2007). Hair loss pattern due to chemotherapy-induced anagen effluvium: A cross-sectional observation. *Dermatology, 215*(1), 36–40. https://doi.org/10.1159/000102031

CHAPTER 8

XEROSTOMIA AND ORAL MUCOSITIS

XEROSTOMIA

Introduction

Xerostomia is the sensation of a dry mouth caused by a significant decrease in the amount of saliva or the thickening of the saliva. Radiation therapy for the treatment of head or neck cancer is the main cause of this condition that has an impact on speech and swallowing as well as on the health of the oral cavity. Xerostomia is usually an acute side effect of radiation but one that may persist for years (Burlage et al., 2001).

Prevalence

Of the patients on conventional radiation therapy for treatment of head and neck cancers, 60% to 75% experience xerostomia; this is reduced to 40% with intensity modulated radiation therapy (IMRT; Strojan et al., 2017). However, despite improvement in radiation techniques, the risk of developing xerostomia remains due to the challenges of sparing the salivary glands in the mouth.

Contributing Factors

Gender, age, smoking, type of chemotherapy prescribed, and alcohol-based mouthwash are additional contributing factors; however, the dose of radiation to the parotid glands is the major cause of this condition. Chemotherapy regimens that include cisplatin, carboplatin, fluorouracil, paclitaxel, and docetaxel increase the risk of xerostomia, and also when administered concurrently with radiation.

Assessment

Patient reports of dry mouth are the most common method to identify this condition. Sialometry measures salivary flow but is used only in research. Figure 8.1 identifies the objective measures that may be useful clinically.

> - Xerostomia Inventory (Thomson, Chalmers, Spencer, & Williams, 1999)
> - Groningen Radiotherapy-Induced Xerostomia Questionnaire (Beetz et al., 2010)
> - Treatment of Cancer Quality of Life Questionnaire, and Head and Neck Module (QLQ-H&N35) (Singer et al., 2013; contains one question about dry mouth).

Figure 8.1 Objective measures of dry mouth.

Management

Prevention of xerostomia may not be possible given the need for radiation and chemotherapy to treat cancer; however, IMRT appears to show some benefit in reducing this symptom (De Felice et al., 2020; Ge et al., 2020). Symptomatic treatment starts with efforts to increase saliva, such as chewing gum (Kaae et al., 2020).

- Acid-tasting candies and fruits or vegetables may also be helpful in stimulating the production of saliva. Saliva substitutes or lubricants are frequently recommended; however, these usually last for a short time only (Strojan et al., 2017) and patients may prefer to sip water constantly.

- Cholinergic agents, such as pilocarpine or cevimeline, have shown some effectiveness. These agents, however, have significant side effects and may not be tolerated, especially if used long term (Brimhall et al., 2013; Cheng et al., 2016).

- Hyperbaric oxygen treatment may also have a role to play in improving saliva production and decreasing xerostomia (Forner et al., 2011).

- Acupuncture has been shown to be effective in preventing and limiting the severity of radiation-induced xerostomia (Garcia et al., 2019).

- Transcutaneous electrostimulation and bethanechol may be offered; however, the evidence on their efficacy is low (Mercadante et al., 2021).

Involvement of a multidisciplinary team, including speech and language therapists, nutritionists, and nurses, in addition to radiation oncologists and surgeons, is key to helping patients deal with this unpleasant symptom that impacts negatively on quality of life.

Guidelines

- **Multinational Association of Supportive Care in Cancer/International Society of Oral Oncology/American Society of Clinical Oncology (ISOO/MASCC/ASCO)**

   ISOO/MASCC/ASCO: Salivary Gland Hypofunction and/or Xerostomia Induced by Nonsurgical Cancer Therapies (Mercadante et al., 2021)

Provides recommendations for the prevention and management of xerostomia after nonsurgical treatment

CASE STUDY

A 74-year-old man is halfway through treatment for cancer of the tongue. He complains that his mouth is always dry and that drinking water frequently has made his nocturia worse.

1. What can you suggest to help him?

He tells you that he cannot chew gum because of his false teeth. His daughter suggested that he should try acupuncture, but he is not sure if this will work; it also costs a lot of money.

2. What other low-cost suggestions might help?

ORAL MUCOSITIS

Introduction

Oral mucositis is a common side effect of radiation therapy to the head and neck, chemotherapy to treat this cancer, as well as concurrent chemoradiation therapy (Elad et al., 2020). It is characterized by erythema and ulceration of the mucous membranes and is the cause of pain, difficulty eating and drinking, and anorexia leading to weight loss, as well as compromised quality of life.

Prevalence

Of the patients, 20% to 40% of those receiving standard chemotherapy and 80% receiving high-dose chemotherapy as conditioning for stem cell transplant will develop mucositis of the oral cavity (Vera-Llonch et al., 2007). In 83% of patients, the use of radiation for treatment of head and neck cancer results in this symptom (Vera-Llonch et al., 2006).

Contributing Factors

Radiation therapy, chemotherapy, and concurrent use of these treatments are the major contributing factors. In addition, age, sex, smoking and alcohol usage, body mass index, low leukocytes, poor dental hygiene and dental disease, and changes in salivary flow are suggested to increase the risk (Vera-Llonch et al., 2006).

Assessment

Patients will report pain caused by inflammation of the mucous membranes, as well as difficulty chewing, swallowing, and/or loss of appetite. Figure 8.2 details the core symptoms that should be assessed in patients with head and neck cancer.

- The Oral Mucositis Assessment Scale (OMAS) assesses ulceration and erythema on the lips, tongue, hard and soft palate, and buccal mucosa (Sonis, 1998; Figure 8.3).

- The World Health Organization (WHO) Oral Toxicity Scale measures mucositis from grade 0 (none), grade 1 (soreness and erythema), grade 2 (erythema and ulcers; patient able to swallow solid diet), grade 3 (ulcers and extensive erythema; patient cannot swallow solid diet), to grade 4 (mucositis to the extent that eating is not possible).

- The OM Daily Questionnaire (OMDQ) (Stiff et al., 2006) assesses six areas of functioning, including mouth and throat soreness, over the past 24 hours and how this limits daily activities.

- The MD Anderson Head and Neck Module of the MD Anderson Symptom Inventory assesses nine specific symptoms including the presence of mouth or throat sores. (www.mdanderson.org/research/departments-labs-institutes/departments-divisions/symptom-research/symptom-assessment-tools/md-anderson-symptom-inventory-head-and-neck-cancer-module.html)

De Sanctis et al. note that no single assessment tool is superior to another and that patient-reported symptoms as well as objective

• Swallowing	• Trismus
• Oral pain	• Taste
• Skin changes	• Excess/thick mucus or saliva
• Dry mouth	• Shoulder motion
• Dental health	

Figure 8.2 Recommended core symptoms that should be assessed in patients with head and neck cancer.

Source: From Falchook, A. D., Green, R., Knowles, M. E., Amdur, R. J., Mendenhall, W., Hayes, D. N., Grilley-Olson, J. E., Weiss, J., Reeve, B., Mitchell, S. A., Basch, E. M., & Chera, B. S. (2016). Comparison of patient- and practitioner-reported toxic effects associated with chemoradiotherapy for head and neck cancer. *JAMA Otolaryngology—Head & Neck Surgery, 142*(6), 517–523. https://doi.org/10.1001/jamaoto.2016.0656.

Grade 1	Grade 2	Grade 3	Grade 4
Erythema	Patchy mucositis <1.5 cm Noncontiguous	Organized mucositis >1.5 cm Contiguous	Necrosis Ulceration Hemorrhage

Figure 8.3 The Radiation-Induced Oral Mucositis Grading Scale.

Source: From Rao, D., Behzadi, F., Le, R. T., Dagan, R., & Fiester, P. (2021). Radiation induced mucositis: What the radiologist needs to know. *Current Problems in Diagnostic Radiology, 50*(6), 899–904. https://doi.org/10.1067/j.cpradiol.2020.10.006.

grading should be used (De Sanctis et al., 2016) because the impact of mucositis may be worse than suggested by examination of the mouth (Chung & Pui, 2017).

Management

PREVENTION: Prevention of mucositis remains key in the management of patients with head and neck cancer undergoing radiation therapy, chemotherapy, and concurrent chemoradiation therapy. The following preventive measures are recommended by the MASCC and the ISOO (Elad et al., 2020):

- Multiagent combination oral care protocols (bland mouth rinses, toothbrushes, and flossing) are recommended for patients undergoing chemotherapy, radiation, and stem cell transplantation.

- Benzydamine mouthwash is recommended for patients receiving >50 Gy and for those receiving chemoradiation.

- Intraoral low-level laser therapy (photobiomodulation) is recommended for patients receiving high-dose chemotherapy for conditioning prior to stem cell transplant, patients receiving radiation therapy alone for head and neck cancer, as well as those receiving chemoradiation for head and neck cancer.

- Cryotherapy is recommended for those undergoing high-dose melphalan as part of conditioning before stem cell transplant, as well as for those who are given a bolus of 5-Fluorouracil chemotherapy.

- Honey may prevent mucositis in patients treated with radiation therapy alone or in combination with chemotherapy.

- Topical morphine 0.2% mouthwash can be used to treat pain from mucositis.

- Oral indomethacin spray also relieves pain from mucositis (Momo et al., 2017).

- Sucralfate should NOT be used to prevent or treat pain in patients with head and neck cancer who are treated with radiation therapy.

- Parenteral glutamine should not be used for prevention in patients undergoing stem cell transplant.

NONPHARMACEUTICAL INTERVENTIONS: There is a paucity of evidence to support the role of vitamins in either the prevention or mitigation of mucositis in this population (García-Gozalbo & Cabañas-Alite, 2021). There is some evidence that zinc sulfate tablets may help reduce both the incidence and severity of mucositis in patients with leukemia treated with chemotherapy (Rambod et al., 2018). Topical zinc has also shown some benefit to patients during radiation therapy (Chaitanya et al., 2020).

Probiotics also show promise (Jiang et al., 2019; Xia et al., 2021) and propolis for women treated with doxorubicin and cyclophosphamide (Piredda et al., 2017) has also shown efficacy; however, these studies are small and more research is needed. A honey mouthwash provided relief for some and prevented weight loss due to anorexia (Charalambous et al., 2018; Khanjani Pour-Fard-Pachekenari et al., 2019). Black mulberry molasses has also been shown to prevent mucositis (Demir Doğan et al., 2017).

Patient education about oral care, including brushing teeth and correct flossing, can improve the quality of life of patients receiving chemotherapy for head and neck cancer (Yüce & Yurtsever, 2019).

Severe oral mucositis may require treatment breaks or admission to hospital for tube feeding or parenteral infusion (Vera-Llonch et al., 2006).

Guidelines

- **Multinational Association of Supportive Care in Cancer/International Society of Oral Oncology (MASCC/ISOO)**

    MASCC/ISOO Clinical Practice Guidelines for the Management of Mucositis Secondary to Cancer Therapy (Elad et al., 2020; Lalla et al., 2014)

    It presents evidence-based recommendations for the management of oral mucositis.

    Guidelines published by other institutions (The European Society for Medical Oncology [ESMO]; National Comprehensive Cancer Network [NCCN]) are adaptations of this guideline.

SUMMARY

Oral mucositis has a significant impact on the quality of life due to pain, as well as difficulty eating and drinking leading to weight loss. There are a number of pharmaceutical and nonpharmaceutical interventions that provide relief; patient education about oral care is also very important to prevent exacerbation or physical damage to the teeth and gums.

A robust set of instructor resources designed to supplement this text is located at http://connect.springerpub.com/content/reference-book/978-0-8261-8524-2. Qualifying Instructors may request access by emailing **textbook@springerpub.com**.

REFERENCES

Brimhall, J., Jhaveri, M. A., & Yepes, J. F. (2013). Efficacy of cevimeline vs. pilocarpine in the secretion of saliva: A pilot study. *Special Care in Dentistry*, *33*(3), 123–127. https://doi.org/10.1111/scd.12010

Burlage, F. R., Coppes, R. P., Meertens, H., Stokman, M. A., & Vissink, A. (2001). Parotid and submandibular/sublingual salivary flow during high dose radiotherapy. *Radiotherapy and Oncology*, *61*(3), 271–274. https://doi.org/10.1016/S0167-8140(01)00427-3

Chaitanya, N., Badam, R., Aryasri, A. S., Pallarla, S., Garlpati, K., Akhila, M., Soni, P., Gali, S., Inamdar, P., Parinita, B., Zaheer, K., Prabhath, T., & Swetha, A. (2020). Efficacy of improvised topical zinc (1%) oral-base on oral mucositis during cancer chemo-radiation—a randomized study. *Journal of Nutritional Science and Vitaminology (Tokyo)*, *66*(2), 93–97. https://doi.org/10.3177/jnsv.66.93

Charalambous, M., Raftopoulos, V., Paikousis, L., Katodritis, N., Lambrinou, E., Vomvas, D., Georgiou, M., & Charalambous, A. (2018). The effect of the use of thyme honey in minimizing radiation—Induced oral mucositis in head and neck cancer patients: A randomized controlled trial. *European Journal of Oncology Nursing*, *34*, 89–97. https://doi.org/10.1016/j.ejon.2018.04.003

Cheng, C.-Q., Xu, H., Liu, L., Wang, R.-N., Liu, Y.-T., Li, J., & Zhou, X.-K. (2016). Efficacy and safety of pilocarpine for radiation-induced xerostomia in patients with head and neck cancer: A systematic review and meta-analysis. *The Journal of the American Dental Association*, *147*(4), 236–243. https://doi.org/10.1016/j.adaj.2015.09.014

Chung, Y. L., & Pui, N. N. M. (2017). Confounding factors associated with oral mucositis assessment in patients receiving chemoradiotherapy for head and neck cancer. *Supportive Care in Cancer*, *25*(9), 2743–2751. https://doi.org/10.1007/s00520-017-3684-x

Demir Doğan, M., Can, G., & Meral, R. (2017). Effectiveness of black mulberry molasses in prevention of radiotherapy-induced oral mucositis: A randomized controlled study in head and neck cancer patients. *Journal of Alternative and Complementary Medicine*, *23*(12), 971–979. https://doi.org/10.1089/acm.2016.0425

De Felice, F., Pranno, N., Papi, P., Brugnoletti, O., Tombolini, V., & Polimeni, A. (2020). Xerostomia and clinical outcomes in definitive intensity modulated radiotherapy (IMRT) versus three-dimensional conformal radiotherapy (3D-CRT) for head and neck squamous cell carcinoma: A meta-analysis. *In Vivo*, *34*(2), 623–629. https://doi.org/10.21873/invivo.11816

De Sanctis, V., Bossi, P., Sanguineti, G., Trippa, F., Ferrari, D., Bacigalupo, A., Ripamonti, C. I., Buglione, M., Pergolizzi, S., Langendjik, J. A., Murphy, B., Raber-Durlacher, J., Russi, E. G., & Lalla, R. V. (2016). Mucositis in head and neck cancer patients treated with radiotherapy and systemic therapies: Literature review and consensus statements. *Critical Reviews in Oncology/Hematology*, *100*, 147–166. https://doi.org/10.1016/j.critrevonc.2016.01.010

Elad, S., Cheng, K. K. F., Lalla, R. V., Yarom, N., Hong, C., Logan, R. M., Bowen, J., Gibson, R., Saunders, D. P., Zadik, Y., Ariyawardana, A., Correa, M. E., Ranna, V., Bossi, P., & Oncology, I. S. o. O. (2020). MASCC/ISOO clinical practice guidelines for the management of mucositis secondary to cancer therapy. *Cancer, 126*(19), 4423–4431. https://doi.org/10.1002/cncr.33100

Falchook, A. D., Green, R., Knowles, M. E., Amdur, R. J., Mendenhall, W., Hayes, D. N., Grilley-Olson, J. E., Weiss, J., Reeve, B., Mitchell, S. A., Basch, E. M., & Chera, B. S. (2016). Comparison of patient- and practitioner-reported toxic effects associated with chemoradiotherapy for head and neck cancer. *JAMA Otolaryngology–Head & Neck Surgery, 142*(6), 517–523. https://doi.org/10.1001/jamaoto.2016.0656

Forner, L., Hyldegaard, O., von Brockdorff, A. S., Specht, L., Andersen, E., Jansen, E. C., Hillerup, S., Nauntofte, B., & Jensen, S. B. (2011). Does hyperbaric oxygen treatment have the potential to increase salivary flow rate and reduce xerostomia in previously irradiated head and neck cancer patients? A pilot study. *Oral Oncology, 47*(6), 546–551. https://doi.org/10.1016/j.oraloncology.2011.03.021

Garcia, M. K., Meng, Z., Rosenthal, D. I., Shen, Y., Chambers, M., Yang, P., Hu, C., Wu, C., Bei, W., Prinsloo, S., Chiang, J., Lopez, G., & Cohen, L. (2019). Effect of true and Sham acupuncture on radiation-induced xerostomia among patients with head and neck cancer: A randomized clinical trial. *JAMA Netw ork Open, 2*(12), e1916910. https://doi.org/10.1001/jamanetwo rkopen.2019.16910

García-Gozalbo, B., & Cabañas-Alite, L. (2021). A narrative review about nutritional management and prevention of oral mucositis in haematology and oncology cancer patients undergoing antineoplastic treatments. *Nutrients, 13*(11), 4075. https://doi.org/10.3390/nu13114075

Ge, X., Liao, Z., Yuan, J., Mao, D., Li, Y., Yu, E., Wang, X., & Ding, Z. (2020). Radiotherapy-related quality of life in patients with head and neck cancers: A meta-analysis. *Supportive Care in Cancer, 28*(6), 2701–2712. https://doi.org/10.1007/s00520-019-05077-5

Jiang, C., Wang, H., Xia, C., Dong, Q., Chen, E., Qiu, Y., Yong, S., Xie, H., Zeng, L., Kuang, J., Ao, F., Gong, X., Li, J., & Chen, T. (2019). A randomized, double-blind, placebo-controlled trial of probiotics to reduce the severity of oral mucositis induced by chemoradiotherapy for patients with nasopharyngeal carcinoma. *Cancer, 125*(7), 1081–1090. https://doi.org/10.1002/cncr.31907

Kaae, J. K., Stenfeldt, L., Hyrup, B., Brink, C., & Eriksen, J. G. (2020). A randomized phase III trial for alleviating radiation-induced xerostomia with chewing gum. *Radiotherapy and Oncology, 142*, 72–78. https://doi.org/10.1016/j.radonc.2019.09.013

Khanjani Pour-Fard-Pachekenari, A., Rahmani, A., Ghahramanian, A., Asghari Jafarabadi, M., Onyeka, T. CA., & Davoodi, A. (2019). The effect of an oral care protocol and honey mouthwash on mucositis in acute myeloid leukemia patients undergoing chemotherapy: A single-blind clinical trial. *Clinical Oral Investigations, 23*(4), 1811–1821. https://doi.org/10.1007/s00784-018-2 621-9

Lalla, R. V., Bowen, J., Barasch, A., Elting, L., Epstein, J., Keefe, D. M., Lalla, R. V., Bowen, J., Barasch, A., Elting, L., Epstein, J., Keefe, D. M., McGuire, D. B., Migliorati, C., Nicolatou-Galitis, O., Peterson, D. E., Raber-Durlacher, J. E., Sonis, S. T., Elad, S., & I. S, o. O. O. (2014). MASCC/ISOO clinical practice guidelines for the management of mucositis secondary to cancer therapy. *Cancer, 120*(10), 1453–1461. https://doi.org/10.1002/cncr.28592

Mercadante, V., Jensen, S. B., Smith, D. K., Bohlke, K., Bauman, J., Brennan, M. T., Coppes, R. P., Jessen, N., Malhotra, N. K., Murphy, B., Rosenthal, D. I., Vissink, A., Wu, J., Saunders, D. P., & Peterson, D. E. (2021). Salivary gland hypofunction and/or xerostomia induced by nonsurgical cancer therapies: ISOO/MASCC/ASCO guideline. *Journal of Clinical Oncology, 39*(25), 2825–2843. https://doi.org/10.1200/jco.21.01208

Momo, K., Nagaoka, H., Kizawa, Y., Bukawa, H., Chiba, S., Kohda, Y., & Homma, M. (2017). Assessment of indomethacin oral spray for the treatment of oropharyngeal mucositis-induced pain during anticancer therapy. *Supportive Care in Cancer, 25*(10), 2997–3000. https://doi.org/10.1007/s00520-017-3817-2

Piredda, M., Facchinetti, G., Biagioli, V., Giannarelli, D., Armento, G., Tonini, G., & De Marinis, M. G. (2017). Propolis in the prevention of oral mucositis in breast cancer patients receiving adjuvant chemotherapy: A pilot randomised controlled trial. *European Journal of Cancer Care (England), 26*(6), e12757. https://doi.org/10.1111/ecc.12757

Rambod, M., Pasyar, N., & Ramzi, M. (2018). The effect of zinc sulfate on prevention, incidence, and severity of mucositis in leukemia patients undergoing chemotherapy. *European Journal of Oncology Nursing, 33*, 14–21. https://doi.org/10.1016/j.ejon.2018.01.007

Rao, D., Behzadi, F., Le, R. T., Dagan, R., & Fiester, P. (2021). Radiation induced mucositis: What the radiologist needs to know. *Current Problems in Diagnostic Radiology, 50*(6), 899–904. https://doi.org/10.1067/j.cpradiol.2020.10.006

Sonis, S. T. (1998). Mucositis as a biological process: A new hypothesis for the development of chemotherapy-induced stomatotoxicity. *Oral Oncology, 34*(1), 39–43. https://doi.org/10.1016/S1368-8375(97)00053-5

Stiff, P. J., Erder, H., Bensinger, W. I., Emmanouilides, C., Gentile, T., Isitt, J., Lu, Z. J., & Spielberger, R. (2006). Reliability and validity of a patient self-administered daily questionnaire to assess impact of oral mucositis (OM) on pain and daily functioning in patients undergoing autologous hematopoietic stem cell transplantation (HSCT). *Bone Marrow Transplant, 37*(4), 393–401. https://doi.org/10.1038/sj.bmt.1705250

Strojan, P., Hutcheson, K. A., Eisbruch, A., Beitler, J. J., Langendijk, J. A., Lee, A. W. M., Corry, J., Mendenhall, W. M., Smee, R., Rinaldo, A., & Ferlito, A. (2017). Treatment of late sequelae after radiotherapy for head and neck cancer. *Cancer Treatment Reviews, 59*, 79–92. https://doi.org/10.1016/j.ctrv.2017.07.003

Vera-Llonch, M., Oster, G., Ford, C. M., Lu, J., & Sonis, S. (2007). Oral mucositis and outcomes of allogeneic hematopoietic stem-cell transplantation in patients with hematologic malignancies. *Supportive Care in Cancer*, *15*(5), 491–496. https://doi.org/10.1007/s00520-006-0176-9

Vera-Llonch, M., Oster, G., Hagiwara, M., & Sonis, S. (2006). Oral mucositis in patients undergoing radiation treatment for head and neck carcinoma. *Cancer*, *106*(2), 329–336. https://doi.org/10.1002/cncr.21622

Xia, C., Jiang, C., Li, W., Wei, J., Hong, H., Li, J., Feng, L., Wei, H., Xin, H., & Chen, T. (2021). A Phase II randomized clinical trial and mechanistic studies using improved probiotics to prevent oral mucositis induced by concurrent radiotherapy and chemotherapy in nasopharyngeal carcinoma. *Frontiers in Immunology*, *12*, 618150. https://doi.org/10.3389/fimmu.2021.618150

Yüce, U., & Yurtsever, S. (2019). Effect of education about oral mucositis given to the cancer patients having chemotherapy on life quality. *Journal of Cancer Education*, *34*(1), 35–40. https://doi.org/10.1007/s13187-017-1262-z

CHAPTER 9

FEVER

INTRODUCTION

Fever in people with cancer needs rapid evaluation because, if associated with neutropenia, it may be life-threatening and will necessitate urgent treatment. The definition of *fever* in a patient with neutropenia is a single oral temperature of ≥38.3°C or 101°F (Freifeld et al., 2011). Oral or axillary temperature measurement is recommended rather than rectal due to the risk of translocation of bacterial infection following insertion of the probe into the rectum (White & Ybarra, 2017).

PREVALENCE

Fever is common in the cancer population, with 10% to 50% of patients with solid tumors and more than 80% of those occurring in hematologic cancer (Klastersky, 2004).

CONTRIBUTING FACTORS

Chemotherapy is the most common risk factor for fever in people with cancer. In addition to chemotherapy, medications affecting the immune system, including psychotropic drugs and anticonvulsants, may suppress bone marrow production of neutrophils (White & Ybarra, 2017). The use of immune checkpoint inhibitors has also been implicated in the development of febrile neutropenia (Boegeholz et al., 2020). Oral mucositis is an additional contributing factor; assessment of the mouth, including the salivary glands, is important to identify the source of infection leading to fever (Zecha et al., 2019).

CASE STUDY

You are working as the triage nurse practitioner at the ED of a rural hospital. A 36-year-old woman presents with a temperature of 39°C

(continued)

SECTION II • GENERAL SYMPTOMS

CASE STUDY (*CONTINUED*)

(102°F); she is shivering and her partner who is with her says that she had chemotherapy 1 week ago.

1. What should you assess before beginning treatment?

2. What investigations should you order?

She is otherwise healthy and she states that she wants to go home because she has children that she cannot leave with her parents for any length of time.

3. What would determine if she can avoid hospitalization?

ASSESSMENT

An absolute neutrophil count (ANC) of less than 500 cells/mm^3 indicates severe neutropenia. Moderate neutropenia is defined as between 500 and 999 cells/mm^3 and mild neutropenia between 1,000 and 1,500 cells/mm^3 (Freifeld et al., 2011).

Laboratory assessment includes a complete blood cell (CBC) count and a platelet count, as well as creatinine and blood urea, electrolytes, hepatic transaminase enzymes, and total bilirubin. In addition, two sets of blood cultures from different venipuncture sites or from two lumens of a central line should be procured. If respiratory symptoms are present, a chest x-ray should be done (Freifeld et al., 2011).

The Multinational Association of Supportive Care in Cancer (MASCC) Risk Index for Febrile Neutropenia (www.mdcalc.com/calc/3913/mascc-risk-index-febrile-neutropenia) identifies those who are at low risk of poor outcome and suggests management strategies where outpatient antibiotics may be appropriate.

MANAGEMENT

Primary prevention in those at risk of neutropenia involves prophylactic antimicrobials. Similarly, antimicrobials should be prescribed to prevent recurrent infections. For patients treated for hematologic cancer, prophylaxis and treatment of fungal infections are vital. Increasingly, granulocyte-colony stimulating factor (G-CSF) is used to prevent febrile neutropenia (Hoshina & Takei, 2021). Patients at low risk can be treated with oral agents, while those at high risk require hospital admission (Klastersky, 2004).

A complete guide to antimicrobial, antifungal, and antiviral therapy is presented in the *Clinical Practice Guideline for the Use of Antimicrobial Agents in Neutropenic Patients With Cancer* (Freifeld et al., 2011). The American Society of Clinical Oncology (Taplitz et al., 2018) recommends that intravenous therapy with broad-spectrum antibiotics begins within 1 hour of triage ("door to needle") and that patients should be monitored for 4 or more hours before discharge. Outpatient oral therapy may be considered and has been shown to be as effective as inpatient therapy (Rivas-Ruiz et al., 2019); however, if the fever continues after 2 to 3 days of oral therapy, inpatient treatment should be considered.

GUIDELINES

- **American Society of Clinical Oncology (ASCO) and Infectious Diseases Society of America**

    Outpatient Management of Fever and Neutropenia in Adults Treated for Malignancy: American Society of Clinical Oncology and Infectious Diseases Society of America Clinical Practice Guideline Update (Taplitz et al., 2018)

    Provides consensus recommendations for outpatient management of fever and neutropenia

- **Infectious Diseases Society of America**

    Clinical Practice Guideline for the Use of Antimicrobial Agents in Neutropenic Patients With Cancer: 2010 Update by the Infectious Diseases Society of America (Freifeld et al., 2011)

    Comprehensive guide to the evaluation and treatment of febrile neutropenia, including recommendations for antimicrobial, antifungal, and antiviral therapies

SUMMARY

Fever and febrile neutropenia in all patients on chemotherapy require immediate assessment and treatment. Patients at high risk for neutropenia require inpatient treatment, while those at low risk may be treated as outpatients.

A robust set of instructor resources designed to supplement this text is located at http://connect.springerpub.com/content/reference-book/978-0-8261-8524-2. Qualifying Instructors may request access by emailing **textbook@springerpub.com**.

REFERENCES

Boegeholz, J., Brueggen, C. S., Pauli, C., Dimitriou, F., Haralambieva, E., Dummer, R., Manz, M. G., & Widmer, C. C. (2020). Challenges in diagnosis and management of neutropenia upon exposure to immune-checkpoint inhibitors: Meta-analysis of a rare immune-related adverse side effect. *BMC Cancer*, 20(1), 300. https://doi.org/10.1186/s12885-020-06763-y

Freifeld, A. G., Bow, E. J., Sepkowitz, K. A., Boeckh, M. J., Ito, J. I., Mullen, C. A., Raad, I. I., Rolston, K. V., Young, J-A H., & Wingard, J. R. (2011). Clinical practice guideline for the use of antimicrobial agents in neutropenic patients with cancer: 2010 update by the infectious diseases society of America. *Clinical Infectious Diseases, 52*(4), e56–e93. https://doi.org/10.1093/cid/cir073

Hoshina, H., & Takei, H. (2021). Granulocyte-colony stimulating factor-associated aortitis in cancer: A systematic literature review. *Cancer Treatment and Research Communications, 29*, 100454. https://doi.org/10.1016/j.ctarc.2021.1 00454

Klastersky, J. (2004). Management of fever in neutropenic patients with different risks of complications. *Clinical Infectious Diseases, 39*(Suppl. 1), S32–S37. https://doi.org/10.1086/383050

Rivas-Ruiz, R., Villasis-Keever, M., Miranda-Novales, G., Castelán-Martínez, O. D., & Rivas-Contreras, S. (2019). Outpatient treatment for people with cancer who develop a low-risk febrile neutropaenic event. *Cochrane Database of Systematic Reviews, 3*(3), Cd009031. https://doi.org/10.1002/14651858.C D009031.pub2

Taplitz, R. A., Kenned., E. B., Bow, E. J., Crews, J., Gleason, C., Hawley, D. K., Langston, A. A., Nastoupil, L. J., Rajotte, M., Rolston, K., Strasfeld, L., & Flowers, C. R. (2018). Outpatient management of fever and neutropenia in adults treated for malignancy: American society of clinical oncology and infectious diseases society of A merica clinical practice guideline update. *Journal of Clinical Oncology, 36*(14), 1443–1453. https://doi.org/10.1200/jco. 2017.77.6211

White, L., & Ybarra, M. (2017). Neutropenic fever. *Hematology/Oncology Clinics of North America, 31*(6), 981–993. https://doi.org/10.1016/j.hoc.2017.08.004

Zecha, J., Raber-Durlacher, J. E., Laheij, A., Westermann, A. M., Epstein, J. B., de Lange, J., & Smeele, L. E. (2019). The impact of the oral cavity in febrile neutropenia and infectious complications in patients treated with myelosuppressive chemotherapy. *Supportive Care in Cancer, 27*(10), 3667–3679. http s://doi.org/10.1007/s00520-019-04925-8

CHAPTER 10

HOT FLASHES

INTRODUCTION

Hot flashes, a subjective feeling of heat that is associated with objective signs of vasodilation and a drop in core temperature, are a distressing symptom of cancer treatment. Often accompanied by sweating and flushing, hot flashes have a negative effect on quality of life (Kadakia et al., 2012). They occur in both women and men as a result of endocrine disruption.

PREVALENCE IN WOMEN

Hot flashes are a side effect of estrogen deprivation in women treated for hormone-sensitive cancers; they occur with varying intensity and frequency and affect more than 90% of women with breast cancer (Vincent, 2015), especially those with ovarian suppression added to tamoxifen or aromatase inhibitors (Pagani et al., 2014).

CONTRIBUTING FACTORS

The pathophysiology of this phenomenon is not well-understood, but dysregulation in the hypothalamus as well as neurotransmitter involvement are thought to be important (Leon-Ferre et al., 2017). Triggers of hot flashes include hot beverages and spicy foods, caffeine, and alcohol (Kaplan & Mahon, 2014). More than 90% of premenopausal women with breast cancer on exemestane or tamoxifen and ovarian suppression report severe hot flashes (Pagani et al., 2014).

ASSESSMENT

The Hot Flash Related Daily Interference Scale (Carpenter, 2001) contains 10 items that measure interference on daily life during the past week on a scale from 0 to 10. It has been validated in women with breast cancer (Figure 10.1).

- Work (outside the home and housework)
- Social activities (time spent with family and friends)
- Leisure activities (e.g., relaxing, hobbies)
- Sleep
- Mood
- Concentration
- Relaxation with others
- Sexuality
- Enjoyment of life
- Overall quality of life

Figure 10.1 Items measured on the Hot Flash Related Daily Interference Scale.

MANAGEMENT

It is important to manage this symptom because experiencing hot flashes when taking endocrine manipulation medications leads to discontinuation of therapy and poor outcomes (Zeng et al., 2022).

Pharmaceutical Interventions

There are a number of evidence-based interventions that have been shown to reduce the frequency of hot flashes in women.

ANTIDEPRESSANTS

Both selective serotonin reuptake inhibitors and serotonin–norepinephrine reuptake inhibitors have shown to improve hot flashes (Dos Santos et al., 2021). These include the following:

- venlafaxine 75 mg/d
- desvenlafaxine 100 to 150 mg/d
- paroxetine 10 to 15 mg/d
- escitalopram 10 to 20 mg/d
- citalopram 10 to 20 mg/d
- fluoxetine 20 mg/d
- sertraline 50 mg/d

Caution should be used when prescribing these medications to women taking tamoxifen due to interference with tamoxifen metabolism, inhibiting the effect on CYP2D6 enzyme, reducing the bioavailability of tamoxifen (Franzoi et al., 2021). Fluoxetine and paroxetine are the medications of highest concern. Selective serotonin–norepinephrine reuptake inhibitors are the safest drugs for women on tamoxifen (Stubbs et al., 2017).

Bupropion has been shown to be minimally effective in reducing hot flashes, but it does have the advantage of not causing the sexual side effects of the other antidepressants (Nuñez et al., 2013).

ANTICONVULSANTS

Gabapentin has been shown to reduce the frequency and duration of hot flashes, although with side effects such as dizziness and unsteadiness (Yoon et al., 2020). Dosage should start at 300 mg at night and then increased every 4 to 7 days until the total dose is 900 mg/d in divided doses (Eden, 2016). Pregabalin has been shown to reduce hot flashes but with limited evidence due to the small number of studies using this treatment (Shan et al., 2020).

ALPHA-ADRENERGIC AGONISTS

Clonidine has been tested to see if its usage reduces hot flashes; a small decrease in occurrence of hot flashes (one per day) has been reported, but side effects are common (Barba et al., 2014). The usual starting dose is half a tablet twice a day and the dose increased to a full tablet once a day; this may cause a small decrease in blood pressure, leading to dizziness. Other side effects include dry mouth, constipation, and headache (Szabo et al., 2019). Stellate ganglion block, while invasive, has been shown to be more effective in reducing hot flashes than pregabalin (Othman & Zaky, 2014). While severe complications are rare, temporary hoarseness and neuralgia on the chest wall have been reported.

Nonpharmaceutical Interventions

For mild hot flashes, behavioral changes can be suggested (Kaplan & Mahon, 2014; Pinkerton & Santen, 2019; Figure 10.2).

- Weight loss of more than 10% of baseline body weight or more than 10 lb has been shown to reduce or even eliminate hot flashes (Pinkerton & Santen, 2019).

- Yoga appears to be effective in reducing hot flashes in menopausal women based on a systematic review and meta-analysis and has benefits for other menopausal symptoms (Cramer et al., 2018).

- Hypnosis is supported by the International Menopause Society to reduce hot flashes (Baber et al., 2016), and a randomized trial showed a 68% reduction in frequency and intensity (Elkins et al., 2008).

- Wearing breathable clothing and dressing in layers
- Avoiding down comforters
- Placing reusable cold packs under pillows
- Taking a cold shower before bed
- Using fans and keeping the temperature cool in the house or office
- Eliminating common triggers for hot flashes such as hot beverages, caffeine, alcohol, and spicy foods to reduce the frequency and/or intensity of hot flashes

Figure 10.2 Managing mild hot flashes.

- Acupuncture may be helpful in alleviating hot flashes, but the evidence on its effectiveness is mixed (Jang et al., 2020; Kim et al., 2018). Because it has few, if any, side effects, it may be suggested for use in women (Wang et al., 2018) as it may provide some improvement (Yuanqing et al., 2020). Acupuncture has been shown to improve other symptoms such as pain, fatigue, and depression and therefore may be of benefit overall in women with multiple symptoms (Li et al., 2021).

- Cognitive behavioral therapy has some effects on the perception and appraisal of hot flashes in women (Atema et al., 2019; Franzoi et al., 2021).

- Lack of effectiveness has been shown for mindfulness/relaxation or exercise (McCormick et al., 2020).

- A cool pad pillow topper helps reduce the frequency and severity of hot flashes at night, and importantly has a positive impact on sleep disturbance (Marshall-McKenna et al., 2016).

- The placebo effect has been shown to impact on the perception of hot flashes in women using supplements such as black cohosh and red clover (Pinkerton & Santen, 2019), homeopathy, paced respiration, evening primrose oil, and omega-3 (Vincent, 2015).

CASE STUDY

Your patient, a 47-year-old woman with ER/PR/Her 2-neu breast cancer, is considering to stop tamoxifen just 3 months after starting the medication. She says that the hot flashes are interfering with her sleep, and this is impacting on her ability to do her job.

1. What suggestion could you make to assess her symptoms?

Two weeks later, she repeats her intention to stop taking tamoxifen. She has had to take a 4-week leave from her work and is worried that she might lose her job if she has to take more time off.

2. What should you offer her at this point in time?

3. She is reluctant to take anything that might impact on her already poor quality of life. What side effects of the interventions do you suggest should be discussed with her?

PREVALENCE IN MEN

Up to 80% of men on androgen deprivation therapy (ADT) experience hot flashes (Ahmadi & Daneshmand, 2013). As with women, hot flashes are distressing, cause sleep disturbance, and have a negative impact on quality of life. This symptom contributes to discontinuation of therapy (Allan et al., 2014) despite the promise of extended survival in men with advanced or recurrent prostate cancer.

CONTRIBUTING FACTORS

Alcohol, hot beverages, and spicy foods may trigger hot flashes; however, it is the decrease in testosterone levels caused by the therapy (luteinizing hormone antagonists or agonists) that is responsible.

ASSESSMENT

The Hot Flush Beliefs and Behavior Scale for Men (Hunter et al., 2014) measures cognitive appraisal and behavioral strategies used by men with prostate cancer. It contains 17 items and may be too long for clinical use.

MANAGEMENT

Pharmaceutical Management

Most of the research into the interventions for this symptom has occurred in women with breast cancer, with a limited evidence base for men with prostate cancer on androgen suppression. Men whose disease status makes them eligible for intermittent ADT experience a reduction in hot flashes (Jaswal & Crook, 2015).

HORMONAL THERAPIES: Cyproterone acetate (100 mg daily) is highly effective in reducing hot flashes in men but interferes with ADT (Ahmadi & Daneshmand, 2013). Use of megestrol acetate or medroxyprogesterone acetate has been studied, with medroxyprogesterone acetate showing the greatest benefit with minimal side effects (Irani et al., 2010).

NONHORMONAL THERAPIES: A moderate effect on hot flashes is seen with use of selective serotonin and serotonin–norepinephrine reuptake inhibitors (Fankhauser et al., 2020). Paroxetine may be the most effective of this class of medication (Hutton et al., 2020), but venlafaxine has also shown greater efficacy than hormonal therapies (Irani et al., 2010). Gabapentin at doses up to 900 mg/d has been shown to be effective, with minimal side effects, in men with prostate cancer experiencing hot flashes (Moraska et al., 2010).

Nonpharmaceutical Management

Traditional acupuncture and electroacupuncture have shown efficacy in reducing hot flashes in this population (Hutton et al., 2020). Maintenance of a healthy body weight, regular exercise (Allan et al., 2014), and lifestyle modification, as suggested for women, may also be helpful.

GUIDELINES

- **National Comprehensive Cancer Network (NCCN)**

    NCCN Guidelines Version 1.2022 Survivorship: Hormone-Related Symptoms

    SMP-4 for Vasomotor Symptoms in Women

    https://www.nccn.org/professionals/physician_gls/pdf/survivorship.pdf

    NCCN Guidelines Version 1.203 Prostate Cancer

    PROS-1 Principle of Androgen Deprivation Therapy: Monitor/Surveillance

    https://www.nccn.org/professionals/physician_gls/pdf/prostate.pdf

- **Oncology Nursing Society (ONS)**

    Oncology Nursing Society Guidelines for Cancer Treatment-Related Hot Flashes in Women With Breast Cancer and Men With Prostate Cancer (Kaplan et al., 2020)

SUMMARY

Hot flashes are a significant side effect of endocrine manipulation in both men and women and may be a reason for discontinuation of therapy. There are both pharmaceutical and nonpharmaceutical interventions for this condition, and a staged approach, starting with lifestyle modification, can be helpful in reducing its frequency and severity.

 A robust set of instructor resources designed to supplement this text is located at http://connect.springerpub.com/content/reference-book/978-0-8261-8524-2. Qualifying Instructors may request access by emailing **textbook@springerpub.com**.

REFERENCES

Ahmadi, H., & Daneshmand, S. (2013). Androgen deprivation therapy: Evidence-based management of side effects. *BJU International*, *111*(4), 543–548. https://doi.org/10.1111/j.1464-410X.2012.11774.x

Allan, C. A., Collins, V. R., Frydenberg, M., McLachlan, R. I., & Matthiesson, K. L. (2014). Androgen deprivation therapy complications. *Endocrine-Related Cancer*, *21*(4), T119–129. https://doi.org/10.1530/erc-13-0467

Atema, V., van Leeuwen, M., Kieffer, J. M., Oldenburg, H. S. A., van Beurden, M., Gerritsma, M. A., Kuenen, M. A., Plaisier, P. W., Lopes Cardozo, A. M. F., van Riet, Y. E. A., Heuff, G., Rijna, H., van der Mejj, S., Noorda, E. M., Timmers, G.-J., Vrouenraets, B. C., Bollen, M., van der Veen, H., Bijker, N., . . . Aaronson, N. K. (2019). Efficacy of internet-based cognitive behavioral therapy for treatment-induced menopausal symptoms in breast cancer survivors: Results of a randomized controlled trial. *Journal of Clinical Oncology, 37*(10), 809–822. https://doi.org/10.1200/jco.18.00655

Baber, R. J., Panay, N., & Fenton, A. (2016). 2016 IMS Recommendations on women's midlife health and menopause hormone therapy. *Climacteric, 19*(2), 109–150. https://doi.org/10.3109/13697137.2015.1129166

Barba, M., Pizzuti, L., Sergi, D., Maugeri-Saccà, M., Vincenzoni, C., Conti, F., Tomao, F., Vizza, E., Di Lauro, L., Di Filippo, F., Carpano, S., Mariani, L., & Vici, P. (2014). Hot flushes in women with breast cancer: State of the art and future perspectives. *Expert Review of Anticancer Therapy, 14*(2), 185–198. https://doi.org/10.1586/14737140.2013.856271

Carpenter, J. S. (2001). The hot flash related daily interference scale: A tool for assessing the impact of hot flashes on quality of life following breast cancer. *Journal of Pain and Symptom Management, 22*(6), 979–989. https://doi.org/10.1016/S0885-3924(01)00353-0

Cramer, H., Peng, W., & Lauche, R. (2018). Yoga for menopausal symptoms—A systematic review and meta-analysis. *Maturitas, 109*, 13–25. https://doi.org/10.1016/j.maturitas.2017.12.005

Dos Santos, B. S., Bordignon, C., & Rosa, D. D. (2021). Managing common estrogen deprivation side effects in HR+ breast cancer: An evidence-based review. *Current Oncology Reports, 23*(6), 63. https://doi.org/10.1007/s11912-021-01055-5

Eden, J. (2016). Endocrine dilemma: Managing menopausal symptoms after breast cancer. *European Journal of Endocrinology, 174*(3), R71–R77. https://doi.org/10.1530/eje-15-0814

Elkins, G., Marcus, J., Stearns, V., Perfect, M., Rajab, M. H., Ruud, C., Palamara, L., & Keith, T. (2008). Randomized trial of a hypnosis intervention for treatment of hot flashes among breast cancer survivors. *Journal of Clinical Oncology, 26*(31), 5022–5026. https://doi.org/10.1200/jco.2008.16.6389

Fankhauser, C. D., Wettstein, M. S., Reinhardt, M., Gessendorfer, A., Mostafid, H., & Hermanns, T. (2020). Indications and complications of androgen deprivation therapy. *Seminars in Oncology Nursing, 36*(4), 151042. https://doi.org/10.1016/j.soncn.2020.151042

Franzoi, M. A., Agostinetto, E., Perachino, M., Del Mastro, L., de Azambuja, E., Vaz-Luis, I., Partridge, A. H., & Lambertini, M. (2021). Evidence-based approaches for the management of side-effects of adjuvant endocrine therapy in patients with breast cancer. *Lancet Oncology, 22*(7), e303–e313. https://doi.org/10.1016/s1470-2045(20)30666-5

Hunter, M. S., Sharpley, C. F., Stefanopoulou, E., Yousaf, O., Bitsika, V., & Christie, D. R. H. (2014). The hot flush beliefs and behaviour scale for men (HFBBS-Men) undergoing treatment for prostate cancer. *Maturitas, 79*(4), 464–470. https://doi.org/10.1016/j.maturitas.2014.09.014

Hutton, B., Hersi, M., Cheng, W., Pratt, M., Barbeau, P., Mazzarello, S., Ahmadzai, N., Skidmore, B., Morgan, S. C., Bordeleau, L., Ginex, P. K., Sadeghirad, B., Morgan, R. L., Marie Cole, K., & Clemons, M. (2020). Comparing interventions for management of hot flashes in patients with breast and prostate cancer: A systematic review with meta-analyses. *Oncology Nursing Forum*, *47*(4), E86–E106. https://doi.org/10.1188/20.Onf.E86-e106

Irani, J., Salomon, L., Oba, R., Bouchard, P., & Mottet, N. (2010). Efficacy of venlafaxine, medroxyprogesterone acetate, and cyproterone acetate for the treatment of vasomotor hot flushes in men taking gonadotropin-releasing hormone analogues for prostate cancer: A double-blind, randomised trial. *The Lancet Oncology*, *11*(2), 147–154. https://doi.org/10.1016/S1470-2045(09)70338-9

Jang, S., Ko, Y., Sasaki, Y., Park, S., Jo, J., Kang, N. H., Yoo, E-S., Park, N.-C., Cho, S. H., Jang, H., Jang, B.-H., Hwang, D.-S., & Ko, S. G. (2020). Acupuncture as an adjuvant therapy for management of treatment-related symptoms in breast cancer patients: Systematic review and meta-analysis (PRISMA-compliant). *Medicine (Baltimore)*, *99*(50), e21820. https://doi.org/10.1097/md.0000000000021820

Jaswal, J., & Crook, J. (2015). The role of intermittent androgen deprivation therapy in the management of biochemically recurrent or metastatic prostate cancer. *Current Urology Reports*, *16*(3), 11. https://doi.org/10.1007/s11934-015-0481-2

Kadakia, K. C., Loprinzi, C. L., & Barton, D. L. (2012). Hot flashes: The ongoing search for effective interventions. *Menopause (New York N.Y.)*, *19*(7), 719–721. https://doi.org/10.1097/gme.0b013e3182578d31

Kaplan, M., Ginex, P. K., Michaud, L. B., Fernández-Ortega, P., Leibelt, J., Mahon, S., Rapoport, B. L., Robinson, V., Maloney, C., Moriarty, K. A., Vrabel, M., & Morgan, R. L. (2020). ONS Guidelines™ for cancer treatment-related hot flashes in women with breast cancer and men with prostate cancer. *Oncology Nursing Forum*, *47*(4), 374–399. https://doi.org/10.1188/20.Onf.374-399

Kaplan, M., & Mahon, S. (2014). Hot flash management: Update of the evidence for patients with cancer. *Clinical Journal of Oncology Nursing*, (18 Suppl), 59–67. https://doi.org/10.1188/14.Cjon.S3.59-67

Kim, T. H., Kang, J. W., & Lee, M. S. (2018). Current evidence of acupuncture for symptoms related to breast cancer survivors: A PRISMA-compliant systematic review of clinical studies in Korea. *Medicine (Baltimore)*, *97*(32), e11793. https://doi.org/10.1097/md.0000000000011793

Leon-Ferre, R. A., Majithia, N., & Loprinzi, C. L. (2017). Management of hot flashes in women with breast cancer receiving ovarian function suppression. *Cancer Treatment Reviews*, *52*, 82–90. https://doi.org/10.1016/j.ctrv.2016.11.012

Li, H., Schlaeger, J. M., Jang, M. K., Lin, Y., Park, C., Liu, T., Sun, M., & Doorenbos, A. Z. (2021). acupuncture improves multiple treatment-related symptoms in breast cancer survivors: A systematic review and meta-analysis. *Journal of Alternative and Complementary Medicine*, *27*(12), 1084–1097. https://doi.org/10.1089/acm.2021.0133

Marshall-McKenna, R., Morrison, A., Stirling, L., Hutchison, C., Rice, A. M., Hewitt, C., Paul, L., Rodger, M., Macpherson, I. R., & McCartney, E. (2016). A randomised trial of the cool pad pillow topper versus standard care for sleep disturbance and hot flushes in women on endocrine therapy for breast cancer. *Supportive Care in Cancer*, 24(4), 1821–1829. https://doi.org/10.1007/s00520-015-2967-3

McCormick, C. A., Brennan, A., & Hickey, M. (2020). Managing vasomotor symptoms effectively without hormones. *Climacteric*, 23(6), 532–538. https://doi.org/10.1080/13697137.2020.1789093

Moraska, A. R., Atherton, P. J., Szydlo, D. W., Barton, D. L., Stella, P. J., Rowland Jr, K. M., Schaefer, P. L., Krook, J., Bearden, J. D., & Loprinzi, C. L. (2010). Gabapentin for the management of hot flashes in prostate cancer survivors: A longitudinal continuation Study—NCCTG Trial N00CB. *Journal of Supportive Oncology*, 8(3), 128.

Nuñez, G. R., Pinczowski, H., Zanellato, R., Tateyama, L., Schindler, F., Fonseca, F., & Del Giglio, A. (2013). Bupropion for control of hot flashes in breast cancer survivors: A prospective, double-blind, randomized, crossover, pilot phase II trial. *Journal of Pain and Symptom Management*, 45(6), 969–979. https://doi.org/10.1016/j.jpainsymman.2012.06.011

Othman, A. H., & Zaky, A. H. (2014). Management of hot flushes in breast cancer survivors: Comparison between stellate ganglion block and pregabalin. *Pain Medicine*, 15(3), 410–417. https://doi.org/10.1111/pme.12331

Pagani, O., Regan, M. M., Walley, B. A., Fleming, G. F., Colleoni, M., Láng, I., Gomez, H. L., Tondini, C., Burstein, H. J., Perez, E. A., Ciruelos, E., Stearns, V., Bonnefoi, H., Martino, S., Geyer, C. E., Pinotti, G., Puglisi, F., Crivellari, D., Ruhstaller, T., & Francis, P. A. (2014). Adjuvant exemestane with ovarian suppression in premenopausal breast cancer. *New England Journal of Medicine*, 371(2), 107–118. https://doi.org/10.1056/NEJMoa1404037

Pinkerton, J. V., & Santen, R. J. (2019). Managing vasomotor symptoms in women after cancer. *Climacteric*, 22(6), 544–552. https://doi.org/10.1080/13697137.2019.1600501

Shan, D., Zou, L., Liu, X., Shen, Y., Cai, Y., & Zhang, J. (2020). Efficacy and safety of gabapentin and pregabalin in patients with vasomotor symptoms: A systematic review and meta-analysis. *American Journal of Obstetrics & Gynecology*, 222(6), 564–579.e512. https://doi.org/10.1016/j.ajog.2019.12.011

Stubbs, C., Mattingly, L., Crawford, S. A., Wickersham, E. A., Brockhaus, J. L., & McCarthy, L. H. (2017). Do SSRIs and SNRIs reduce the frequency and/or severity of hot flashes in menopausal women. *Journal of the Oklahoma State Medical Association*, 110(5), 272–274.

Szabo, R. A., Marino, J. L., & Hickey, M. (2019). Managing menopausal symptoms after cancer. *Climacteric*, 22(6), 572–578. https://doi.org/10.1080/13697137.2019.1646718

Vincent, A. J. (2015). Management of menopause in women with breast cancer. *Climacteric, 18*(5), 690–701. https://doi.org/10.3109/13697137.2014.996749

Wang, X. P., Zhang, D. J., Wei, X. D., Wang, J. P., & Zhang, D. Z. (2018). Acupuncture for the relief of hot flashes in breast cancer patients: A systematic review and meta-analysis of randomized controlled trials and observational studies. *Journal of Cancer Research and Therapies, 14,* S600–S608. https://doi.org/10.4103/0973-1482.183174

Yoon, S. H., Lee, J. Y., Lee, C., Lee, H., & Kim, S. N. (2020). Gabapentin for the treatment of hot flushes in menopause: A meta-analysis. *Menopause, 27*(4), 485–493. https://doi.org/10.1097/gme.0000000000001491

Yuanqing, P., Yong, T., Haiqian, L., Gen, C., Shen, X., Dong, J., & Miaomiao, Q. (2020). Acupuncture for hormone therapy-related side effects in breast cancer patients: A GRADE-assessed systematic review and updated meta-analysis. *Integrative Cancer Therapies, 19.*https://doi.org/10.1177/1534735420940394

Zeng, E., He, W., Smedby, K. E., & Czene, K. (2022). Adjuvant hormone therapy — related hot flashes predict treatment discontinuation and worse breast cancer prognosis. *Journal of the National Comprehensive Cancer Network, 20*(6), 683–689.e682. https://doi.org/10.6004/jnccn.2021.7116

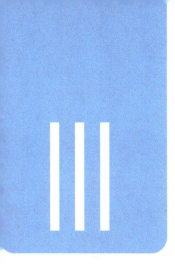

Gastrointestinal Symptoms

CHAPTER 11

CONSTIPATION

INTRODUCTION

Opioid-induced bowel dysfunction (OIBD) describes a distressing syndrome of which constipation and straining to have a bowel movement are most distressing (Bell et al., 2009). Other symptoms in this syndrome include fatigue, reflux, bloating, passing gas, and lower abdominal pain. These symptoms may lead to patients underdosing or refusing pain medication. *Opioid-induced constipation* is defined as reduced frequency of bowel movements (less than 3 per week), development or worsening of straining to pass stool, a sense of incomplete emptying of the bowels, harder stools, or distress with bowel function (Gaertner et al., 2015).

PREVALENCE

Of the patients who are prescribed opioids for pain relief, 60% to 90% experience constipation (Bell et al., 2009; Katakami et al., 2017a). Constipation is also experienced by patients treated with certain chemotherapy agents, including vinca alkaloids, and those with reduced oral intake.

CONTRIBUTING FACTORS

Beyond opioid medications, chemotherapy itself can cause constipation (Hanai et al., 2016). Radiation therapy can sometimes cause constipation (Efverman, 2020), and patients who have an ostomy may also experience this symptom (Vonk-Klaassen et al., 2016). The use of antiemetics is also a contributing factor (Hanai et al., 2016).

ASSESSMENT

Physical examination of the abdomen may reveal a distended and palpable bowel.

- The Patient Assessment of Constipation (PAC) Symptoms Questionnaire is a self-reported questionnaire that uses a Likert scale to assess 12 symptoms in three domains (abdominal, rectal, and stool;

- www.content-eu-1.content-cms.com/2b02a3e0-0b88-47df-ad46-d72278932bc/dxdam/eb/eb692116-c54b-4a1d-a5e6-b44c524aadf5/NL_Target%20OIC_PAC_SYM%20Vragenlist.pdf).

- The Bristol Stool Chart is a tool that depicts seven different types of stools in pictures to help patients describe the appearance of their stools. Type 1 shows hard lumps and type 7 describes stools that are entirely liquid (www.continence.org.au/bristol-stool-chart).

- The Bowel Function Index (BFI) is a clinician-administered scale of three items (ease of defecation, feeling of incomplete bowel evacuation, and personal judgment of constipation; Ducrotté & Caussé, 2012).

MANAGEMENT

Management of constipation may start with suggesting lifestyle interventions, such as increasing fluid intake, participating in regular exercise, and responding to the urge to defecate promptly (Crockett et al., 2019). However, opioid-induced constipation generally requires more intensive intervention and/or switching to a different, less constipating analgesic agent (Figure 11.1).

- Stool softeners (docusate sodium)
- Osmotic laxatives (polyethylene glycol, magnesium citrate, lactulose)
- Lubricants (mineral oil)
- Stimulant laxatives (bisacodyl, senna, sodium picosulfate)
- Soluble fiber (oats, certain fruits and vegetables, psyllium, methylcellulose, calcium polycarbophil)
- May use enemas as rescue therapy, but often not preferred by patients

Figure 11.1 First-line agents for management of constipation.

Source: From Crockett, S., Greer, K., Heidelbaugh, J., Falk-Ytter, Y., Hanson, B., & Sultan, S. (2019). American Gastroenterological Association Institute guideline on the medical management of opioid-induced constipation. *Gastroenterology, 156,* 218–226. https://doi.org/10.1053/gastro.2018.07.016.

CASE STUDY

Your patient is taking oxycodone for pain relief and, other than some drowsiness, is happy with pain control. His wife asks you for a referral to a nutritionist.

1. Before making the referral, what should you ask her?

(continued)

> ### CASE STUDY (*CONTINUED*)
>
> She responds that her husband is not eating much and she is concerned about the amount of weight he has lost.
>
> 2. What information would be helpful to assess his gastrointestinal health?
>
> He admits that he is having hard stools ("like nuts") every other day.
>
> 3. What would you suggest to this couple?

Pharmaceutical Management of Opioid-Induced Constipation

First-, second-, and third-line interventions for the management of constipation are available.

SECOND-LINE AGENTS

Prescription strength laxatives such as prucalopride and lubiprostone have been shown to be moderately effective (Nee et al., 2018).

THIRD-LINE AGENTS

Peripherally acting mu-opioid receptor antagonists (PAMORAs) are highly effective in restoring bowel function but should be used with caution due to the potential for adverse events. These agents include naloxegol for the treatment of laxative-refractory, opioid-induced constipation (Crockett et al., 2019), methylnaltrexone (Mori et al., 2017), and naldemedine (0.2 mg once per day; Katakami et al., 2017b).

Fixed-dose oxycodone/naloxone prolonged-release tablets (OXN PR) have been shown to provide pain relief and improve bowel function in patients in whom other laxatives have not been effective in managing constipation (Morlion et al., 2018).

Nonpharmaceutical Management of Constipation

Acupuncture using transcutaneous electrical nerve stimulation has shown efficacy in managing opioid-induced constipation (Cai et al., 2019). Similarly, acupuncture with electrostimulation relieves postoperative constipation in patients with brain cancer (Li et al., 2020).

Nonpharmaceutical Management of Antiemetic-Induced Constipation

Self-management of antiemetic-induced constipation has shown efficacy in women with breast cancer (Hanai et al., 2016). The protocol involves abdominal massage stretching of abdominal muscles and education on the correct position for defecation. Education about nutrition and instruction to eat a diet with 12% to 15% protein, 30% to 35% fats, and 55% to 60% carbohydrates in the form of grains also reduced the occurrence of constipation in women with breast cancer receiving chemotherapy (Abdollahi et al., 2019). Auricular acupressure also relieved constipation in women with breast cancer receiving chemotherapy with no reported side effects (Shin & Park, 2018). A small study in patients with leukemia found that consuming 200 g of sweet potato daily prevented constipation in patients hospitalized for administration of chemotherapy (Zou et al., 2016).

GUIDELINES

- **American Gastroenterological Association Institute**

    American Gastroenterological Association Institute Guideline on the Medical Management of Opioid-Induced Constipation (Crockett et al., 2019)

- **Oncology Nursing Society (ONS)**

    ONS Guidelines™ for Opioid-Induced and Non–Opioid-Related Cancer Constipation (Ginex et al., 2020)

SUMMARY

Constipation, often caused by antiemetic medications or opioids, impacts negatively on quality of life and is a source of distress. Interventions range from lifestyle and dietary interventions to medications that should be used with caution as they can interfere with pain control.

A robust set of instructor resources designed to supplement this text is located at http://connect.springerpub.com/content/reference-book/978-0-8261-8524-2. Qualifying Instructors may request access by emailing **textbook@springerpub.com**.

REFERENCES

Abdollahi, R., Najafi, S., Razmpoosh, E., Shoormasti, R. S., Haghighat, S., Raji Lahiji, M., Chamari, M., Asgari, M., Cheshmazar, E., & Zarrati, M. (2019). The effect of dietary intervention along with nutritional education on reducing the gastrointestinal side effects caused by chemotherapy among women with breast cancer. *Nutrition and Cancer, 71*(6), 922–930. https://doi.org/10.1080/01635581.2019.1590608

Bell, T. J., Panchal, S. J., Miaskowski, C., Bolge, S. C., Milanova, T., & Williamson, R. (2009). The prevalence, severity, and impact of opioid-induced bowel dysfunction: Results of a US and European patient survey (PROBE 1). *Pain Medicine, 10*(1), 35–42. https://doi.org/10.1111/j.1526-4637.2008.00495.x

Cai, H., Zhou, Q., Bao, G., Kong, X., & Gong, L. Y. (2019). Transcutaneous electrical nerve stimulation of acupuncture points enhances therapeutic effects of oral lactulose solution on opioid-induced constipation. *Journal of International Medical Research, 47*(12), 6337–6348. https://doi.org/10.1177/0300060519874539

Crockett, S., Greer, K., Heidelbaugh, J., Falk-Ytter, Y., Hanson, B., & Sultan, S. (2019). American gastroenterological association institute guideline on the medical management of opioid-induced constipation. *Gastroenterology, 156,* 218–226. https://doi.org/10.1053/gastro.2018.07.016

Ducrotté, P., & Caussé, C. (2012). The Bowel Function Index: A new validated scale for assessing opioid-induced constipation. *Current Medical Research and Opinion, 28,* 457–466. https://doi.org/10.1185/03007995.2012.657301

Efverman, A. (2020). Treatment expectations seem to affect bowel health when using acupuncture during radiotherapy for cancer: Secondary outcomes from a clinical randomized sham-controlled trial. *Complementary Therapies in Medicine, 52,* 102404. https://doi.org/10.1016/j.ctim.2020.102404

Gaertner, J., Siemens, W., Camilleri, M., Davies, A., Drossman, D., Webster, L., & Becker, G. (2015). Definitions and outcome measures of clinical trials regarding opioid-induced constipation: A systematic review. *Journal of Clinical Gastroenterology, 49*(1), 9–16. https://doi.org/10.1097/MCG.000000 0000000246

Ginex, P., Hanson, B., LeFebvre, K., Lin, Y., Moriarty, K., Maloney, C., Vrabel, M., & Morgan, R. (2020). Management of opioid-induced and non–opioid-related constipation in patients with cancer: Systematic review and meta-analysis. *Oncology Nursing Forum, 47*(6), E211–E224. https://doi.org/10.1188/20.ONF.E211-E224

Hanai, A., Ishiguro, H., Sozu, T., Tsuda, M., Arai, H., Mitani, A., & Tsuboyama, T. (2016). Effects of a self-management program on antiemetic-induced constipation during chemotherapy among breast cancer patients: A randomized controlled clinical trial. *Breast Cancer Research and Treatment, 155*(1), 99–107. https://doi.org/10.1007/s10549-015-3652-4

Katakami, N., Harada, T., Murata, T., Shinozaki, K., Tsutsumi, M., Yokota, T., Arai, M., Tada, Y., Narabayashi, M., & Boku, N. (2017a). Randomized phase III and extension studies of naldemedine in patients with opioid-induced constipation and cancer. *Journal of Clinical Oncology, 35*(34), 3859–3866. https://doi.org/10.1200/jco.2017.73.0853

Katakami, N., Oda, K., Tauchi, K., Nakata, K., Shinozaki, K., Yokota, T., Suzuki, Y., Narabayashi, M., & Boku, N. (2017b). Phase IIb, randomized, double-blind, placebo-controlled study of naldemedine for the treatment of opioid-induced constipation in patients with cancer. *Journal of Clinical Oncology, 35*(17), 1921–1928. https://doi.org/10.1200/jco.2016.70.8453

Li, D., Li, H., Liu, H., Bao, H., Zhu, T., Tian, J., Li, H., Li, J., Guo, X., Zhuang, Z., Cai, G., & Yang, Y. (2020). Impact of electroacupuncture stimulation on postoperative constipation for patients undergoing brain tumor surgery. *Journal of Neuroscience Nursing, 52*(5), 257–262. https://doi.org/10.1097/jnn.000000 0000000531

Mori, M., Ji, Y., Kumar, S., Ashikaga, T., & Ades, S. (2017). Phase II trial of subcutaneous methylnaltrexone in the treatment of severe opioid-induced constipation (OIC) in cancer patients: An exploratory study. *International Journal of Clinical Oncology, 22*(2), 397–404. https://doi.org/10.1007/s1014 7-016-1041-6

Morlion, B. J., Mueller-Lissner, S. A., Vellucci, R., Leppert, W., Coffin, B. C., Dickerson, S. L., & O'Brien, T. (2018). Oral prolonged-release oxycodone/naloxone for managing pain and opioid-induced constipation: A review of the evidence. *Pain Practice, 18*(5), 647–665. https://doi.org/10.1111/papr.12646

Nee, J., Zakari, M., Sugarman, M. A., Whelan, J., Hirsch, W., Sultan, S., Ballou, S., Iturrino, J., & Lembo, A. (2018). Efficacy of treatments for opioid-induced constipation: Systematic review and meta-analysis. *Clinical Gastroenterology and Hepatology, 16*(10), 1569–1584.e1562. https://doi.org/10.1016/j.cgh.2018.01.021

Shin, J., & Park, H. (2018). Effects of auricular acupressure on constipation in patients with breast cancer receiving chemotherapy: A randomized control trial. *Western Journal of Nursing Research, 40*(1), 67–83. https://doi.org/10.1177/0193945916680362

Vonk-Klaassen, S. M., de Vocht, H. M., den Ouden, M. E., Eddes, E. H., & Schuurmans, M. J. (2016). Ostomy-related problems and their impact on quality of life of colorectal cancer ostomates: A systematic review. *Quality of Life Research, 25*(1), 125–133. https://doi.org/10.1007/s11136-015-1050-3

Zou, J. Y., Xu, Y., Wang, X. H., Jiang, Q., & Zhu, X. M. (2016). Improvement of constipation in leukemia patients undergoing chemotherapy using sweet potato. *Cancer Nursing, 39*(3), 181–186. https://doi.org/10.1097/ncc.0000000000000257

CHAPTER 12

DIARRHEA

INTRODUCTION

Diarrhea is common in people with cancer due to a variety of factors, including systemic chemotherapy and newer anticancer therapies, as well as radiation to the pelvis. It is defined as the frequent passage of loose stools with urgency, or more frequent loose stools than is normal for the individual (Bossi et al., 2018). While people frequently adjust to this symptom, it has a negative impact on quality of life and may limit activities (Fernandes & Jervoise, 2020), as well as lead to discontinuation of therapy. The gut microbiome is thought to play a key role in the development of diarrhea, including after both radiation therapy (Bai et al., 2021; Tonneau et al., 2021) and chemotherapy (Secombe et al., 2019).

PREVALENCE

Between 5% and 47% of patients receiving chemotherapy have experienced diarrhea (Andreyev et al., 2014). Of patients on immune checkpoint inhibitors (ICIs), 20% to 30% will develop diarrhea despite only 5% or less showing evidence of colitis (Tang et al., 2021). When combined with chemotherapy or tyrosine kinase inhibitors, ICIs cause diarrhea in 17% to 56% of patients (Nielsen et al., 2022). Capecitabine plus irinotecan has the highest risk for grades 3 and 4 diarrhea at 47%, and FOLFOXIRI causes diarrhea in 20% of patients (Bossi et al., 2018).

Of patients undergoing radiation to the pelvis, 60% will experience temporary mild diarrhea (Bossi et al., 2018). Of patients with head and neck cancer, 42% have reported experiencing diarrhea when chemotherapy was delivered concurrently with radiation compared with 29% of those treated with radiation alone, demonstrating that toxicity may occur distantly from the target tumor(s) (Sonis et al., 2015). Intensity-modulated radiation therapy reduces the risk of diarrhea (Lawrie et al., 2018).

SECTION III • GASTROINTESTINAL SYMPTOMS

CONTRIBUTING FACTORS

Patient-related factors for chemotherapy-induced diarrhea (CID) include female sex, colorectal cancer, lactose intolerance, older age, and poor performance status (Smith et al., 2020). Treatment-related factors include a range of medications (see Figure 12.1).

ASSESSMENT

Evaluation of the history of onset, stool composition, and number of stools is the first step in assessment. Assessment of other systemic symptoms (fever, dehydration, pain/cramping, dizziness) and medications, as well as food intake (Benson et al., 2004), can provide additional information about potentially modifying factors. The grade of the diarrhea according to the Common Terminology Criteria for Adverse Events (CTCAE) classification (see Figure 12.2) helps dictate management.

Physical examination should include abdominal assessment and hydration status; electrolytes should also be measured (O'Brien et al., 2005).

Human epidermal growth factor receptor 2 (HER-2)—targeted agents (Li & Gu, 2019)	Afatinib, neratinib—high risk of all-grade diarrhea Trastuzumab—lowest risk of diarrhea
Immune checkpoint inhibitors (Gong & Wang, 2020)	Ipilimumab, nivolumab, pembrolizumab
Tyrosine kinase inhibitors (Tang et al., 2021)	Erlotinib, gefitinib, vandetanib, dacomitinib, lapatinib
Cytotoxic drugs (Bossi et al., 2018)	5-Flouracil, irinotecan, capecitabine, taxanes, anthracyclines, cisplatin, carboplatin
Surgery for colorectal cancer (Yde et al., 2018)	Bile acid malabsorption, small intestine bacterial overgrowth, disruption of the ileal brake
Pelvic radiation therapy (Bossi et al., 2018)	

Figure 12.1 Causes of treatment-related diarrhea.

Grade 1	Increase of <4 stools per day over baseline
Grade 2	Increase of 4–6 stools per day over baseline; limits activities of daily living
Grade 3	Increase of 7 or more loose stools per day; admittance to hospital indicated
Grade 4	Urgent intervention required; life-threatening consequences

Figure 12.2 Common Terminology Criteria for Adverse Events grades of diarrhea.

Source: From Common Terminology Criteria for Adverse Events (CTCAE) Version 5.0 Published: November 27, 2017. U.S. Department of Health and Human Services National Institutes of Health National Cancer Institute. https://ctep.cancer.gov/protocoldevelopment/electronic_applications/docs/ctcae_v5_quick_reference_8.5x11.pdF.

CHAPTER 12 • DIARRHEA **109**

- The Systemic Therapy-Induced Assessment Tool (STIDAT; Lui et al., 2017), a patient-reported questionnaire, assesses a number of factors, including the number of bowel movements per day, the number of diarrhea episodes, antidiarrhea medications, urgency, pain, fecal incontinence, perception of diarrhea severity, and quality of life.

- The Bristol Stool Scale can also be used by patients to describe the type of bowel movement they are having (www.continence.org. au/bristol-stool-chart).

CASE STUDY

You are seeing a 35-year-old woman in the survivorship clinic. She was diagnosed with cervical cancer 3 months ago and treated with both brachytherapy and chemotherapy. She reports that she continues to have burning with urination. You ask permission to do a visual examination of her vulva and perineum and you notice that there is irritation to the tissues that extends to the perianal area.

1. What else should you ask her?

She says that she is having five or sometimes six loose bowel movements a day and she thinks this is due to the plant-based diet she started after her diagnosis.

2. Could the change in her diet be a cause of the loose stools?

3. What other advice could you offer her?

MANAGEMENT

Patient education should include foods and medications to avoid (see Figure 12.3). These may cause or contribute to loose bowel movements.

Foods/Beverages
Milk and dairy products
Alcohol
Caffeine
Spicy foods
High-fiber and high-fat foods
Prune and orange juice

Medications
Bulk laxatives and stool softeners
Drugs that promote motility, e.g., metoclopramide

Figure 12.3 Foods and medications to avoid.

Pharmaceutical Management

Loperamide is the only agent that has shown effectiveness in managing diarrhea in this population, with a maximum dose of 24 mg/d (de Lemos et al., 2018). The very low risk of cardiac events with chronic, high-dose use is balanced by the benefit of controlling diarrhea in this population. Patients should be advised to ignore the instructions on the package about maximum dose (Andreyev et al., 2014).

Nonpharmaceutical Management

Probiotics may reduce CID in patients with cancer; however, the evidence on their efficacy and safety is limited (Hassan et al., 2018). Efficacy has been shown in a small study of women treated with radiation for gynecologic cancer (Ahrén et al., 2022) and they may prevent radiation-induced diarrhea in this population (Qiu et al., 2019).

A high-fiber diet may be helpful in patients with diarrhea after pelvic radiation (Allenby et al., 2020). For severe diarrhea, a clear liquid diet or the BRAT diet (bananas, rice, apple sauce, and toast) may help. Oral rehydration with fluids that contain salt and sugar, broth, or Gatorade may be suggested. If the patient becomes severely dehydrated, admission to hospital may be needed for intravenous rehydration. Early evidence suggests that hyperbaric oxygen may also be of benefit (Yuan et al., 2020).

GUIDELINES

- **American Cancer Society (ACS)**

  American Cancer Society Colorectal Cancer Survivorship Care Guidelines (El-Shami et al., 2015)

- **American Society of Clinical Oncology (ASCO)**

  ASCO Recommended Guidelines for the Treatment of Cancer Treatment-Induced Diarrhea (Benson et al., 2004)

- **British Society of Gastroenterology**

  British Society of Gastroenterology Endorsed Guidance for the Management of ICI-Induced Enterocolitis (Powell et al., 2020)

- **European Society for Medical Oncology (ESMO)**

  ESMO Clinical Practice Guidelines: Diarrhea in Adult Cancer Patients (Bossi et al., 2018)

SUMMARY

Treatment-induced diarrhea is a serious side effect of chemotherapy and radiation to the pelvis. Newer agents, including Her2-targeted agents, tyrosine uptake inhibitors, and ICIs, also cause this symptom. Diarrhea has a negative impact on quality of life and may necessitate cessation of treatment.

A robust set of instructor resources designed to supplement this text is located at http://connect.springerpub.com/content/reference-book/978-0-8261-8524-2. Qualifying Instructors may request access by emailing **textbook@springerpub.com**.

REFERENCES

Ahrén, I. L., Bjurberg, M., Steineck, G., Bergmark, K., & Jeppsson, B. (2022). Decreasing the adverse effects in pelvic radiotherapy: A randomized controlled trial evaluating the use of probiotics. *Advances in Radiation Oncology*, 8(1), 101089. https://doi.org/10.1016/j.adro.2022.101089

Allenby, T. H., Crenshaw, M. L., Mathis, K., Champ, C. E., Simone, N. L., Schmitz, K. H., Tchelebi, L. T., & Zaorsky, N. G. (2020). A systematic review of home-based dietary interventions during radiation therapy for cancer. *Technical Innovations & Patient Support in Radiation Oncology*, 16, 10–16. https://doi.org/10.1016/j.tipsro.2020.08.001

Andreyev, J., Ross, P., Donnellan, C., Lennan, E., Leonard, P., Waters, C., Wedlake, L., Bridgewater, J., Glynne-Jones, R., Allum, W., Chau, I., Wilson, R., & Ferry, D. (2014). Guidance on the management of diarrhoea during cancer chemotherapy. *The Lancet Oncology*, 15(10), e447–e460. https://doi.org/10.1016/S1470-2045(14)70006-3

Bai, J., Barandouzi, Z. A., Rowcliffe, C., Meador, R., Tsementzi, D., & Bruner, D. W. (2021). Gut microbiome and its associations with acute and chronic gastrointestinal toxicities in cancer patients with pelvic radiation therapy: A systematic review. *Frontiers in Oncology*, 11, 745262. https://doi.org/10.3389/fonc.2021.745262

Benson, A. B., Ajani, J. A., Catalano, R. B., Engelking, C., Kornblau, S. M., Martenson, J. A., McCallum, R., Mitchell, E. P., O'Dorisio, T. M., Vokes, E. E., & Wadler, S. (2004). Recommended guidelines for the treatment of cancer treatment-induced diarrhea. *Journal of Clinical Oncology*, 22(14), 2918–2926. https://doi.org/10.1200/JCO.2004.04.132

Bossi, P., Antonuzzo, A., Cherny, N. I., Rosengarten, O., Pernot, S., Trippa, F., Schuler, U., Snegovoy, A., Jordan, K., Ripamonti, C. I., & ESMO, Guidelines Committee. (2018). Diarrhoea in adult cancer patients: ESMO clinical practice guidelines. *Annals of Oncology*, 29(Suppl 4), iv126–iv142. https://doi.org/10.1093/annonc/mdy145

de Lemos, M. L., Guenter, J., & Kletas, V. (2018). Loperamide and cardiac events: Is high-dose use still safe for chemotherapy-induced diarrhea? *Journal of Oncology Pharmacy Practice*, 24(8), 634–636. https://doi.org/10.1177/1078155217718384

El-Shami, K., Oeffinger, K. C., Erb, N. L., Willis, A., Bretsch, J. K., Pratt-Chapman, M. L., Cannady, R. S., Wong, S. L., Rose, J., Barbour, A. L., Stein, K. D., Sharpe, K. B., Brooks, D. D., & Cowens-Alvarado, R. L. (2015). American Cancer Society colorectal cancer survivorship care guidelines. *CA: A Cancer Journal for Clinicians*, 65(6), 427–455. https://doi.org/10.3322/caac.21286

Fernandes, D. C., & Jervoise, N. A. H. (2020). Chronic diarrhoea in an oncology patient—clinical assessment and decision making. *Best Practice and Research in Clinical Gastroenterology, 48–49*, 101708. https://doi.org/10.1016/j.bpg.2020.101708

Hassan, H., Rompola, M., Glaser, A. W., Kinsey, S. E., & Phillips, R. S. (2018). Systematic review and meta-analysis investigating the efficacy and safety of probiotics in people with cancer. *Supportive Care in Cancer, 26*(8), 2503–2509. https://doi.org/10.1007/s00520-018-4216-z

Lam, D., & Jones, O. (2020). Changes to gastrointestinal function after surgery for colorectal cancer. *Best Practice and Research in Clinical Gastroenterology, 48–49*, 101705. https://doi.org/10.1016/j.bpg.2020.101705

Lawrie, T. A., Green, J. T., Beresford, M., Wedlake, L., Burden, S., Davidson, S. E., Henson, C. C., & Andreyev, H. J. N. (2018). Interventions to reduce acute and late adverse gastrointestinal effects of pelvic radiotherapy for primary pelvic cancers. *Cochrane Database of Systematci Reviews, 1*(1), Cd012529. https://doi.org/10.1002/14651858.CD012529.pub2

Lui, M., Gallo-Hershberg, D., & DeAngelis, C. (2017). Development and validation of a patient-reported questionnaire assessing systemic therapy induced diarrhea in oncology patients. *Health and Quality of Life Outcomes, 15*(1), 249–249. https://doi.org/10.1186/s12955-017-0794-6

Nielsen, D. L., Juhl, C. B., Chen, I. M., Kellermann, L., & Nielsen, O. H. (2022). Immune checkpoint inhibitor-induced diarrhea and colitis: Incidence and management. A systematic review and meta-analysis. *Cancer Treatment Reviews, 109*, 102440. https://doi.org/10.1016/j.ctrv.2022.102440

O'Brien, B. E., Kaklamani, V. G., & Benson, A. B., 3rd. (2005). The assessment and management of cancer treatment-related diarrhea. *Clinical Colorectal Cancer, 4*(6), 375–381. https://doi.org/10.3816/ccc.2005.n.009 discussion 382–373

Powell, N., Ibraheim, H., Raine, T., Speight, R. A., Papa, S., Brain, O., Green, M., Samaan, M. A., Spain, L., Yousaf, N., Hunter, N., Eldridge, L., Pavlidis, P., Irving, P., Hayee, B., Turajlic, S., Larkin, J., Lindsay, J. O., & Gore, M. (2020). British Society of Gastroenterology endorsed guidance for the management of immune checkpoint inhibitor-induced enterocolitis. *The Lancet Gastroenterology and Hepatology, 5*(7), 679–697. https://doi.org/10.1016/s2468-1253(20)30014-5

Qiu, G., Yu, Y., Wang, Y., & Wang, X. (2019). The significance of probiotics in preventing radiotherapy-induced diarrhea in patients with cervical cancer: A systematic review and meta-analysis. *International Journal of Surgery, 65*, 61–69. https://doi.org/10.1016/j.ijsu.2019.03.015

Secombe, K. R., Coller, J. K., Gibson, R. J., Wardill, H. R., & Bowen, J. M. (2019). The bidirectional interaction of the gut microbiome and the innate immune system: Implications for chemotherapy-induced gastrointestinal toxicity. *International Journal of Cancer, 144*(10), 2365–2376. https://doi.org/10.1002/ijc.31836

Smith, P., Lavery, A., & Turkington, R. C. (2020). An overview of acute gastrointestinal side effects of systemic anti-cancer therapy and their management. *Best Practice & Research Clinical Gastroenterology*, *48–49*, 101691. https://doi.org/10.1016/j.bpg.2020.101691

Sonis, S., Elting, L., Keefe, D., Nguyen, H., Grunberg, S., Randolph-Jackson, P., & Brennan, M. (2015). Unanticipated frequency and consequences of regimen-related diarrhea in patients being treated with radiation or chemoradiation regimens for cancers of the head and neck or lung. *Supportive Care in Cancer*, *23*(2), 433–439. https://doi.org/10.1007/s00520-014-2395-9

Tang, L., Wang, J., Lin, N., Zhou, Y., He, W., Liu, J., & Ma, X. (2021). Immune checkpoint inhibitor-associated colitis: From mechanism to management. *Frontiers in Immunology*, *12*, 800879. https://doi.org/10.3389/fimmu.2021.800879

Tonneau, M., Elkrief, A., Pasquier, D., Paz Del Socorro, T., Chamaillard, M., Bahig, H., & Routy, B. (2021). The role of the gut microbiome on radiation therapy efficacy and gastrointestinal complications: A systematic review. *Radiotherap y and Oncology*, *156*, 1–9. https://doi.org/10.1016/j.radonc.2020.10.033

Yuan, J. H., Song, L. M., Liu, Y., Li, M. W., Lin, Q., Wang, R., Zhang, C.-S., & Dong, J. (2020). The effects of hyperbaric oxygen therapy on pelvic radiation induced gastrointestinal complications (rectal bleeding, diarrhea, and pain): A meta-analysis. *Frontiers in Oncology*, *10*, 390. https://doi.org/10.3389/fonc.2020.00390

CHAPTER 13

NAUSEA AND VOMITING

INTRODUCTION

Nausea and vomiting are two of the most feared side effects of cancer treatment. Chemotherapy-induced nausea and vomiting (CINV) is highly distressing and often very severe. Nausea and vomiting are also associated with opiates, surgery, and importantly radiation therapy-induced nausea and vomiting (RINV). The occurrence of this impacts negatively on quality of life, may reduce adherence to treatment, and may require breaks in treatment regimens.

There are different types of CINV: acute (within 24 hours of chemotherapy), delayed (between 2 and 5 days after treatment), and breakthrough nausea and vomiting (within 5 days of receiving antiemetics; Razvi et al., 2019). Prevention of CINV is key in the management of this symptom.

Anticipatory nausea (less often vomiting) is a conditioned response after a prior chemotherapy treatment that involved severe nausea and vomiting. An important cause of nausea and vomiting in this patient population is the use of opioid analgesia. Other causes include bowel obstruction, infections, and certain antibiotics.

PREVALENCE

CINV and RINV occur in 40% to 80% of patients receiving treatment for cancer (Vidall et al., 2016). Anticipatory nausea and vomiting occurs in up to 30% of patients by the fourth chemotherapy cycle (Morrow, Roscoe, Kirshner et al., 1998). Of patients with cancer on opioids for chronic pain, 25% will experience nausea and 17% will have emesis (Sande et al., 2019).

CONTRIBUTING FACTORS

The type of chemotherapeutic agent, the route and rate of administration, as well as the dose influence emetogenicity. The target for radiation therapy predicts the risk of nausea and vomiting (see the "Assessment" section for more details).

A prior history of receiving chemotherapy and experiencing emesis increases the risk of emesis with subsequent treatment (Morrow, Roscoe, Hickok, et al., 1998). Women are more likely to experience CINV and younger patients more likely than older adults. Other patient factors include little or no alcohol use, a history of morning sickness in pregnancy, and being prone to motion sickness (NCCN Guidelines Version 2.2023; https://www.nccn.org/professionals/physician_gls/pdf/antiemesis.pdf).

ASSESSMENT

There are several assessment tools available for this patient population:

- The Multinational Association of Supportive Care in Cancer (MASCC) Antiemesis Tool (MAT) is an eight-item questionnaire that should be completed by the patient on the day following chemotherapy, as well as from the day after treatment up to 4 days after (Molassiotis et al., 2007).

- The Memorial Symptom Assessment Scale has one item for nausea and one for vomiting. This scale assesses the frequency, severity, and distress/bother with each symptom (http://www.npcrc.org/files/news/memorial_symptom_assessment_scale.pdf).

- The Functional Assessment of Cancer Therapy (FACT-G) has one item that assesses nausea on a five-item Likert scale from not at all to very much in the past 7 days (https://www.facit.org/_files/ugd/626819_acb819ba51fd4552807feef38250db3f.pdf).

Assessment of Chemotherapy Agents

Chemotherapy agents are classified based on the risk of emesis (see Figure 13.1).

High	>90% risk of emesis
Moderate	>30%–90% risk of emesis
Low	10%–30% risk of emesis
Minimal	<10% risk of emesis

Figure 13.1 Risk categories for emesis.

Source: From Roila, F., Molassiotis, A., Herrstedt, J., Aapro, M., Gralla, R. J., Bruera, E., Clark-Snow, R. A., Dupuis, L. L., Einhorn, L. H., Feyer, P., Hesketh, P. J., Jordan, K., Olver, I., Rapoport, B. L., Roscoe, J., Ruhlmann, C. H., Walsh, D., Warr, D., van de Wetering, M., & Participants of the MASCC/ESMO Consensus Conference Copenhagen 2015. (2016). 2016 MASCC and ESMO guideline update for the prevention of chemotherapy- and radiotherapy-induced nausea and vomiting and of nausea and vomiting in advanced cancer patients. *Participants of the MASCC/ESMO Consensus Conference Copenhagen 2015, 27*(Suppl 5), v119–v133. https://doi.org/10.1093/annonc/mdw270.

High emetogenic agents include combination anthracycline/cyclo-phosphamide, cisplatin, carmustine, high dose (>1,500 g/m²) dacar-bazine, mechlorethamine, and streptozocin.

There is a very long list of agents that have a *moderate risk of CINV*, including most of the epidermal growth factor receptor (EGFR) inhibi-tor agents, taxanes, gemcitabine, 5-fluorouracil, methotrexate, and mito-mycin, among others. Oral agents including tyrosine kinase inhibitors, capecitabine, etoposide, and everolimus are also included in this category.

Agents with a *low risk of CINV* include bleomycin, fludarabine, nivolumab, and bevacizumab, among others. Oral agents that are included in this category include gefitinib, methotrexate, and chlo-rambucil (Box 13.1).

Box 13.1 Emetogenic Agents

A full list of emetogenic agents can be found in the 2016 Multinational Association of Supportive Care in Cancer (MASCC) and European Society of Medical Oncology (ESMO) guideline (Roila et al., 2016), as well as the National Comprehensive Cancer Network (NCCN) guidelines, which are regularly updated (https://www.nccn.org/guidelines/guidelines-detail?category=3&id = 1415).

Assessment of Radiation Therapy Agents

The risk for *RINV* is classified as high (total body radiation), moder-ate (upper abdominal radiation and craniospinal), low (cranium, head and neck, thorax, pelvis), and low (breast and limbs; Roila et al., 2016).

MANAGEMENT

Prevention of Acute and Delayed Chemotherapy-Induced Nausea and Vomiting

There are a number of treatment regimens to prevent acute and delayed emesis for highly emetogenic, moderately emetogenic, and low/mini-mal emetogenic chemotherapy. They should be started before treatment, with continued use for 2 to 3 or 4 days to prevent delayed CINV. These regimens contain different combinations of NK1 receptor agonists, sero-tonin 5-HT3 agonists, dexamethasone, and olanzapine (Figure 13.2).

- MASCC and ESMO guidelines (Roila et al., 2016)
- ASCO, NCCN, MASCC/ESMO guidelines (Razvi et al., 2019)
- NCCN guidelines Version 2, 2022 (AE 1–AE 11)
  https://www.nccn.org/professionals/physician_gls/pdf/antiemesis.pdf

The guidelines also provide information about managing nausea and vomiting with oral chemotherapies and radiation-induced emesis.

These guidelines are very similar with differences based on the literature available for review at the time of development.

Figure 13.2 Detailed recommendations for prevention and treatment of nausea and vomiting. ASCO, American Society of Clinical Oncology; ESMO, European Society for Medical Oncology; MASCC, Multinational Association of Supportive Care in Cancer; NCCN, National Comprehensive Cancer Network.

A study found that a minority of advanced practice clinicians follow the guidelines for prevention of CINV (Mellin et al., 2018). There has been a slow uptake of the recommendations to prescribe olanzapine prophylaxis to patients on highly emetogenic chemotherapy (Childs et al., 2022).

Breakthrough Chemotherapy-Induced Nausea and Vomiting

If a patient experiences breakthrough CINV while on appropriate management, a reevaluation of the patient's disease status, chemotherapy regimen, any other concurrent medications, and medications should be performed.

If olanzapine was not included in the preventive regimen of antiemetics, it should be added (Vig et al., 2014). A 5-mg dose is as effective as 10-mg with less somnolence (Yanai et al., 2018).

The American Society of Clinical Oncology (ASCO) 2020 guidelines (Hesketh et al., 2020) suggest that, for breakthrough CINV in patients who have received olanzapine, an NK1 receptor agonist, lorazepam or alprazolam, an alternative serotonin 5-HT3 agonist, or a dopaminergic antagonist may be offered.

Synthetic cannabinoids (dronabinol) can be used as a rescue emetic or for refractory CINV (Hesketh et al., 2020); however, medical marijuana is not recommended.

Anticipatory Nausea

This occurs in almost a third of patients already on treatment and may also occur in chemotherapy-naïve patients who anticipate that they are going to experience CINV (Roscoe et al., 2004). Other than ensuring that patients receive effective prevention for all chemotherapy cycles, complementary therapies along with behavioral therapy with desensitization may be helpful. Hypnosis, progressive muscle relaxation, music, and cognitive distraction (e.g., video games) may also be helpful.

Opioid-Induced Nausea and Vomiting

Despite the relatively high proportion of patients with cancer who experience chronic pain requiring opioids, there is little high-level evidence for managing these distressing symptoms. There is weak evidence for switching opioids, changing the route of administration, or using antiemetics (Sande et al., 2019). Taking opioids with food does not reduce nausea and vomiting and may increase the occurrence of these symptoms (Raffa et al., 2017).

Complementary Therapies

Patients may prefer to take complementary therapies in addition to pharmaceutical interventions. There is only weak evidence to support these interventions, but they are unlikely to cause harm. Additionally, education about CINV and support from a dietitian who provides a personalized meal plan are effective in reducing the severity of nausea (Gala et al., 2022). There is a suggestion that a diet with sufficient protein and fat may also lower the incidence of CINV (Figure 13.3).

- Acupuncture (Jang et al., 2020)
- Aromatherapy (Toniolo et al., 2021)
- Ginger (Borges et al., 2020; Chang & Peng, 2019; Saneei Totmaj et al., 2019)
- Music (Kiernan et al., 2018; Wei et al., 2020)
- Reflexology (Wanchai & Armer, 2020)

Figure 13.3 Complementary therapies for chemotherapy-induced nausea and vomiting.

Cannabis and Cannabinoids

CASE STUDY

Your patient is a 24-year-old man with acute myeloid leukemia. He is an inpatient who will start high-dose chemotherapy in preparation for a stem cell transplant. He has been badgering the unit nurses for a pass to see his friends before his transplant. The nurses call you to "talk some sense into him."

1. What question(s) would you ask him?

He says that he "smokes weed" regularly and he is scared that he is going to be sick from the chemotherapy.

2. How would you respond to this?

He insists that he wants to use cannabis during the induction chemotherapy, and he is going to sign himself out against medical advice if you do not allow him to do this.

3. What are your next steps in this situation?

Despite patient interest in and use of medical cannabis to control nausea (Raghunathan et al., 2022), there is weak evidence to support its use (Pratt et al., 2019; Sawtelle & Holle, 2021). There is a limited number of randomized clinical trials of cannabinoids in this population (Chow et al., 2020). A 2015 Cochrane review concluded that while cannabinoids may be useful in the refractory CINV scenario, methodologic issues in the studies reviewed limit the conclusions (Smith et al., 2015). A more recent review suggests that cannabis may be helpful in nausea and vomiting with only mild side effects (Kleckner et al., 2019). There may be a role for the use of these substances in the palliative setting (Turgeman & Bar-Sela, 2019). Inhalation of cannabis is not supported due to the risk of adverse effects on the respiratory tract; however, there is no support for this in the literature (Abrams, 2019).

GUIDELINES

- **American Society of Clinical Oncology (ASCO)**

  American Society of Clinical Oncology (2020) Guidelines on Antiemetics, Update (Hesketh et al., 2020)

- **Multinational Association of Supportive Care in Cancer (MASCC)**

  MASCC Guidelines—Antiemetic Study Group (all under revision)

  https://mascc.org/resources/mascc-guidelines/

- **Multinational Association of Supportive Care in Cancer (MASCC) and European Society for Medical Oncology (ESMO)**

  2016 MASCC and ESMO Guideline Update for the Prevention of Chemotherapy- and Radiotherapy-Induced Nausea and Vomiting and of Nausea and Vomiting in Advanced Cancer Patients (Roila et al., 2016)

- **National Cancer Institute (NCI)**

  National Cancer Institute (2022). Nausea and Vomiting Related to Cancer Treatment (PDQ®)—Health Professional Version

  https://www.cancer.gov/about-cancer/treatment/side-effects/nausea/nausea-hp-pdq#_189

- **National Comprehensive Cancer Network (NCCN)**

  NCCN Guidelines Version 2.2023 Antiemesis

  https://www.nccn.org/professionals/physician_gls/pdf/antiemesis.pdf

- **Oncology Nursing Society (ONS)**

  Oncology Nursing Society (2018). Antiemetic Guidelines: Using Education to Improve Adherence and Reduce Incidence of CINV in Patients Receiving Highly Emetogenic Chemotherapy (Mellin et al., 2018)

SUMMARY

Nausea and vomiting remain two of the most feared side effects of cancer treatment. CINV is categorized by how likely these side effects will occur, with highly emetogenic drugs causing the most distress, but moderate- or low/minimal-risk therapies as well as oral agents also causing these symptoms and associated distress. Guidelines from a variety of sources provide evidence-based interventions for both prevention and management. There is limited evidence for nonpharmaceutical interventions.

A robust set of instructor resources designed to supplement this text is located at http://connect.springerpub.com/content/reference-book/978-0-8261-8524-2. Qualifying Instructors may request access by emailing **textbook@springerpub.com**.

REFERENCES

Abrams, D. I. (2019). Should oncologists recommend cannabis? *Current Treatment Options in Oncology, 20*(7), 59. https://doi.org/10.1007/s11864-019-0659-9

Borges, D. O., Freitas, K., Minicucci, E. M., & Popim, R. C. (2020). Benefits of ginger in the control of chemotherapy-induced nausea and vomiting. *Revista Brasileria de Enfermagem, 73*(2), e20180903. https://doi.org/10.1590/0034-7167-2018-0903

Chang, W. P., & Peng, Y. X. (2019). Does the oral administration of ginger reduce chemotherapy-induced nausea and vomiting? A meta-analysis of 10 randomized controlled trials. *Cancer Nursing, 42*(6), E14–E23. https://doi.org/10.1097/ncc.0000000000000648

Childs, D. S., Jr, D. A. H., Sangaralingham, L., Orme, J. J., O'Sullivan, C. C., Loprinzi, C. L., & Ruddy, K. J. (2022). Slow uptake of an effective therapy: Patterns of olanzapine prescribing for those receiving highly emetogenic chemotherapy. *JCO Oncology Practice, 18*(12), e1953–e1960. https://doi.org/10.1200/op.22.00389

Childs, D. S., Jr, D. A. H., Sangaralingham, L., Orme, J. J., O'Sullivan, C. C., Loprinzi, C. L., & Ruddy, K. J. (2022). Slow uptake of an effective therapy: Patterns of olanzapine prescribing for those receiving highly emetogenic chemotherapy. *JCO Oncology Practice, 18*(12), e1953–e1960. https://doi.org/10.1200/op.22.00389

Chow, R., Valdez, C., Chow, N., Zhang, D., Im, J., Sodhi, E., & Lock, M. (2020). Oral cannabinoid for the prophylaxis of chemotherapy-induced nausea and vomiting-a systematic review and meta-analysis. *Supportive Care in Cancer, 28*(5), 2095–2103. https://doi.org/10.1007/s00520-019-05280-4

Gala, D., Wright, H. H., Zigori, B., Marshall, S., & Crichton, M. (2022). Dietary strategies for chemotherapy-induced nausea and vomiting: A systematic review. *Clinical Nutrition, 41*(10), 2147–2155. https://doi.org/10.1016/j.clnu.2022.08.003

Hesketh, P. J., Kris, M. G., Basch, E., Bohlke, K., Barbour, S. Y., Clark-Snow, R. A., Danso, M. A., Dennis, K., Dupuis, L. L., Dusetzina, S. B., Eng, C., Feyer, P. C., Jordan, K., Noonan, K., Sparacio, D., & Lyman, G. H. (2020). Antiemetics: ASCO guideline update. *Journal of Clinical Oncology, 38*(24), 2782–2797. https://doi.org/10.1200/jco.20.01296

Jang, S., Ko, Y., Sasaki, Y., Park, S., Jo, J., Kang, N. H., Yoo, E.-S., Park, N.-C., Cho, S. H., Jang, H., Jang, B.-H., Hwang, D.-S., & Ko, S. G. (2020). Acupuncture as an adjuvant therapy for management of treatment-related symptoms in breast cancer patients: Systematic review and meta-analysis

(PRISMA-compliant). *Medicine (Baltimore), 99*(50), e21820. https://doi.org/10.1097/md.0000000000021820

Kiernan, J. M., Conradi Stark, J., & Vallerand, A. H. (2018). Chemotherapy-induced nausea and vomiting mitigation with music interventions. *Oncology Nursing Forum, 45*(1), 88–95. https://doi.org/10.1188/18.Onf.88-95

Kleckner, A. S., Kleckner, I. R., Kamen, C. S., Tejani, M. A., Janelsins, M. C., Morrow, G. R., & Peppone, L. J. (2019). Opportunities for cannabis in supportive care in cancer. *Therapeutic Advances in Medical Oncology, 11*, 1758835919866362. https://doi.org/10.1177/1758835919866362

Mellin, C., Lexa, M., Leak Bryant, A., Mason, S., & Mayer, D. (2018). Antiemetic guidelines: Using education to improve adherence and reduce incidence of CINV in patients receiving highly emetogenic chemotherapy. *Clinical Journal of Oncology Nursing, 22*(3), 297–303. https://doi.org/10.1188/18.CJON.297-303

Molassiotis, A., Coventry, P. A., Stricker, C. T., Clements, C., Eaby, B., Velders, L., Rittenberg, C., & Gralla, R. J. (2007). Validation and psychometric assessment of a short clinical scale to measure chemotherapy-induced nausea and vomiting: The MASCC antiemesis tool. *Journal of Pain and Symptom Management, 34*(2), 148–159. https://doi.org/10.1016/j.jpainsymman.2006.10.018

Morrow, G. R., Roscoe, J. A., Hickok, J. T., Stern, R. M., Pierce, H. I., King, D. B., Banerjee, T. K., & Weiden, P. (1998). Initial control of chemotherapy-induced nausea and vomiting in patient quality of life. *Oncology (Williston Park), 12*(3 Suppl 4), 32–37.

Morrow, G. R., Roscoe, J. A., Kirshner, J. J., Hynes, H. E., & Rosenbluth, R. J. (1998). Anticipatory nausea and vomiting in the era of 5-HT3 antiemetics. *Supportive Care in Cancer, 6*(3), 244–247. https://doi.org/10.1007/s005200050161

Pratt, M., Stevens, A., Thuku, M., Butler, C., Skidmore, B., Wieland, L. S., Clemons, M., Kanji, S., & Hutton, B. (2019). Benefits and harms of medical cannabis: A scoping review of systematic reviews. *Systematic Reviews, 8*(1), 320. https://doi.org/10.1186/s13643-019-1243-x

Raffa, R. B., Colucci, R., & Pergolizzi, J. V. (2017). The effects of food on opioid-induced nausea and vomiting and pharmacological parameters: A systematic review. *Postgraduate Medicine, 129*(7), 698–708. https://doi.org/10.1080/00325481.2017.1345282

Raghunathan, N. J., Brens, J., Vemuri, S., Li, Q. S., Mao, J. J., & Korenstein, D. (2022). In the weeds: A retrospective study of patient interest in and experience with cannabis at a cancer center. *Supportive Care in Cancer, 30*(9), 7491–7497. https://doi.org/10.1007/s00520-022-07170-8

Razvi, Y., Chan, S., McFarlane, T., McKenzie, E., Zaki, P., DeAngelis, C., Pidduck, W., Bushehri, A., Chow, E., & Jerzak, K. J. (2019). ASCO, NCCN, MASCC/ESMO: A comparison of antiemetic guidelines for the treatment of chemotherapy-induced nausea and vomiting in adult patients.

Supportive Care in Cancer, 27(1), 87–95. https://doi.org/10.1007/s00520-0 18-4464-y

Roila, F., Molassiotis, A., Herrstedt, J., Aapro, M., Gralla, R. J., Bruera, E., Clark-Snow, R. A., Dupuis, L. L., Einhorn, L. H., Feyer, P., Hesketh, P. J., Jordan, K., Olver, I., Rapoport, B. L., Roscoe, J., Ruhlmann, C. H., Walsh, D., Warr, D., van de Wetering, M., & Participants of the MASCC/ESMO Consensus Conference Copenhagen 2015. (2016). 2016 MASCC and ESMO guideline update for the prevention of chemotherapy- and radiotherapy-induced nausea and vomiting and of nausea and vomiting in advanced cancer patients. *Participants of the MASCC/ESMO Consensus Conference Copenhagen 2015, 27*(Suppl 5), v119–v133. https://doi.org/10.1093/anno nc/mdw270

Roscoe, J. A., Bushunow, P., Morrow, G. R., Hickok, J. T., Kuebler, P. J., Jacobs, A., & Banerjee, T. K. (2004). Patient expectation is a strong predictor of severe nausea after chemotherapy: A University of Rochester Community Clinical Oncology Program study of patients with breast carcinoma. *Cancer, 101*(11), 2701–2708. https://doi.org/10.1002/cncr.20718

Sande, T. A., Laird, B. J. A., & Fallon, M. T. (2019). The management of opioid-induced nausea and vomiting in patients with cancer: A systematic review. *Journal of Palliative Medicine, 22*(1), 90–97. https://doi.org/10.1089 /jpm.2018.0260

Saneei Totmaj, A., Emamat, H., Jarrahi, F., & Zarrati, M. (2019). The effect of ginger (Zingiber officinale) on chemotherapy-induced nausea and vomiting in breast cancer patients: A systematic literature review of randomized controlled trials. *Phytotherapy Research, 33*(8), 1957–1965. https://doi.org/10.10 02/ptr.6377

Sawtelle, L., & Holle, L. M. (2021). Use of cannabis and cannabinoids in patients with cancer. *Annals of Pharmacotherapy, 55*(7), 870–890. https://doi. org/10.1177/1060028020965224

Smith, L. A., Azariah, F., Lavender, V. T., Stoner, N. S., & Bettiol, S. (2015). Cannabinoids for nausea and vomiting in adults with cancer receiving chemotherapy. *Cochrane Database of Systematic Reviews, 2015*(11), Cd009464. http s://doi.org/10.1002/14651858.CD009464.pub2

Toniolo, J., Delaide, V., & Beloni, P. (2021). Effectiveness of inhaled aromatherapy on chemotherapy-induced nausea and vomiting: A systematic review. *The Journal of Alternative and Complementary Medicine, 27*(12), 1058–1069. http s://doi.org/10.1089/acm.2021.0067

Turgeman, I., & Bar-Sela, G. (2019). Cannabis for cancer—illusion or the tip of an iceberg: A review of the evidence for the use of cannabis and synthetic cannabinoids in oncology. *Expert Opinion on Investigational Drugs, 28*(3), 285–296. https://doi.org/10.1080/13543784.2019.1561859

Vidall, C., Sharma, S., & Amlani, B. (2016). Patient–practitioner perception gap in treatment-induced nausea and vomiting. *British Journal of Nursing*

(Mark Allen Publishing), 25(16), S4–S11. https://doi.org/10.12968/bjon.2016.25.S4

Vig, S., Seibert, L., & Green, M. R. (2014). Olanzapine is effective for refractory chemotherapy-induced nausea and vomiting irrespective of chemotherapy emetogenicity. *Journal of Cancer Research and Clinical Oncology, 140*(1), 77–82. https://doi.org/10.1007/s00432-013-1540-z

Wanchai, A., & Armer, J. M. (2020). A systematic review association of reflexology in managing symptoms and side effects of breast cancer treatment. *Complement Therapies in Clinical Practice, 38*, 101074. https://doi.org/10.1016/j.ctcp.2019.101074

Wei, T. T., Tian, X., Zhang, F. Y., Qiang, W. M., & Bai, A. L. (2020). Music interventions for chemotherapy-induced nausea and vomiting: A systematic review and meta-analysis. *Supportive Care in Cancer, 28*(9), 4031–4041. https://doi.org/10.1007/s00520-020-05409-w

Yanai, T., Iwasa, S., Hashimoto, H., Ohyanagi, F., Takiguchi, T., Takeda, K., Nakao, M., Sakai, H., Nakayama, T., Minato, K., Arai, T., Suzuki, K., Shimada, Y., Nagashima, K., Terakado, H., & Yamamoto, N. (2018). A double-blind randomized phase II dose-finding study of olanzapine 10 mg or 5 mg for the prophylaxis of emesis induced by highly emetogenic cisplatin-based chemotherapy. *International Journal of Clinical Oncology, 23*(2), 382–388. https://doi.org/10.1007/s10147-017-1200-4

CHAPTER 14

ANOREXIA AND CACHEXIA

INTRODUCTION

Anorexia or loss of appetite is common in advanced cancer and is a major factor in the development of cachexia. It is distressing to family caregivers as they may perceive this as their fault (Poole & Froggatt, 2002). Cancer cachexia is a multifactorial syndrome where there is ongoing loss of muscle mass, with or without loss of body fat, that cannot be fully reversed by nutritional interventions and leads to functional impairment (Fearon et al., 2011). Cachexia is different from malnutrition or sarcopenia; both of these conditions are either precursors or contributing factors to cachexia (Meza-Valderrama et al., 2021). Cachexia is unfortunately not assessed consistently and has a negative impact on health-related quality of life, and its management is challenging.

PREVALENCE

Approximately 50% of people with cancer, especially advanced cancer, experience the weight and skeletal muscle mass loss that defines cachexia (Suzuki et al., 2013).

CONTRIBUTING FACTORS

Cachexia has several contributing factors:

- Cytokines and inflammation are major contributors to cachexia. Specifically, the cytokines interleukin-6 (IL-6), tumor necrosis factor-alpha (TNF-alpha), and interleukin-8 (IL-8) are associated with the development of cachexia because they increase basal metabolic rate and induce anorexia (Paval et al., 2022).

- Reduced dietary intake or malabsorption due to pain, ascites, dysphagia, xerostomia, depression, constipation, nausea or vomiting, and fatigue are important factors (Del Fabbro et al., 2011; Kwang & Kandiah, 2010).

- The presence of tumor(s) in the gastrointestinal tract, especially in the pancreas, causes malabsorption of nutrients, leading to weight loss and cachexia (Danai et al., 2018).

- Treatment can also be a contributing factor. Chemotherapy and its impact on taste and smell contributes to weight loss (Bernhardson et al., 2008; Steinbach et al., 2009). In men with advanced prostate cancer who are prescribed androgen deprivation therapy, muscle wasting occurs that may lead to cachexia (Smith et al., 2012). Sorafenib prescribed to patients with renal cell cancer (Antoun et al., 2010) and also bevacizumab cause symptoms such as anorexia and nausea and vomiting, leading to cachexia (Poterucha et al., 2012). There is limited evidence to support other potential contributing factors, including high-dose corticosteroids, hypogonadism, or insulin resistance (Fearon et al., 2011).

ASSESSMENT

Grading Systems

Involuntary weight loss is the key criterion for cachexia and is included in the Common Terminology Criteria for Adverse Events (CTCAE; ctep.cancer.gov/protocoldevelopment/electronic_applications/docs/ctcae_v5_quick_reference_8.5x11.pdf).

According to this document, percentage weight loss (%WL) indicates the severity:

- Grade 1 is described as 5% to 10% weight loss with no intervention necessary.

- Grade 2 is weight loss of 10% to <20% from baseline with nutritional support indicated.

- Grade 3 is ≥20% weight loss from baseline with tube feeding or total parenteral nutrition suggested.

Fearon et al. (2011) suggest that there are three distinct stages in the cachexia spectrum:

- Precachexia reflects weight loss of ≤5%.

- Cachexia reflects weight loss >5% or body mass index (BMI) <20; or sarcopenia with >2% weight loss.

- Refractory cachexia reflects a variable degree of cachexia with disease not responsive to cancer treatment.

Assessment using the Fearon criteria (Fearon et al., 2011) is more accurate than clinical assessment (van der Werf et al., 2018). However, an assessment of the patient at risk for cachexia includes risk factors for weight loss and symptoms that impact on the patient's ability to eat or drink (Dev, 2018). Physical examination should include assessment of subcutaneous adipose tissue, muscle wasting, ascites or edema, as well as physical functioning. Assessing the quality of life is also very important. The Anorexia/Cachexia Subscale (A/CS) of the Functional Assessment of Anorexia/Cachexia Therapy (FAACT) questionnaire with a cutoff of ≤37 can be used in the diagnosis of cachexia, in addition to the Visual Analog Scale (VAS) for appetite with a cutoff of ≤70 (Blauwhoff-Buskermolen et al., 2016). Dietary intake can be challenging to measure; however, it does provide information related to caloric intake.

Measurement Tools

ASSESSMENT OF ANOREXIA: The A/CS of the FAACT questionnaire as well as the VAS for appetite may be used. The cutoff value for the FAACT-A/CS scale is ≤37 and for the VAS ≤70 (Blauwhoff-Buskermolen et al., 2016).

There are a number of tools that assess malnutrition in patients but none that address cachexia specifically.

- Patient-Generated Subjective Global Assessment (PG-SGA; Bauer et al., 2002; Thoresen et al., 2002)

- Mini Nutritional Assessment (MNA; Guigoz, 2006)

- Malnutrition Universal Screening Tool (MUST; Boléo-Tomé et al., 2012)

- Simplified Nutritional Appetite Questionnaire (SNAQ; Lau et al., 2020)

- Nutrition Risk Screening 2022 (Deer et al., 2019)

The PG-SGA appears to be the most appropriate tool as it contains items that reflect the domains of cachexia, including depletion of nutritional stores, muscle mass (by physical examination), anorexia or reduced food intake, catabolic drivers (fever and corticosteroids), and functional and psychosocial effects (Blum & Strasser, 2011).

To increase accuracy in diagnosing cachexia, criteria for the classification of cancer-related weight loss have been created. The addition of BMI allows for greater accuracy in prognosis (Martin et al., 2015; Figure 14.1).

In an analysis of the accuracy of the Weight Loss Grading System (WLGS), adding Karnofsky Performance Status findings, the presence of anorexia, as well as measurement of physical and emotional functioning to the WLGS improves the accuracy of prognosis (Vagnildhaug et al., 2017). An important finding is that the grade of weight loss has predicted the likelihood of progression of cachexia; grade 2 cachexia predicts greater risk of progression than grade 0 or 1, suggesting that it is at this grade that interventions should be initiated.

Grade 0	Weight-stable patients (i.e., weight loss $\pm2.4\%$) with BMI ≥25.0 kg/m^2 (with the longest survival, up to 29 months)
Grade 1	BMI 20–25 kg/m^2 and weight loss $\leq2.4\%$, or BMI ≥28 kg/m^2 and weight loss 2.5%–6% (median survival 14.6 months)
Grade 2	BMI 20–28 kg/m^2 and weight loss 2.5%–6%, or BMI ≥28 kg/m^2 and weight loss 6%–11% (median survival 10.8 months)
Grade 3	BMI ≤20 and weight stable or loss of $<6\%$, BMI 20–28 kg/m^2 and weight loss 6%–11%, BMI 22 to >28 kg/m^2 and weight loss 11%–15%, or BMI ≥28.0 kg/m^2 and weight loss $>15\%$ (median survival 7.6 months)
Grade 4	BMI ≤20 kg/m^2 and weight loss 6%–11%, BMI ≤22 kg/m^2 and weight loss 11%–15%, or BMI ≤28 kg/m^2 and weight loss $>15\%$ (median survival 4.3 months)

Figure 14.1 Weight Loss Grading System. BMI, body mass index.

Source: From Martin, L., Senesse, P., Gioulbasanis, I., Antoun, S., Bozzetti, F., Deans, C., Strasser, F., Thoresen, L., Jagoe, R. T., Chasen, M., Lundholm, K., Bosaeus, I., Fearon, K. H., & Baracos, V. E. (2015). Diagnostic criteria for the classification of cancer-associated weight loss. *Journal of Clinical Oncology, 33*(1), 90–99. https://doi.org/10.1200/jco.2014.56.1894.

BIOLOGICAL MARKERS: Catabolism may occur in cachexia due to tumor metabolism or inflammation. Inflammation may be confirmed by serum C-reactive protein; however, inflammation may not be present.

FUNCTIONAL AND PSYCHOSOCIAL EFFECTS: Functional status can be assessed by the European Organisation for Research and Treatment of Cancer (EORTC) Quality of Life Questionnaire (QLQ)-C30 (https://qol.eortc.org/questionnaire/eortc-qlq-c30), as well as by the Karnofsky score. To assess psychosocial effects, asking about the amount of distress caused by the inability to eat or how the patient feels (guilt, pressure, or stress in relationships) about their food intake and/or weight loss (Fearon et al., 2011) may help identify sources of distress.

MANAGEMENT

Anorexia and weight loss are distressing to the patient and their family members/caregivers. Food holds emotional weight, and the changes in appearance of the patient as the cachexia continues can cause guilt among caregivers as these may suggest that they are not providing the best care. It is important to advise the patient and their caregivers that, in advanced cancer, anorexia is common, and that forcing the patient to eat is counterproductive and may result in choking and/or aspiration. Food and fluids can be provided as requested by the patient, but it is important that the family/caregiver does not pressure the patient to eat (Orrevall, 2015).

Referral to a registered dietitian/nutritionist may be helpful; providing guidance on how to optimize nutrition and avoiding harmful supplements can be constructive and may help alleviate guilt. While increasing nutritional intake may improve the patient's quality of life, mortality is not improved (Baldwin et al., 2012).

The European Society for Medical Oncology (ESMO) guidelines (Arends et al., 2021) suggest a multimodal approach that includes the following:

- During anticancer treatment for patients who are expected to live more than a few months (3–6 months), interventions should be used to prevent further deterioration of body weight and muscle loss and to alleviate symptoms such as nausea and vomiting.

- If life expectancy is less than 3 to 6 weeks, the focus should be on alleviating symptoms such as thirst, dysphagia, and nausea and vomiting. Existential distress of both the patient and the family members should also be addressed and referral to appropriate sources made, for example, spiritual care and psychosocial support.

- Anticachexia interventions may be considered for a limited period to see whether they are effective.

Pharmaceutical Interventions

The American Society of Clinical Oncology (ASCO) guidelines advise that pharmaceutical interventions have limited evidence; however, *progesterone analogs* (megestrol acetate) and *short-term corticosteroids* may be prescribed (Roeland et al., 2020).

- A Cochrane review (Ruiz Garcia et al., 2013) found that *megestrol acetate* improves appetite in patients with cancer and also promotes slight weight gain. However, there is uncertainty about the optimal dose for this medication, with higher doses presenting greater benefit but with an increased risk of adverse events, including death, edema, and thrombotic events (Roeland et al., 2020).

- Megestrol acetate is not Food and Drug Administration (FDA)-approved for people with cancer (Garcia & Shamliyan, 2018), but off-label use is not uncommon (Brown et al., 2021).

- *Corticosteroids* should only be used for a short period of time (weeks); they act mainly on reduction of inflammation. While in the short term they increase appetite and well-being, this effect is transient and longer term use may cause adverse events that result in the deterioration of patients who are cachexic (Schakman et al., 2013).

- *Anamorelin*, a ghrelin receptor agonist, has shown some efficacy in improving body weight, lean body mass, and quality of life in patients with cachexia (Zhang et al., 2018); however, it is not approved by the FDA.

- *Olanzapine* shows limited effectiveness in preventing ongoing weight loss (Naing et al., 2015). When used in combination with megestrol acetate, weight gain of ≥5% over 8 weeks was seen in a small study ($N = 80$; Navari & Brenner, 2010).

- *Cannabinoids* including nabilone (Turcott et al., 2018) may have a role to play in increasing appetite; however, there is insufficient evidence to recommend these agents and safety concerns remain (Roeland et al., 2020).

Other pharmaceutical agents with little to no evidence in managing cachexia include nonsteroidal anti-inflammatory agents, androgens, prokinetics (metoclopramide, domperidone; Arends et al., 2021), and thalidomide (Roeland et al., 2020).

Tube feeding is recommended for patients receiving anticancer treatment who cannot tolerate oral nutrition for more than a few days; a percutaneous endoscopic gastrostomy is preferred to a nasogastric tube if support is needed for more than 4 weeks. Parenteral nutrition may be offered to a select group of patients but is not recommended for those who are malnourished while receiving chemotherapy (Arends et al., 2021).

Nonpharmaceutical Interventions

Exercise: Small studies have shown that 3 months of resistance exercise improved muscle strength and lean body mass in patients with pancreatic cancer who had cachexia (Kamel et al., 2020). Progressive resistance exercise showed some improvement in the quality of life of cachectic patients with head and neck cancer undergoing radiation therapy but no improvement in cachexia (Grote et al., 2018). A Cochrane review of exercise interventions (Grande et al., 2021) questioned their safety, effectiveness, and acceptability for patients with cachexia.

Acupuncture: Men with cachexia experienced a decrease in leptin levels along with increased appetite and weight gain in a study of patients with gastrointestinal cancer who received targeted acupuncture to traditional acupuncture points for systemic inflammation, anorexia, and loss of muscle mass (Yoon et al., 2020). A similar study in the same patient population suggested that targeted acupuncture resulted in weight gain by normalizing metabolism (Grundmann et al., 2019). Another very small study ($N = 7$) showed that acupuncture improved appetite and slowed weight loss in patients with gastrointestinal cancer (Yoon et al., 2015).

Mindfulness: In a small study ($N = 53$) of patients with cachexia who were on active treatment, the intervention (mindfulness workshops, and alternating dietary and psychosocial sessions) showed an increase in weight and improvement in fatigue (Focan et al., 2015). The authors caution that this intensive intervention may not be reproducible on a larger scale.

CASE STUDY

Mr. S. is a 47-year-old man with gastric cancer. He was treated with surgery, radiation, and chemotherapy, but the cancer has remained

(continued)

CASE STUDY (*CONTINUED*)

out of control, and based on clinical assessment he has developed cachexia.

1. What would you expect to observe in this man?

2. What other criteria would you assess to gain an accurate picture of his condition?

He has lost 20 lb (>5% of his body weight) and refuses to get out of bed as he feels "too weak." He is refusing to eat or drink, and his wife and sister are very worried that he is avoiding the treatment for his condition.

3. What advice would you give them?

His wife is demanding that some treatment is offered. His sister has contacted a lawyer about declaring him incompetent.

4. What are your next steps?

Dietary supplements including vitamins and minerals: There is limited evidence to support the use of protein supplements in the management of cachexia, and vitamins and mineral supplements are also lacking in evidence (Mochamat et al., 2017); however, they appear to be safe and many patients may be willing to try these in the absence of other effective interventions.

GUIDELINES

- **American Society of Clinical Oncology (ASCO)**

    ASCO Guideline: Management of Cancer Cachexia (Roeland et al., 2020)

- **European Society for Medical Oncology (EMSO)**

    ESMO Clinical Practice Guidelines: Cancer Cachexia in Adult Patients (Arends et al., 2021)

SUMMARY

Cachexia is common in those with advanced cancer. Patients experience weight loss, loss of muscle mass, and anorexia, and these symptoms have an impact on both physical and emotional functioning. It also causes distress, especially to family members/caregivers, who may feel guilty about the care they provide. Management includes multimodality interventions with patient and family/caregiver counseling about the inevitability of ongoing symptoms.

A robust set of instructor resources designed to supplement this text is located at http://connect.springerpub.com/content/reference-book/978-0-8261-8524-2.
Qualifying Instructors may request access by emailing **textbook@springerpub.com**.

REFERENCES

Antoun, S., Baracos, V. E., Birdsell, L., Escudier, B., & Sawyer, M. B. (2010). Low body mass index and sarcopenia associated with dose-limiting toxicity of sorafenib in patients with renal cell carcinoma. *Annals of Oncology, 21*(8), 1594–1598. https://doi.org/10.1093/annonc/mdp605s

Arends, J., Strasser, F., Gonella, S., Solheim, T. S., Madeddu, C., Ravasco, P., Buonaccorso, L., de van der Schueren, M. A. E., Baldwin, C., Chasen, M., & Ripamonti, C. I. (2021). Cancer cachexia in adult patients: ESMO Clinical Practice Guidelines(✩). *ESMO Open, 6*(3), 100092. https://doi.org/10.1016/j.esmoop.2021.100092

Baldwin, C., Spiro, A., Ahern, R., & Emery, P. W. (2012). Oral nutritional interventions in malnourished patients with cancer: A systematic review and meta-analysis. *Journal of the National Cancer Institute, 104*(5), 371–385. https://doi.org/10.1093/jnci/djr556

Bauer, J., Capra, S., & Ferguson, M. (2002). Use of the scored patient-generated subjective global assessment (PG-SGA) as a nutrition assessment tool in patients with cancer. *European Journal of Clinical Nutrition, 56*(8), 779–785. https://doi.org/10.1038/sj.ejcn.1601412

Bernhardson, B. M., Tishelman, C., & Rutqvist, L. E. (2008). Self-reported taste and smell changes during cancer chemotherapy. *Supportive Care in Cancer, 16*(3), 275–283. https://doi.org/10.1007/s00520-007-0319-7

Blauwhoff-Buskermolen, S., Ruijgrok, C., Ostelo, R. W., de Vet, H. C. W., Verheul, H. M. W., de van der Schueren, M. A. E., & Langius, J. A. E. (2016). The assessment of anorexia in patients with cancer: Cut-off values for the FAACT–A/CS and the VAS for appetite. *Supportive Care in Cancer, 24*(2), 661–666. https://doi.org/10.1007/s00520-015-2826-2

Blum, D., & Strasser, F. (2011). Cachexia assessment tools. *Current Opinion in Supportive & Palliative Care, 5*(4), 350–355. https://doi.org/10.1097/SPC.0b013e32834c4a05

Boléo-Tomé, C., Monteiro-Grillo, I., Camilo, M., & Ravasco, P. (2012). Validation of the malnutrition universal screening tool (MUST) in cancer. *British Journal of Nutrition, 108*(2), 343–348. https://doi.org/10.1017/S000711451100571X

Brown, T. J., Gandhi, S., Smith, T. J., & Gupta, A. (2021). Lessons from spending on megestrol for cancer cachexia. *Supportive Care in Cancer, 29*(10), 5553–5555. https://doi.org/10.1007/s00520-021-06240-7

Danai, L. V., Babic, A., Rosenthal, M. H., Dennstedt, E. A., Muir, A., Lien, E. C., Mayers, J. R., Tai, K., Lau, A. N., Jones-Sali, P., Prado, C. M., Petersen, G. M.,

Takahashi, N., Sugimoto, M., Yeh, J. J., Lopez, N., Bardeesy, N., Castillo, C. F., Liss, A. S. ... Vander Heiden, M. G. (2018). Altered exocrine function can drive adipose wasting in early pancreatic cancer. *Nature, 558*(7711), 600–604. https://doi.org/10.1038/s41586-018-0235-7

Deer, R., McCall, M., & Volpi, E. (2019). Comparison of malnutrition screening tools for use in hospitalized older adults (OR36-02-19). *Current Developments in Nutrition, 3*(Suppl. 1). https://doi.org/10.1093/cdn/nzz035.OR36-02-19

Del Fabbro, E., Hui, D., Dalal, S., Dev, R., Nooruddin, Z. I., & Bruera, E. (2011). Clinical outcomes and contributors to weight loss in a cancer cachexia clinic. *Journal of Palliative Medicine, 14*(9), 1004–1008. https://doi.org/10.1089/jpm .2011.0098

Dev, R. (2018). Measuring cachexia—diagnostic criteria. *Annals of Palliative Medicine, 8*(1), 24–32. https://apm.amegroups.com/article/view/21146

Fearon, K., Strasser, F., Anker, S. D., Bosaeus, I., Bruera, E., Fainsinger, R. L., Jatoi, A., Loprinzi, C., MacDonald, N., Mantovani, G., Davis, M., Muscaritoli, M., Ottery, F., Radbruch, L., Ravasco, P., Walsh, D., Wilcock, A., Kaasa, S., & Baracos, V. E. (2011). Definition and classification of cancer cachexia: An international consensus. *The Lancet Oncology, 12*(5), 489–495. https://doi.or g/10.1016/S1470-2045(10)70218-7

Focan, C., Houbiers, G., Gilles, L., Van Steeland, T., Georges, N., Maniglia, A., Lobelle, J.-P., Baro, V., & Graas, M. P. (2015). Dietetic and psychological mindfulness workshops for the management of cachectic cancer patients. A randomized study. *Anticancer Research, 35*(11), 6311–6315.

Garcia, J. M., & Shamliyan, T. A. (2018). Off-Label megestrol in patients with anorexia-cachexia syndrome associated with malignancy and its treatments. *The American Journal of Medicine, 131*(6), 623–629.e621. https://doi.org/10.1 016/j.amjmed.2017.12.028

Grande, A. J., Silva, V., Sawaris Neto, L., Teixeira Basmage, J. P., Peccin, M. S., & Maddocks, M. (2021). Exercise for cancer cachexia in adults. *Cochrane Database of Systematic Reviews, 3*(3), Cd010804. https://doi.org/10.1002/146 51858.CD010804.pub3

Grote, M., Maihöfer, C., Weigl, M., Davies-Knorr, P., & Belka, C. (2018). Progressive resistance training in cachectic head and neck cancer patients undergoing radiotherapy: A randomized controlled pilot feasibility trial. *Radiation Oncology, 13*(1), 215. https://doi.org/10.1186/s13014-018-1157-0

Grundmann, O., Yoon, S. L., Williams, J. J., Gordan, L., & George, T. J., Jr. (2019). Augmentation of cancer cachexia components with targeted acupuncture in patients with gastrointestinal cancers: A randomized controlled pilot study. *Integrative Cancer Therapies, 18*, 1534735418823269. https://doi.org/10.1177 /1534735418823269

Guigoz, Y. (2006). The mini nutritional assessment (MNA®) review of the literature-what does it tell us? *Journal of Nutrition Health and Aging, 10*(6), 466.

Kamel, F. H., Basha, M. A., Alsharidah, A. S., & Salama, A. B. (2020). Resistance training impact on mobility, muscle strength and lean mass in pancreatic cancer cachexia: A randomized controlled trial. *Clinical Rehabilitation, 34*(11), 1391–1399. https://doi.org/10.1177/0269215520941912

Kwang, A. Y., & Kandiah, M. (2010). Objective and subjective nutritional assessment of patients with cancer in palliative care. *American Journal of Hospice and Palliative Medicine, 27*(2), 117–126. https://doi.org/10.1177/1049909109353900

Lau, S., Pek, K., Chew, J., Lim, J. P., Ismail, N. H., Ding, Y. Y., Cesari, M., & Lim, W. S. (2020). The simplified nutritional appetite questionnaire (SNAQ) as a screening tool for risk of malnutrition: Optimal cutoff, factor structure, and validation in healthy community-dwelling older adults. *Nutrients, 12*(9), 2885. https://www.mdpi.com/2072-6643/12/9/2885

Martin, L., Senesse, P., Gioulbasanis, I., Antoun, S., Bozzetti, F., Deans, C., Strasser, F., Thoresen, L., Jagoe, R. T., Chasen, M., Lundholm, K., Bosaeus, I., Fearon, K. H., & Baracos, V. E. (2015). Diagnostic criteria for the classification of cancer-associated weight loss. *Journal of Clinical Oncology, 33*(1), 90–99. https://doi.org/10.1200/jco.2014.56.1894

Meza-Valderrama, D., Marco, E., Dávalos-Yerovi, V., Muns, M. D., Tejero-Sánchez, M., Duarte, E., & Sánchez-Rodríguez, D. (2021). Sarcopenia, malnutrition, and cachexia: Adapting definitions and terminology of nutritional disorders in older people with cancer. *Nutrients, 13*(3). https://doi.org/10.3390/nu13030761

Mochamat, C. H., Marinova, M., Kaasa, S., Stieber, C., Conrad, R., Radbruch, L., & Mücke, M. (2017). A systematic review on the role of vitamins, minerals, proteins, and other supplements for the treatment of cachexia in cancer: A European Palliative Care Research Centre cachexia project. *Journal of Cachexia, Sarcopenia and Muscle, 8*(1), 25–39. https://doi.org/10.1002/jcsm.12127

Naing, A., Dalal, S., Abdelrahim, M., Wheler, J., Hess, K., Fu, S., Hong, D. S., Janku, F., Falchook, G. S., Ilustre, I., Ouyang, F., & Kurzrock, R. (2015). Olanzapine for cachexia in patients with advanced cancer: An exploratory study of effects on weight and metabolic cytokines. *Supportive Care in Cancer, 23*(9), 2649–2654. https://doi.org/10.1007/s00520-015-2625-9

Navari, R. M., & Brenner, M. C. (2010). Treatment of cancer-related anorexia with olanzapine and megestrol acetate: A randomized trial. *Supportive Care in Cancer, 18*(8), 951–956. https://doi.org/10.1007/s00520-009-0739-7

Orrevall, Y. (2015). Nutritional support at the end of life. *Nutrition, 31*(4), 615–616. https://doi.org/10.1016/j.nut.2014.12.004

Paval, D. R., Patton, R., McDonald, J., Skipworth, R. J. E., Gallagher, I. J., & Laird, B. J. (2022). A systematic review examining the relationship between cytokines and cachexia in incurable cancer. *Journal of Cachexia, Sarcopenia and Muscle, 13*(2), 824–838. https://doi.org/10.1002/jcsm.12912

Poole, K., & Froggatt, K. (2002). Loss of weight and loss of appetite in advanced cancer: A problem for the patient, the carer, or the health professional?

Palliative Medicine, 16(6), 499–506. https://doi.org/10.1191/0269216302pm 593oa

Poterucha, T., Burnette, B., & Jatoi, A. (2012). A decline in weight and attrition of muscle in colorectal cancer patients receiving chemotherapy with bevacizumab. *Medical Oncology, 29*(2), 1005–1009. https://doi.org/10.1007/s120 32-011-9894-z

Roeland, E. J., Bohlke, K., Baracos, V. E., Bruera, E., Del Fabbro, E., Dixon, S., Fallon, M., Herrstedt, J., Lau, H., Platek, M., Rugo, H. S., Schnipper, H. H., Smith, T. J., Tan, W., & Loprinzi, C. L. (2020). Management of cancer cachexia: ASCO guideline. *Journal of Clinical Oncology, 38*(21), 2438–2453. https://doi.org/10.1200/jco.20.00611

Ruiz Garcia, V., López-Briz, E., Carbonell Sanchis, R., Gonzalvez Perales, J. L., & Bort-Marti, S. (2013). Megestrol acetate for treatment of anorexia-cachexia syndrome. *Cochrane Database of Systematic Reviews, 2013*(3), Cd004310. https://doi.org/10.1002/14651858.CD004310.pub3

Schakman, O., Kalista, S., Barbé, C., Loumaye, A., & Thissen, J. P. (2013). Glucocorticoid-induced skeletal muscle atrophy. *The International Journal of Biochemistry & Cell Biology, 45*(10), 2163–2172. https://doi.org/10.1016/j.biocel.2013.05.036

Smith, M. R., Saad, F., Egerdie, B., Sieber, P. R., Tammela, T. L., Ke, C., Leder, B. Z., & Goessl, C. (2012). Sarcopenia during androgen-deprivation therapy for prostate cancer. *Journal of Clinical Oncology, 30*(26), 3271–3276. https://doi.org/10.1200/jco.2011.38.8850

Steinbach, S., Hummel, T., Böhner, C., Berktold, S., Hundt, W., Kriner, M., Heinrich, P., Sommer, H., Hanusch, C., Prechtl, A., Schmidt, B., Bauerfeind, I., Seck, K., Jacobs, V. R., Schmalfeldt, B., & Harbeck, N. (2009). Qualitative and quantitative assessment of taste and smell changes in patients undergoing chemotherapy for breast cancer or gynecologic malignancies. *Journal of Clinical Oncology, 27*(11), 1899–1905. https://doi.org/10.1200/jco.2008.19.2690

Suzuki, H., Asakawa, A., Amitani, H., Nakamura, N., & Inui, A. (2013). Cancer cachexia—Pathophysiology and management. *Journal of Gastroenterology, 48*(5), 574–594. https://doi.org/10.1007/s00535-013-0787-0

Thoresen, L., Fjeldstad, I., Krogstad, K., Kaasa, S., & Falkmer, U. G. (2002). Nutritional status of patients with advanced cancer: The value of using the subjective global assessment of nutritional status as a screening tool. *Palliative Medicine, 16*(1), 33–42. https://doi.org/10.1191/0269216302pm 486oa

Turcott, J. G., Del Rocío Guillen Núñez, M., Flores-Estrada, D., Oñate-Ocaña, L. F., Zatarain-Barrón, Z. L., Barrón, F., & Arrieta, O. (2018). The effect of nabilone on appetite, nutritional status, and quality of life in lung cancer patients: A randomized, double-blind clinical trial. *Supportive Care in Cancer, 26*(9), 3029–3038. https://doi.org/10.1007/s00520-018-4154-9

Vagnildhaug, O. M., Blum, D., Wilcock, A., Fayers, P., Strasser, F., Baracos, V. E., Hjermstad, M. J., Kaasa, S., Laird, B., & Solheim, T. S. (2017). The applicability of a weight loss grading system in cancer cachexia: A longitudinal analysis. *Journal of Cachexia, Sarcopenia and Muscle, 8*(5), 789–797. https://doi.org/10.1002/jcsm.12220

van der Werf, A., van Bokhorst, Q. N. E., de van der Schueren, M. A. E., Verheul, H. M. W., & Langius, J. A. E. (2018). Cancer cachexia: Identification by clinical assessment versus international consensus criteria in patients with metastatic colorectal cancer. *Nutrition and Cancer, 70*(8), 1322–1329. https://doi.org/10.1080/01635581.2018.1504092

Yoon, S. L., Grundmann, O., Williams, J. J., & Carriere, G. (2015). Novel intervention with acupuncture for anorexia and cachexia in patients with gastrointestinal tract cancers: A feasibility study. *Oncology Nursing Forum, 42*(2), E102–E109. https://doi.org/10.1188/15.Onf.E102-e109

Yoon, S. L., Grundmann, O., Williams, J. J., Wu, S. S., Leeuwenburgh, C., Huo, Z., & George, T. J., Jr. (2020). Differential response to targeted acupuncture by gender in patients with gastrointestinal cancer cachexia: Secondary analysis of a randomized controlled trial. *Acupuncture in Medicine, 38*(1), 53–60. https://doi.org/10.1177/0964528419873670

Zhang, F., Shen, A., Jin, Y., & Qiang, W. (2018). The management strategies of cancer-associated anorexia: A critical appraisal of systematic reviews. *BMC Complementary and Alternative Medicine, 18*(1), 236. https://doi.org/10.1186/s12906-018-2304-8

CHAPTER 15

DYSPHAGIA

INTRODUCTION

Dysphagia is the subjective sensation of having difficulty swallowing. A tumor in the esophagus will cause rapidly progressive difficulty swallowing, initially for solids and then later for liquids. Treatment for this cancer as well as treatment for cancer of the head or neck also cause dysphagia. Both surgery and organ-sparing chemoradiation cause difficulty swallowing, and this has a significant impact on quality of life. For patients, being able to swallow is of high priority (Wilson et al., 2011).

PREVALENCE

The incidence of human papillomavirus (HPV)-related head and neck cancer has increased in recent years, affecting younger people who do not have a history of tobacco or alcohol use (Li et al., 2020). The severity of this symptom is in part associated with treatment modality, with intensity-modulated radiation therapy having the least impact on swallowing (Roets et al., 2018).

Dysphagia is not uncommon in all kinds of cancer, with 20% of patients reporting problems swallowing liquids and 46% swallowing solids (Frowen et al., 2020). However, the prevalence is much higher (79%) in patients with head and neck cancer treated with chemoradiation (Rinkel et al., 2016). Improvement may be seen between 6 months and 5 years after chemoradiation, but up to 24% of patients continue to have dysphagia at 5 years after treatment (Frowen et al., 2016). Dysphagia may persist with 54% of patients unable to tolerate a normal diet for 10 or more years (Kraaijenga et al., 2015).

CONTRIBUTING FACTORS

Concurrent chemoradiation and fractionated radiation are linked to the development of acute dysphagia (Crowder et al., 2018). Age, advanced stage of cancer, site of tumor, and radiation dose to the tumor are major contributing factors to late dysphagia (Jiang et al., 2016). Preexisting

138 SECTION III • GASTROINTESTINAL SYMPTOMS

dysphagia at baseline due to the presence of a tumor predisposes the patient to worse posttreatment problems (Crowder et al., 2018).

CASE STUDY

Your patient is a 38-year-old man with no history of smoking or alcohol use. He has been diagnosed with an aggressive oral tumor and you are seeing him for his pretreatment physical examination. He will receive concurrent chemoradiation therapy prior to eventual surgery to remove the tumor on his tongue.

1. He asks you why this has happened given that he does not have any risk factors. What is your response?

His body mass index (BMI) is 19 kg/m^2; he runs four to five times a week and has been training for an ultra-marathon in the summer. He asks you what he can do to maintain his training.

2. What are your concerns for him and what advice would you give him?

He is shocked by what you tell him. He asks if there is anything he can do to prevent this.

3. What should you do now?

ASSESSMENT

Swallowing is a complex process, and because the available measures assess different domains, more than one measure is needed for accuracy (Pedersen et al., 2016).

The Radiation Therapy Oncology Group (RTOG) Dysphagia Grading Scale of swallowing status defines limitations in swallowing (Gaspar et al., 2000; Box 15.1).

Box 15.1 Radiation Therapy Oncology Group Dysphagia Grading Scale

Grade 1	No dysphagia: able to eat any solids
Grade 2	Mild dysphagia: semisolids and liquids
Grade 3	Moderate dysphagia: able to take liquids only
Grade 4	Complete obstruction: unable to take even liquids

The Common Terminology Criteria for Adverse Events (CTCAE) has a similar grading system (see Box 15.2; www.ctep.cancer.gov/protocoldevelopment/electronic_applications/docs/ctcae_v5_quick_reference_8.5x11.pdf).

CHAPTER 15 • DYSPHAGIA 139

Box 15.2 The Common Terminology Criteria for Adverse Events Grading System

Grade 1	Symptomatic but able to eat a regular diet
Grade 2	Symptomatic with altered eating/swallowing
Grade 3	Severely altered eating/swallowing with tube feeding, total parenteral nutrition, or hospitalization indicated
Grade 4	Life-threatening consequences and urgent intervention indicated

There are a number of tools available to measure dysphagia (see Figure 15.1).

MANAGEMENT

Treatment for dysphagia focuses predominately on pain control that may be challenging if oral medications are not tolerated. Alternative methods include transmucosal, transdermal, inhaled, rectal, or intranasal routes (Argoff & Kopecky, 2014). For patients with incurable esophageal cancer, esophageal stenting and radiation therapy may help reduce symptoms. If stenting is not possible, fractionated radiation is the preferred modality as it reduces exposure of adjacent tissues (van der Bogt et al., 2018). While stenting may improve short-term nutritional intake during neoadjuvant treatment, there are concerns about poor oncologic outcomes and they should not be used in patients with potentially curable esophageal cancer who will undergo surgery (Ahmed et al., 2020). There is mixed evidence on the use of therapeutic exercises that improve swallowing (Gillman et al., 2022; Perry et al., 2016), including prehabilitation protocols that are intensive and need to be continued for months after treatment (Duarte et al., 2013).

100 mL water swallow test (Patterson et al., 2011)	Patient drinks 100 mL as quickly as possible and time measured from lips to resting larynx
Normalcy of Diet score (NOD; List et al., 1990)	Scores range for 0 = tube feeding to 100 = full diet with no restrictions
MD Anderson Dysphagia Inventory (Chen et al., 2001)	Likert scale of 20 items experienced over past week
SWAL-QOL Tool (McHorney et al., 2002)	10 items that include physical and psychosocial dimensions
Dysphagia Handicap Index (Silbergleit et al., 2012)	25 items on a 1–7 Likert scale
EORTC–QLQ-0G25 (Lagergren et al., 2007)	25-Item Likert scale to be used with the QLQ-C30
Swallowing Outcome After Laryngectomy (Govender, 2016)	17-Item Likert scale

Figure 15.1 Dysphagia assessment tools.

SUMMARY

Dysphagia has multiple impacts on quality of life as well as functional and psychosocial challenges due to the important role that eating plays. Weight loss and pain are important consequences of the inability to swallow, and unfortunately interventions are limited.

 A robust set of instructor resources designed to supplement this text is located at http://connect.springerpub.com/content/reference-book/978-0-8261-8524-2. Qualifying Instructors may request access by emailing **textbook@springerpub.com**.

REFERENCES

Ahmed, O., Bolger, J. C., O'Neill, B., & Robb, W. B. (2020). Use of esophageal stents to relieve dysphagia during neoadjuvant therapy prior to esophageal resection: A systematic review. *Disease of the Esophagus, 33*(1), doz090. https://doi.org/10.1093/dote/doz090

Argoff, C. E., & Kopecky, E. A. (2014). Patients with chronic pain and dysphagia (CPD): Unmet medical needs and pharmacologic treatment options. *Current Medical Research and Opinion, 30*(12), 2543–2559. https://doi.org/10.1185/03007995.2014.967388

Crowder, S. L., Douglas, K. G., Yanina Pepino, M., Sarma, K. P., & Arthur, A. E. (2018). Nutrition impact symptoms and associated outcomes in post-chemoradiotherapy head and neck cancer survivors: A systematic review. *Journal of Cancer Survivorship, 12*(4), 479–494. https://doi.org/10.1007/s11764-018-0687-7

Duarte, V. M., Chhetri, D. K., Liu, Y. F., Erman, A. A., & Wang, M. B. (2013). Swallow preservation exercises during chemoradiation therapy maintains swallow function. *Otolaryngology—Head and Neck Surgery, 149*(6), 878–884. https://doi.org/10.1177/0194599813502310

Frowen, J., Drosdowsky, A., Perry, A., & Corry, J. (2016). Long-term swallowing after chemoradiotherapy: Prospective study of functional and patient-reported changes over time. *Head & Neck, 38*(S1), E307–E315. https://doi.org/10.1002/hed.23991

Frowen, J., Hughes, R., & Skeat, J. (2020). The prevalence of patient-reported dysphagia and oral complications in cancer patients. *Supportive Care in Cancer, 28*(3), 1141–1150. https://doi.org/10.1007/s00520-019-04921-y

Gaspar, L. E., Winter, K., Kocha, W. I., Coia, L. R., Herskovic, A., & Graham, M. (2000). A Phase I/II study of external beam radiation, brachytherapy, and concurrent chemotherapy for patients with localized carcinoma of the esophagus (Radiation Therapy Oncology Group Study 9207). *Cancer, 88*(5), 988–995. https://doi.org/10.1002/(SICI)1097-0142(20000301)88:5<988::AID-CNCR7>3.0.CO;2-U

Gillman, A., Hayes, M., Sheaf, G., Walshe, M., Reynolds, J. V., & Regan, J. (2022). Exercise-based dysphagia rehabilitation for adults with oesophageal cancer: A systematic review. *BMC Cancer*, 22(1), 53. https://doi.org/10.1186/s12885-021-09155-y

Govender, R., Lee, M. T., Drinnan, M., Davies, T., Twinn, C., & Hilari, K. (2016). Psychometric evaluation of the swallowing outcomes after laryngectomy (SOAL) patient-reported outcome measure. *Head & Neck, 38*(S1), E1639–E1645. https://doi.org/10.1002/hed.24291

Jiang, N., Zhang, L. J., Li, L. Y., Zhao, Y., & Eisele, D. W. (2016). Risk factors for late dysphagia after (chemo)radiotherapy for head and neck cancer: A systematic methodological review. *Head Neck, 38*(5), 792–800. https://doi.org/10.1002/hed.23963

Kraaijenga, S. A. C., Oskam, I. M., van der Molen, L., Hamming-Vrieze, O., Hilgers, F. J. M., & van den Brekel, M. W. M. (2015). Evaluation of long term (10-years+) dysphagia and trismus in patients treated with concurrent chemo-radiotherapy for advanced head and neck cancer. *Oral Oncology, 51*(8), 787–794. https://doi.org/10.1016/j.oraloncology.2015.05.003

Li, P., Constantinescu, G. C., Nguyen, N. A., & Jeffery, C. C. (2020). Trends in reporting of swallowing outcomes in oropharyngeal cancer studies: A systematic review. *Dysphagia, 35*(1), 18–23. https://doi.org/10.1007/s00455-019-09996-7

Pedersen, A., Wilson, J., McColl, E., Carding, P., & Patterson, J. (2016). Swallowing outcome measures in head and neck cancer—How do they compare? *Oral Oncology, 52*, 104–108. https://doi.org/10.1016/j.oraloncology.2015.10.015

Perry, A., Lee, S. H., Cotton, S., & Kennedy, C. (2016). Therapeutic exercises for affecting post-treatment swallowing in people treated for advanced-stage head and neck cancers. *Cochrane Database of Systematic Reviews, 2016*(8), Cd011112. https://doi.org/10.1002/14651858.CD011112.pub2

Rinkel, R. N., Verdonck-de Leeuw, I. M., Doornaert, P., Buter, J., de Bree, R., Langendijk, J. A., Aaronson, N. K., & Leemans, C. R. (2016). Prevalence of swallowing and speech problems in daily life after chemoradiation for head and neck cancer based on cut-off scores of the patient-reported outcome measures SWAL-QOL and SHI. *European Archives of Oto-Rhino-Laryngology, 273*(7), 1849–1855. https://doi.org/10.1007/s00405-015-3680-z

Roets, E., Tukanova, K., Govarts, A., & Specenier, P. (2018). Quality of life in oropharyngeal cancer: A structured review of the literature. *Supportive Care in Cancer, 26*(8), 2511–2518. https://doi.org/10.1007/s00520-018-4227-9

van der Bogt, R. D., Vermeulen, B. D., Reijm, A. N., Siersema, P. D., & Spaander, M. C. W. (2018). Palliation of dysphagia. *Best Practice & Research Clinical Gastroenterology, 36–37*, 97–103. https://doi.org/10.1016/j.bpg.2018.11.010

Wilson, J. A., Carding, P. N., & Patterson, J. M. (2011). Dysphagia after nonsurgical head and neck cancer treatment: Patients' perspectives. *Otolaryngology — Head and Neck Surgery, 145*(5), 767–771. https://doi.org/10.1177/0194599811414506

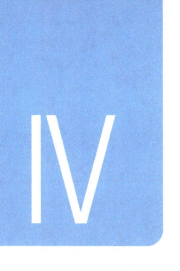

Genitourinary Symptoms

CHAPTER 16

INCONTINENCE

INTRODUCTION

Both urinary and fecal incontinence are side effects of cancer treatment that have a significant impact on quality of life. Urinary incontinence occurs as a result of surgical treatment for prostate cancer in men. Treatment for gynecologic cancer in women and bladder and colorectal cancer treatment in both men and women may result in fecal incontinence.

INCONTINENCE IN MEN

Urinary incontinence is classified as either stress urinary incontinence (SUI) or urge urinary incontinence (UUI) due to overactive bladder syndrome. A combination of stress and urge incontinence is described as mixed urinary incontinence. After treatment for prostate cancer, both stress and urge incontinence may occur due to damage to the urethral sphincter after surgery; irritative symptoms are more likely to be experienced as a side effect of radiation therapy.

Prevalence

The prevalence of incontinence after surgery for prostate cancer varies based on how the condition is defined; the number of pads needed per day is commonly used as a measure (Figure 16.1).

No or occasional pad use	83%
0–1 pad used daily for occasional dribbling	92.3%
0–1 pad used daily	93.4%

Figure 16.1 Incontinence at 24 months after radical prostatectomy.
Source: From Sacco, E., Prayer-Galetti, T., Pinto, F., Fracalanza, S., Betto, G., Pagano, F., & Artibani, W. (2006). Urinary incontinence after radical prostatectomy: Incidence by definition, risk factors and temporal trend in a large series with a long-term follow-up. *BJU International, 97*(6), 1234–1241. https://doi.org/10.1111/j.1464-410X.2006.06185.x.

Incontinence has a negative impact up to 24 months after surgery (Wallerstedt et al., 2019). The rates of incontinence are similar after robotic-assisted radical prostatectomy and open radical prostatectomy (Haglind et al., 2015). Incontinence after high-intensity focused ultrasound occurs in 3% of men with refinement of the technique used (Crouzet et al., 2014). Urinary incontinence with arousal or orgasm is called *climacturia* and occurs in 38% of men after radical prostatectomy (Frey et al., 2017) and 4% of men after external beam radiation (Frey et al., 2017).

Contributing Factors

After treatment for prostate cancer, SUI is due to inadequate urethral sphincter function and UUI is caused by bladder outlet obstruction or overactive bladder. Other contributing factors include nonnerve-sparing radical prostatectomy (Steineck et al., 2015), older age (Lardas et al., 2022), preoperative incontinence (Wei et al., 2000), and prostate volume (Ficarra et al., 2012).

Higher doses of radiation to the bladder during stereotactic body radiation therapy increase the risk of urinary incontinence (Iarrobino et al., 2019).

Assessment

A detailed history from the patient will identify the type of incontinence. Leakage that occurs with movement, laughing, coughing, or sneezing suggests stress incontinence. Leakage with a sudden need to urinate is indicative of urge incontinence. Asking about how many pads per day the man uses as well as how wet the pads are is helpful in identifying the severity and impact of the incontinence.

- *Formal pad testing*, either for 1 hour as a screening test or 24 hours to assess the volume of leakage, may also be used and is the gold standard for assessing the degree of incontinence (Soto González et al., 2018).

- *Urodynamics* may be used to establish the cause of stress incontinence if the history is unclear (Sandhu et al., 2019).

- *Cystoscopy* is used to assess sphincter function as well as the urethra and bladder neck, especially if surgical intervention with an artificial urinary sphincter is planned (King & Almallah, 2012).

Management

Pelvic floor muscle exercises or training: Conservative management with pelvic floor muscle exercises/training is noninvasive, low cost, and has no side effects. These exercises, with or without biofeedback, have shown efficacy in reducing leakage (Aydın Sayılan & Özbaş, 2018; Milios et al.,

Patient Perception of Bladder Condition (PPBC)	Single item
Urogenital Distress Inventory (UDI-6)	6 items
International Consultation on Incontinence Questionnaire—Urinary Incontinence Short Form	4 items
Incontinence Impact Questionnaire	7 items
Incontinence Quality of Life Questionnaire (men)	22 items
King's Health Questionnaire	22 items

Figure 16.2 Incontinence measures.
Source: From Emmons, K. R., & Robinson, J. P. (2013). Urinary incontinence severity and quality-of-life instruments. *Journal of Wound Ostomy & Continence Nursing, 40*(4), 350–354. https://doi.org/10.1097/WON.0b013e318297c766.

2019; Soto González et al., 2020; Zhang et al., 2015). Self-efficacy and social support increase the potential to improve incontinence (Zhang et al., 2020), and decreased leakage as a result of performing these exercises results in less anxiety for men after treatment (Zhang et al., 2019). Pelvic floor muscle training has also shown efficacy in managing climacturia (Geraerts et al., 2016). Men can also be encouraged to void prior to sex or to use a condom, but this may not be possible for men who do not achieve a rigid erection. A tension loop made of silicone tied at the base of the penis has been shown to be effective and noninvasive (Kannady & Clavell-Hernández, 2020; Mehta et al., 2013). Preoperative pelvic muscle training may be of use in men undergoing radiation therapy to prevent incontinence (Kutluturkan et al., 2021), but this may be less successful for those having surgery (de Lira et al., 2019).

Devices: Some men may prefer to use an absorbent pad or device to control incontinence. Absorbent pads may be useful for men during the day; however, when wet, they are uncomfortable and associated with odor. A condom catheter (sheath drainage system) or body worn urinal may be acceptable for some men; however, satisfaction is low with the latter. A penile clamp is least likely to leak, but it is uncomfortable/painful and is mostly used for a limited time, for example, while swimming (Macaulay et al., 2015).

Pharmaceutical agents: If and when conservative management is no longer effective, pharmaceutical agents such as antimuscarinics (e.g., oxybutynin) or beta-3 agonists (e.g., Mirabegron) may be prescribed for urge incontinence (Gandi & Sacco, 2021). However, all of these pharmaceutical agents cause side effects that patients may not tolerate.

Surgery: Artificial urinary sphincters are regarded as the most effective intervention in patients who have the dexterity and cognitive ability to use this device correctly. Male slings can also be considered for those with mild to moderate stress incontinence but not for those with severe SUI. Adjustable balloon devices are approved for use but there is a risk of intraoperative complications when inserted by surgeons with limited training in the use of these devices. Urethral bulking agents are not recommended for men treated for prostate cancer (Sandhu et al., 2019).

CASE STUDY

Jim B. is a 67-year-old man with intermediate-risk prostate cancer who was treated with a radical prostatectomy 3 months ago. He has come to see you because he is experiencing urinary leakage and is angry that he was not informed about this side effect of the treatment. He manages the daily leakage with pads and adult diapers at night.

1. What questions should you ask him?

2. What other assessment(s) should you do?

He tells you that the most distressing side effect is the urinary leakage that occurs when he masturbates.

3. What advice can you give him about this?

He is not interested in taking any medication and he has heard that there are supplements that can help.

4. What nonpharmaceutical options are there for him?

INCONTINENCE IN WOMEN

Almost all the literature on incontinence in women relates to noncancer causes and treatments for both stress and urgency incontinence in older women. There is a small body of literature on cancer-related urinary incontinence in women.

Prevalence

The prevalence of urinary incontinence in women globally ranges from 5% to 70%, with higher prevalence associated with increasing age (Milsom & Gyhagen, 2019). In gynecologic cancer survivors, the prevalence is suggested to range from 7% (Firmeza et al., 2022) to over 60% (Rutledge et al., 2010).

Laparoscopic nerve-sparing radical hysterectomy reduces the risk of incontinence as compared with nonnerve-sparing laparoscopic hysterectomy (Wu et al., 2019). Breast cancer survivors with the genitourinary syndrome of menopause as a result of treatment also experience urinary frequency and dribbling, but with lower prevalence (2.8%; Cook et al., 2017). However, this is likely underreported, as suggested by Colombage et al. (2021) who found that 38% of women with breast cancer reported urinary incontinence.

There is a strong association between urinary incontinence and anxiety and depression (Cheng et al., 2020), as well as health-related quality of life (Aoki et al., 2017). There is also an impact on family caregivers, who experience financial, emotional, and caregiver stress from providing physical support and management to these women (Talley et al., 2021).

Contributing Factors

Multimodality treatments for gynecologic cancers include radical surgery, radiation therapy, and chemotherapy. These treatments all impact on the pelvic floor, causing anatomical changes to the lower urinary tract. Both nerve and vascular supplies are impacted (Rutledge et al., 2014).

Assessment

Similar to the assessment of urinary incontinence in men, assessment in women includes history, physical examination, a voiding diary, pad test, and urodynamic tests for patients before surgical intervention (Aoki et al., 2017). Patient questionnaires for assessment of urinary function for both men and women include those presented in Figure 16.2. Questionnaires specifically for women include the 21-item Bladder Health Survey (Minassian et al., 2016) and the Bristol Female Lower Urinary Tract Symptoms Short Form (12 items; Emmons & Robinson, 2013).

Management

Conservative: Pelvic floor muscle exercises/training for women with incontinence after treatment for gynecologic cancer reduced incontinence in 80% of women (Rutledge et al., 2014). Studies of this intervention have shown effectiveness in community samples of women with incontinence (Bø & Hilde, 2013; Ghaderi et al., 2016; Wu et al., 2020), including in a group setting (Dumoulin et al., 2020). Weight loss has also been shown to be helpful in reducing incontinence (Bascur-Castillo et al., 2022). Continence products such as pads are often used by women, but many do not use appropriate products; menstrual pads are not recommended for incontinence. Nurse continence advisors are helpful in guiding women about the best products to use (Aoki et al., 2017). Continence Product Advisor also provides useful information on their website (continenceproductadvisor.org). Electroacupuncture may be helpful in managing incontinence (Lai et al., 2020; Wang et al., 2019); however, to date, there have been no studies in women with cancer using this intervention.

Devices: Vaginal cones and pessaries have not been shown to be effective (Lipp et al., 2014). CO_2 laser treatment is also not recommended (Alexander et al., 2022).

Pharmacologic: Treatment with antimuscarinics (e.g., oxybutynin) or beta-3 agonists (e.g., mirabegron) is useful in the management of urge incontinence (Bientinesi & Sacco, 2018). Low-dose intravaginal estriol is also suggested (Castellani et al., 2015); however, there is some controversy in women with hormone-dependent breast cancer (see Chapters 17 and 18 on male and female sexual dysfunction).

Surgery: Usually not first-line treatment, suburethral sling surgery is effective for SUI (Franzen et al., 2015). Vaginal mesh surgery has significant side effects, including the onset of urgency incontinence, and should be considered with caution (Aoki et al., 2017).

FECAL INCONTINENCE

Fecal incontinence, the involuntary or uncontrolled passage of liquid or solid feces, may be a side effect of cancer therapies (surgery, chemotherapy, or radiation to the pelvis) in both men and women. Fecal incontinence causes poor quality of life as well as embarrassment and perianal skin problems and itching (Lai et al., 2013).

Prevalence

The prevalence of fecal incontinence in patients with colorectal cancer depends on the type of treatment and time since treatment. After surgery, fecal incontinence peaks at 2 weeks, with up to 96% of patients experiencing incontinence with liquid stools and 56% with solid stools. Three months after surgery, 16% to 55% remain incontinent with liquid stools and 12% to 22% are incontinent with solid stools (Gong et al., 2012). The low anterior resection syndrome (LARS) causes a variety of symptoms including fecal and flatus incontinence in 80% of patients who undergo low or very low anterior resection (Bulfone et al., 2020). Treatment with chemoradiation causes fecal incontinence that is worse 5 years after neoadjuvant therapy (Horisberger et al., 2014); 40% of patients report being incontinent of stool always or most of the time and 68% wore pads all the time.

Contributing Factors

In the context of cancer, surgery, radiation, and adjuvant chemotherapy are most commonly associated with fecal incontinence. Fecal incontinence occurs in 8.39% of community-dwelling adults, with increasing age, diabetes, urinary incontinence, and multiple chronic illnesses as contributing factors (Ditah et al., 2014).

Assessment

There are five established measures of the impact of fecal incontinence on quality of life (Rockwood, 2004):

- Gastrointestinal Quality of Life Index (Eypasch et al., 1995), which contains 36 items

- Fecal Incontinence Quality of Life Scale (Rockwood et al., 2000), which contains 29 items

- Functional Assessment of Cancer Therapy-Colorectal (FACT-C; Ward et al., 1999), which contains 44 items and was designed to assess the quality of life of those with colorectal cancer; a comprehensive questionnaire with only one question specific to fecal incontinence

- Wexner Score, also known as the Cleveland Clinic Fecal Incontinence Severity Scoring System (CCIS), which contains a Likert scale (never, rarely, sometimes, usually, always) for five scenarios; the most closely correlated with patients' subjective perception of severity of incontinence (Seong et al., 2011)

- Manchester Health Questionnaire (Bugg et al., 2001), which is for women only and contains 31 items; can use anorectal manometry to provide an objective measure of anal tone and sphincter weakness (Carrington et al., 2020)

Management

Patient education is the first step in managing fecal incontinence. This includes information about dietary interventions that may be helpful, such as psyllium supplements (Bliss et al., 2014).

Conservative: Pelvic floor muscle exercises are the most effective conservative management for fecal incontinence in patients who have had surgery for colorectal cancer, for anterior resection (Chan et al., 2021), intersphincteric resection (Kuo et al., 2015), and after stoma closure (Lin et al., 2016). Supervised pelvic floor muscle training with biofeedback is optimal (Ussing et al., 2019). Acupuncture may also be helpful (Sipaviciute et al., 2021).

Pharmaceutical: Loperamide is effective in improving stool consistency and frequency (Lal et al., 2019).

Nerve stimulation: Sacral nerve stimulation improves fecal incontinence (Simillis et al., 2018), including in patients with LARS (Bulfone et al., 2020).

GUIDELINES

- **American Society of Colon and Rectal Surgeons**
  The American Society of Colon and Rectal Surgeons' Clinical Practice Guideline for the Treatment of Fecal Incontinence

  https://fascrs.org/ascrs/media/files/downloads/Clinical%20 Practice%20Guidelines/clinical_practice_guideline_for_ the_treatment_of_fecal_incontinence.pdf

- **American Urological Association/Society of Urodynamics, Female Pelvic Medicine and Urogenital Reconstruction (AUA/SUFU)**

Incontinence After Prostate Treatment: AUA/SUFU Guideline (Sandhu et al., 2019)

- **Canadian Urological Association**

    Canadian Urological Association 2012 Update: Guidelines for Adult Urinary Incontinence Collaborative Consensus Document for the Canadian Urological Society (under revision)

    https://www.cua.org/system/files/Guideline-Files/guidelines_for_adult_urinary_incontinence_collaborative_consensus_doc.pdf

- **European Association of Urology (EAU)**
  EAU Guidelines (not specific to cancer)

    uroweb.org/eau-guidelines/discontinued-topics/urinary-incontinence

- Fourth International Consultation on Incontinence Recommendations on the International Scientific Committee: Evaluation and Treatment of Urinary Incontinence, Pelvic Organ Prolapse, and Fecal Incontinence (Abrams et al., 2010)

- Guideline of Guidelines: Urinary Incontinence (not specific to cancer; Syan & Brucker, 2016)

SUMMARY

Both urinary and fecal incontinence have a negative impact on quality of life and are known to cause distress to both men and women. These side effects are common after surgery or radiation for cancers affecting the pelvic organs. There are a range of interventions to mitigate these side effects but patients may be embarrassed to discuss these with healthcare clinicians unless asked directly about their occurrence.

A robust set of instructor resources designed to supplement this text is located at http://connect.springerpub.com/content/reference-book/978-0-8261-8524-2. Qualifying Instructors may request access by emailing **textbook@springerpub.com**.

REFERENCES

Abrams, P., Andersson, K. E., Birder, L., Brubaker, L., Cardozo, L., Chapple, C., Cottenden, A., Davila, W., de Ridder, D., Dmochowski, R., Drake, M., DuBeau, C., Fry, C., Hanno, P., Hay Smith, J., Herschorn, S., Hosker, G., Kelleher, C., Koelbl, H., & Wyndaele, J. J. (2010). Fourth international consultation on incontinence recommendations of the international scientific committee: Evaluation and treatment of urinary incontinence, pelvic organ prolapse, and fecal incontinence. *Neurourology and Urodynamics, 29*(1), 213–240. https://doi.org/10.1002/nau.20870

Alexander, J. W., Karjalainen, P., Ow, L. L., Kulkarni, M., Lee, J. K., Karjalainen, T., Leitch, A., Ryan, G., & Rosamilia, A. (2022). CO(2) surgical laser for treatment of stress urinary incontinence in women: a randomized controlled trial. *American Journal of Obstetrics Gynecology*, 227(3), 473.e471–473.e412. https://doi.org/10.1016/j.ajog.2022.05.054

Aoki, Y., Brown, H. W., Brubaker, L., Cornu, J. N., Daly, J. O., & Cartwright, R. (2017). Urinary incontinence in women. *Nature Reviews Disease Primers, 3*, 17042. https://doi.org/10.1038/nrdp.2017.42

Aydın Sayılan, A., & Özbaş, A. (2018). The effect of pelvic floor muscle training on incontinence problems after radical prostatectomy. *American Journal of Men's Health, 12*(4), 1007–1015. https://doi.org/10.1177/1557988318757242

Bascur-Castillo, C., Carrasco-Portiño, M., Valenzuela-Peters, R., Orellana-Gaete, L., Viveros-Allende, V., & Ruiz Cantero, M. T. (2022). Effect of conservative treatment of pelvic floor dysfunctions in women: An umbrella review. *International Journal of Gynecology & Obstetrics, 159*(2), 372–391. https://doi.org/10.1002/ijgo.14172

Bientinesi, R., & Sacco, E. (2018). Managing urinary incontinence in women—A review of new and emerging pharmacotherapy. *Expert Opinion on Pharmacotherapy, 19*(18), 1989–1997. https://doi.org/10.1080/14656566.2018.1532502

Bliss, D. Z., Savik, K., Jung, H. J., Whitebird, R., Lowry, A., & Sheng, X. (2014). Dietary fiber supplementation for fecal incontinence: A randomized clinical trial. *Research in Nursing & Health, 37*(5), 367–378. https://doi.org/10.1002/nur.21616

Bø, K., & Hilde, G. (2013). Does it work in the long term?—A systematic review on pelvic floor muscle training for female stress urinary incontinence. *Neurourology and Urodynamics, 32*(3), 215–223. https://doi.org/10.1002/nau.22292

Bugg, G. J., Kiff, E. S., & Hosker, G. (2001). A new condition-specific health-related quality of life questionnaire for the assessment of women with anal incontinence. *British Journal of Obstetrics and Gynaecology, 108*(10), 1057–1067. https://doi.org/10.1016/S0306-5456(01)00245-5

Bulfone, G., Del Negro, F., Del Medico, E., Cadorin, L., Bressan, V., & Stevanin, S. (2020). Rehabilitation strategies for low anterior resection syndrome. A systematic review. *Annali dell'Istituto Superiore di Sanità, 56*(1), 38–47. https://doi.org/10.4415/ann_20_01_07

Carrington, E. V., Heinrich, H., Knowles, C. H., Fox, M., Rao, S., Altomare, D. F., Bharucha, A. E., Burgell, R., Chey, W. D., Chiarioni, G., Dinning, P., Emmanuel, A., Farouk, R., Felt-Bersma, R. J. F., Jung, K. W., Lembo, A., Malcolm, A., Mittal, R. K., Mion, F., & Scott, S. M. (2020). The international anorectal physiology working group (IAPWG) recommendations: Standardized testing protocol and the London classification for disorders of anorectal function. *Neurogastroenterology & Motility, 32*(1).https://doi.org/10.1111/nmo.13679

Castellani, D., Saldutto, P., Galica, V., Pace, G., Biferi, D., Paradiso Galatioto, G., & Vicentini, C. (2015). Low-dose intravaginal estriol and pelvic floor rehabilitation in post-menopausal stress urinary incontinence. *Urologia Internationalis, 95*(4), 417–421. https://doi.org/10.1159/000381989

Chan, K. Y. C., Suen, M., Coulson, S., & Vardy, J. L. (2021). Efficacy of pelvic floor rehabilitation for bowel dysfunction after anterior resection for colorectal cancer: A systematic review. *Supportive Care in Cancer, 29*(4), 1795–1809. https://doi.org/10.1007/s00520-020-05832-z

Cheng, S., Lin, D., Hu, T., Cao, L., Liao, H., Mou, X., Zhang, Q., Liu, J., & Wu, T. (2020). Association of urinary incontinence and depression or anxiety: A meta-analysis. *Journal of International Medical Research, 48*(6), 300060520931348. https://doi.org/10.1177/0300060520931348

Colombage, U. N., Lin, K. Y., Soh, S. E., & Frawley, H. C. (2021). Prevalence and impact of bladder and bowel disorders in women with breast cancer: A systematic review with meta-analysis. *Neurourology and Urodynamics, 40*(1), 15–27. https://doi.org/10.1002/nau.24531

Cook, E. D., Iglehart, E. I., Baum, G., Schover, L. L., & Newman, L. L. (2017). Missing documentation in breast cancer survivors: Genitourinary syndrome of menopause. *Menopause, 24*(12), 1360–1364. https://doi.org/10.1097/gme.0000000000000926

Crouzet, S., Chapelon, J. Y., Rouvière, O., Mege-Lechevallier, F., Colombel, M., Tonoli-Catez, H., Martin, X., & Gelet, A. (2014). Whole-gland ablation of localized prostate cancer with high-intensity focused ultrasound: Oncologic outcomes and morbidity in 1002 patients. *European Urology, 65*(5), 907–914. https://doi.org/10.1016/j.eururo.2013.04.039

de Lira, G. H. S., Fornari, A., Cardoso, L. F., Aranchipe, M., Kretiska, C., & Rhoden, E. L. (2019). Effects of perioperative pelvic floor muscle training on early recovery of urinary continence and erectile function in men undergoing radical prostatectomy: A randomized clinical trial. *International Brazilian Journal of Urology, 45*(6), 1196–1203. https://doi.org/10.1590/s1677-5538.ibju.2019.0238

Ditah, I., Devaki, P., Luma, H. N., Ditah, C., Njei, B., Jaiyeoba, C., Salami, A., Ditah, C., Ewelukwa, O., & Szarka, L. (2014). Prevalence, trends, and risk factors for fecal incontinence in United States Adults, 2005–2010. *Clinical Gastroenterology and Hepatology, 12*(4), 636–643.e632. https://doi.org/10.1016/j.cgh.2013.07.020

Dumoulin, C., Morin, M., Danieli, C., Cacciari, L., Mayrand, M. H., Tousignant, M., & Abrahamowicz, M. (2020). Group-Based vs individual pelvic floor muscle training to treat urinary incontinence in older women: A randomized clinical trial. *JAMA Internal Medicine, 180*(10), 1284–1293. https://doi.org/10.1001/jamainternmed.2020.2993

Emmons, K. R., & Robinson, J. P. (2013). Urinary incontinence severity and quality-of-life instruments. *Journal of Wound Ostomy & Continence Nursing, 40*(4), 350–354. https://doi.org/10.1097/WON.0b013e318297c766

Eypasch, E., Williams, J. I., Wood-Dauphinee, S., Ure, B. M., Schmülling, C., Neugebauer, E., & Troidl, H. (1995). Gastrointestinal Quality of Life

Index: Development, validation and application of a new instrument. *British Journal of Surgery, 82*(2), 216–222. https://doi.org/10.1002/bjs.1800820229

Ficarra, V., Novara, G., Rosen, R. C., Artibani, W., Carroll, P. R., Costello, A., Menon, M., Montorsi, F., Patel, V. R., Stolzenburg, J.-U., Van der Poel, H., Wilson, T. G., Zattoni, F., & Mottrie, A. (2012). Systematic review and meta-analysis of studies reporting urinary continence recovery after robot-assisted radical prostatectomy. *European Urology, 62*(3), 405–417. https://doi.org/10.1016/j.eururo.2012.05.045

Firmeza, M. A., Vasconcelos, C. T. M., Vasconcelos Neto, J. A., Brito, L. G. O., Alves, F. M., & Oliveira, N. M. V. (2022). The effects of hysterectomy on urinary and sexual functions of women with cervical cancer: A systematic review. *Revista Brasileira de Ginecologia e Obstetrícia, 44*(8), 790–796. https://doi.org/10.1055/s-0042-1748972

Franzen, K., Andersson, G., Odeberg, J., Midlöv, P., Samuelsson, E., Stenzelius, K., & Hammarström, M. (2015). Surgery for urinary incontinence in women 65 years and older: A systematic review. *International Urogynecology Journal, 26*(8), 1095–1102. https://doi.org/10.1007/s00192-014-2573-9

Frey, A., Pedersen, C., Lindberg, H., Bisbjerg, R., Sønksen, J., & Fode, M. (2017). Prevalence and predicting factors for commonly neglected sexual side effects to external-beam radiation therapy for prostate cancer. *The Journal of Sexual Medicine, 14*(4), 558–565. https://doi.org/10.1016/j.jsxm.2017.01.015

Gandi, C., & Sacco, E. (2021). Pharmacological management of urinary incontinence: Current and emerging treatment. *Clinical Pharmacology, 13,* 209–223. https://doi.org/10.2147/cpaa.S289323

Geraerts, I., Van Poppel, H., Devoogdt, N., De Groef, A., Fieuws, S., & Van Kampen, M. (2016). Pelvic floor muscle training for erectile dysfunction and climacturia 1 year after nerve sparing radical prostatectomy: A randomized controlled trial. *International Journal of Impotence Research, 28*(1), 9–13. https://doi.org/10.1038/ijir.2015.24

Ghaderi, F., Mohammadi, K., Amir Sasan, R., Niko Kheslat, S., & Oskouei, A. E. (2016). Effects of stabilization exercises focusing on pelvic floor muscles on low back pain and urinary incontinence in women. *Urology, 93,* 50–54. https://doi.org/10.1016/j.urology.2016.03.034

Gong, X., Jin, Z., & Zheng, Q. (2012). Anorectal function after partial intersphincteric resection in ultra-low rectal cancer. *Colorectal Disease, 14*(12), e802–e806. https://doi.org/10.1111/j.1463-1318.2012.03177.x

Haglind, E., Carlsson, S., Stranne, J., Wallerstedt, A., Wilderäng, U., Thorsteinsdottir, T., Lagerkvist, M., Damber, J.-E., Bjartell, A., Hugosson, J., Wiklund, P., & Steineck, G. (2015). Urinary incontinence and erectile dysfunction after robotic versus open radical prostatectomy: A prospective, controlled, nonrandomised trial. *European Urology, 68*(2), 216–225. https://doi.org/10.1016/j.eururo.2015.02.029

Horisberger, K., Rothenhoefer, S., Kripp, M., Hofheinz, R. D., Post, S., & Kienle, P. (2014). Impaired continence function five years after intensified chemoradiation in patients with locally advanced rectal cancer. *European Journal of Surgical Oncology, 40*(2), 227–233. https://doi.org/10.1016/j.ejso.2013.11.029

Iarrobino, N. A., Gill, B., Sutera, P. A., Kalash, R., D'Ambrosio, ., & Heron, D. E. (2019). Early exploratory analysis for patient-reported quality of life and dosimetric correlates in hypofractionated stereotactic body radiation therapy (SBRT) for low-risk and intermediate-risk prostate cancer: Interim results from a prospective phase II clinical trial. *American Journal of Clinical Oncology, 42*(11), 856–861. https://doi.org/10.1097/coc.0000000000000586

Kannady, C., & Clavell-Hernández, J. (2020). Orgasm-associated urinary incontinence (climacturia) following radical prostatectomy: A review of pathophysiology and current treatment options. *Asian Journal of Andrology, 22*(6), 549–554. https://doi.org/10.4103/aja.aja_145_19

King, T., & Almallah, Y. Z. (2012). Post-radical-prostatectomy urinary incontinence: The management of concomitant bladder neck contracture. *Advances in Urology, 2012*, 295798. https://doi.org/10.1155/2012/295798

Kuo, L. J., Lin, Y. C., Lai, C. H., Lin, Y. K., Huang, Y. S., Hu, C. C., & Chen, S. C. (2015). Improvement of fecal incontinence and quality of life by electrical stimulation and biofeedback for patients with low rectal cancer after intersphincteric resection. *Archives of Physical Medicine and Rehabilitation, 96*(8), 1442–1447. https://doi.org/10.1016/j.apmr.2015.03.013

Kutluturkan, S., Urvaylioglu, A. E., & Kilic, D. (2021). Effect of Kegel exercises on the prevention of urinary and fecal incontinence in patients with prostate cancer undergoing radiotherapy. *European Journal of Oncology Nursing: The Official Journal of European Oncology Nursing Society, 51*, 101913–101913. https://doi.org/10.1016/j.ejon.2021.101913

Lai, X., Wong, F. K., & Ching, S. S. (2013). Review of bowel dysfunction of rectal cancer patients during the first five years after sphincter-preserving surgery: A population in need of nursing attention. *European Journal of Oncology Nursing, 17*(5), 681–692. https://doi.org/10.1016/j.ejon.2013.06.001

Lai, X., Zhang, J., Chen, J., Lai, C., & Huang, C. (2020). Is electroacupuncture safe and effective for treatment of stress urinary incontinence in women? A systematic review and meta-analysis. *Journal of International Medical Research, 48*(10), 300060520948337. https://doi.org/10.1177/0300060520948337

Lal, N., Simillis, C., Slesser, A., Kontovounisios, C., Rasheed, S., Tekkis, P. P., & Tan, E. (2019). A systematic review of the literature reporting on randomised controlled trials comparing treatments for faecal incontinence in adults. *Acta Chirurgica Belgica, 119*(1), 1–15. https://doi.org/10.1080/00015458.2018.149392

Lardas, M., Grivas, N., Debray, T. P. A., Zattoni, F., Berridge, C., Cumberbatch, M., Van den Broeck, T., Briers, E., De Santis, M., Farolfi, A., Fossati, N., Gandaglia, G., Gillessen, S., O'Hanlon, S., Henry, A., Liew, L., Mason, M., Moris, L., Oprea-Lager, D., & Mottet, N. (2022). Patient-and Tumour-related prognostic factors for urinary incontinence after radical prostatectomy for nonmetastatic prostate cancer: A systematic review and meta-analysis. *European Urology Focus, 8*(3), 674–689. https://doi.org/10.1016/j.euf.2021.04.020

Lin, Y. H., Yang, H. Y., Hung, S. L., Chen, H. P., Liu, K. W., Chen, T. B., & Chi, S. C. (2016). Effects of pelvic floor muscle exercise on faecal incontinence in rectal cancer patients after stoma closure. *European Journal of Cancer Care (England), 25*(3), 449–457. https://doi.org/10.1111/ecc.12292

Lipp, A., Shaw, C., & Glavind, K. (2014). Mechanical devices for urinary incontinence in women. *Cochrane Database of Systematic Reviews, 2014*(12), Cd001756. https://doi.org/10.1002/14651858.CD001756.pub6

Macaulay, M., Broadbridge, J., Gage, H., Williams, P., Birch, B., Moore, K. N., Cottenden, A., & Fader, M. J. (2015). A trial of devices for urinary incontinence after treatment for prostate cancer. *BJU International, 116*(3), 432–442. https://doi.org/10.1111/bju.13016

Mehta, A., Deveci, S., & Mulhall, J. P. (2013). Efficacy of a penile variable tension loop for improving climacturia after radical prostatectomy. *BJU International, 111*(3), 500–504. https://doi.org/10.1111/j.1464-410X.2012.11269.x

Milios, J. E., Ackland, T. R., & Green, D. J. (2019). Pelvic floor muscle training in radical prostatectomy: A randomized controlled trial of the impacts on pelvic floor muscle function and urinary incontinence. *BMC Urology, 19*(1), 116. https://doi.org/10.1186/s12894-019-0546-5

Milsom, I., & Gyhagen, M. (2019). The prevalence of urinary incontinence. *Climacteric, 22*(3), 217–222. https://doi.org/10.1080/13697137.2018.1543263

Minassian, V. A., Yan, X. S., Sun, H., Platte, R. O., & Stewart, W. F. (2016). Clinical validation of the Bladder Health Survey for urinary incontinence in a population sample of women. *International Urogynecology Journal, 27*(3), 453–461. https://doi.org/10.1007/s00192-015-2849-8

Rockwood, T. H. (2004). Incontinence severity and QOL scales for fecal incontinence. *Gastroenterology, 126*, S106–S113. https://doi.org/10.1053/j.gastro.2003.10.057

Rockwood, T. H., Church, J. M., Fleshman, J. W., Kane, R. L., Mavrantonis, C., Thorson, A. G., Wexner, S., Bliss, D., & Lowry, A. C. (2000). Fecal incontinence quality of life scale: Quality of life instrument for patients with fecal incontinence. *Diseases of the Colon & Rectum, 43*(1), 9–16; discussion 16–17. https://doi.org/10.1007/bf02237236

Rutledge, T. L., Heckman, S. R., Qualls, C., Muller, C. Y., & Rogers, R. G. (2010). Pelvic floor disorders and sexual function in gynecologic cancer survivors: A cohort study. *American Journal of Obstetrics and Gynecology, 203*(5), 514.e511–514.e517. https://doi.org/10.1016/j.ajog.2010.08.004

Rutledge, T. L., Rogers, R., Lee, S. J., & Muller, C. Y. (2014). A pilot randomized control trial to evaluate pelvic floor muscle training for urinary incontinence among gynecologic cancer survivors. *Gynecologic Oncology, 132*(1), 154–158. https://doi.org/10.1016/j.ygyno.2013.10.024

Sacco, E., Prayer-Galetti, T., Pinto, F., Fracalanza, S., Betto, G., Pagano, F., & Artibani, W. (2006). Urinary incontinence after radical prostatectomy: Incidence by definition, risk factors and temporal trend in a large series with a long-term follow-up. *BJU International, 97*(6), 1234–1241. https://doi.org/10.1111/j.1464-410X.2006.06185.x

Sandhu, J. S., Breyer, B., Comiter, C., Eastham, J. A., Gomez, C., Kirages, D. J., Kittle, C., Lucioni, A., Nitti, V. W., Stoffel, J. T., Westney, O. L., Murad, M. H., & McCammon, K. (2019). Incontinence after prostate treatment: AUA/SUFU guideline. *The Journal of Urology, 202*(2), 369–378. https://doi.org/10.1097/ju.0000000000000314

Seong, M.-K., Jung, S.-I., Kim, T.-W., & Joh, H.-K. (2011). Comparative analysis of summary scoring systems in measuring fecal incontinence. *Journal of the Korean Surgical Society, 81*(5), 326–331. https://doi.org/10.4174/jkss.2011.81.5.326

Simillis, C., Lal, N., Qiu, S., Kontovounisios, C., Rasheed, S., Tan, E., & Tekkis, P. P. (2018). Sacral nerve stimulation versus percutaneous tibial nerve stimulation for faecal incontinence: A systematic review and meta-analysis. *International Journal of Colorectal Disease, 33*(5), 645–648. https://doi.org/10.1007/s00384-018-2976-z

Sipaviciute, A., Aukstikalnis, T., Samalavicius, N. E., & Dulskas, A. (2021). The role of traditional acupuncture in patients with fecal incontinence-mini-review. *International Journal of Environmental Research and Public Health, 18*(4). https://doi.org/10.3390/ijerph18042112

Soto González, M., Da Cuña Carrera, I., Gutiérrez Nieto, M., López García, S., Ojea Calvo, A., & Lantarón Caeiro, E. M. (2020). Early 3-month treatment with comprehensive physical therapy program restores continence in urinary incontinence patients after radical prostatectomy: A randomized controlled trial. *Neurourology and Urodynamics, 39*(5), 1529–1537. https://doi.org/10.1002/nau.24389

Soto González, M., Da Cuña Carrera, I., Lantarón Caeiro, E. M., Gutiérrez Nieto, M., López García, S., & Ojea Calvo, A. (2018). Correlation between the 1-hour and 24-hour pad test in the assessment of male patients with post-prostatectomy urinary incontinence. *Progrès en Urologie, 28*(11), 536–541. https://doi.org/10.1016/j.purol.2018.06.011

Steineck, G., Bjartell, A., Hugosson, J., Axén, E., Carlsson, S., Stranne, J., Wallerstedt, A., Persson, J., Wilderäng, U., Thorsteinsdottir, T., Gustafsson, O., Lagerkvist, M., Jiborn, T., Haglind, E., & Wiklund, P. (2015). Degree of preservation of the neurovascular bundles during radical prostatectomy and urinary continence 1 year after surgery. *European Urology, 67*(3), 559–568. https://doi.org/10.1016/j.eururo.2014.10.011

Syan, R., & Brucker, B. M. (2016). Guideline of guidelines: Urinary incontinence. *BJU International, 117*(1), 20–33. https://doi.org/10.1111/bju.13187

Talley, K. M. C., Davis, N. J., Peden-McAlpine, C., Martin, C. L., Weinfurter, E. V., & Wyman, J. F. (2021). Navigating through incontinence: A qualitative systematic review and meta-aggregation of the experiences of family caregivers. *International Journal of Nursing Studies, 123*, 104062. https://doi.org/10.1016/j.ijnurstu.2021.104062

Ussing, A., Dahn, I., Due, U., Sørensen, M., Petersen, J., & Bandholm, T. (2019). Efficacy of supervised pelvic floor muscle training and biofeedback vs attention-control treatment in adults with fecal incontinence. *Clinical Gastroenterology and Hepatology, 17*(11), 2253–2261.e2254. https://doi.org/10.1016/j.cgh.2018.12.015

Wallerstedt, A., Nyberg, T., Carlsson, S., Thorsteinsdottir, T., Stranne, J., Tyritzis, S. I., Kollberg, K. S., Hugosson, J., Bjartell, A., Wilderäng, U., Wiklund, P., Steineck, G., & Haglind, E. (2019). Quality of life after open radical prostatectomy compared with robot-assisted radical prostatectomy. *European Urology Focus, 5*(3), 389–398. https://doi.org/10.1016/j.euf.2017.12.010

Wang, W., Liu, Y., Sun, S., Liu, B., Su, T., Zhou, J., & Liu, Z. (2019). Electroacupuncture for postmenopausal women with stress urinary incontinence: Secondary analysis of a randomized controlled trial. *World Journal of Urology, 37*(7), 1421–1427. https://doi.org/10.1007/s00345-018-2521-2

Ward, W. L., Hahn, E. A., Mo, F., Hernandez, L., Tulsky, D. S., & Cella, D. (1999). Reliability and validity of the Functional Assessment of Cancer Therapy-Colorectal (FACT-C) quality of life instrument. *Quality of Life Research, 8*(3), 181–195. https://doi.org/10.1023/A:1008821826499

Wei, J. T., Dunn, R. L., Marcovich, R., Montie, J. E., & Sanda, M. G. (2000). Prospective assessment of patient reported urinary continence after radical prostatectomy. *The Journal of Urology, 164*(3 Pt 1), 744–748. https://doi.org/10.1097/00005392-200009010-00029

Wu, C., Newman, D. K., & Palmer, M. H. (2020). Unsupervised behavioral and pelvic floor muscle training programs for storage lower urinary tract symptoms in women: A systematic review. *International Urogynecology Journal, 31*(12), 2485–2497. https://doi.org/10.1007/s00192-020-04498-9

Wu, J., Ye, T., Lv, J., He, Z., & Zhu, J. (2019). Laparoscopic nerve-sparing radical hysterectomy vs laparoscopic radical hysterectomy in cervical cancer: A systematic review and meta-analysis of clinical efficacy and bladder dysfunction. *Journal of Minimally Invasive Gynecology, 26*(3), 417–426.e416. https://doi.org/10.1016/j.jmig.2018.10.012

Zhang, A. Y., Bodner, D. R., Fu, A. Z., Gunzler, D. D., Klein, E., Kresevic, D., Moore, S., Ponsky, L., Purdum, M., Strauss, G., & Zhu, H. (2015). Effects of patient centered interventions on persistent urinary incontinence after prostate cancer treatment: A randomized, controlled trial. *Journal of Urology, 194*(6), 1675–1681. https://doi.org/10.1016/j.juro.2015.07.090

Zhang, A. Y., Burant, C., Fu, A. Z., Strauss, G., Bodner, D. R., & Ponsky, L. (2020). Psychosocial mechanisms of a behavioral treatment for urinary incontinence of prostate cancer survivors. *Journal of Psychosocial Oncology, 38*(2), 210–227. https://doi.org/10.1080/07347332.2019.1678547

Zhang, A. Y., Ganocy, S., Fu, A. Z., Kresevic, D., Ponsky, L., Strauss, G., Bodner, D. R., & Zhu, H. (2019). Mood outcomes of a behavioral treatment for urinary incontinence in prostate cancer survivors. *Supportive Care in Cancer, 27*(12), 4461–4467. https://doi.org/10.1007/s00520-019-04745-w

CHAPTER 17

SEXUAL DYSFUNCTION IN WOMEN

INTRODUCTION

The sexuality concerns of many women who have been treated for cancer are an unmet need (Stabile et al., 2017) despite recognition that multiple facets of sexual functioning are affected by cancer treatments. Up to a quarter of partnered women are not sexually active and are dissatisfied with the situation (Marino et al., 2017). It is important to recognize that, in women treated for cancer, no single area of sexual function is likely to be effectively targeted for treatment; global sexual function is more often the focus of treatment (Pyke & Clayton, 2019). Loss of libido, arousal difficulties, pain with penetration or sexual touch, and alterations in orgasms, along with body image concerns, are intertwined for these women and a global approach to assessment and treatment is needed. For example, loss of breast sensuality and the subsequent impact on their sexual response are important to women treated for breast cancer.

PREVALENCE

Sexual concerns are a significant issue for women after treatment for cancer; the prevalence of sexual dysfunction overall ranges from 33% to 43%. Of women with breast cancer, 74% qualify for a diagnosis of female sexual dysfunction (Jing et al., 2019).

CONTRIBUTING FACTORS

All treatments for cancer, including surgery, radiation, chemotherapy, and endocrine manipulation therapy, impact on sexual function.

GENERAL ASSESSMENT OF SEXUAL DYSFUNCTION

Oncology care clinicians may not feel comfortable starting the conversation, yet there are models that have been shown to be effective in initiating a conversation about sexual concerns. It is important to ask about any distress associated with sexual symptoms because, if there is no or low distress, the woman may not be interested in doing anything about it. Commonly, distress is related to the impact of problems with sexual functioning on their primary relationship. For women who are not in a sexual relationship, they may be concerned about how this may affect a future relationship or if they are willing to engage in a relationship in the future. There are a number of general assessment models that can be used, as outlined in Figure 17.1.

PLISSIT Model

Permission—give the patient permission to ask questions by introducing the topic.
Limited **I**nformation—most patients want validation.
Specific **S**uggestion—provide guidance based on the concerns of the patient.
Intensive **T**herapy—refer patient to a specialist, e.g., sex therapist, gynecologist (Annon, 1974).

BETTER Model

Bring up the topic—give the patient the opportunity to ask questions or voice their concerns.
Explain that sexuality is part of quality of life—validate the patient's concerns.
Timing may not be right.
Tell the patient that resources will be found.
Educate the patient about the sexual side effects of their treatment.
Record that the conversation has been carried out (Mick et al., 2003).

CARD Model

Cancer treatment can affect sexual health which is important to many women and couples' quality of life.
Ask what concerns the patient has.
Resources/referrals should be provided to the patient.
Document that the conversation has been carried out (Wang et al., 2015).

5 A's Model

Ask whether the patient has any sexuality concerns.
Assess by asking additional questions.
Advise the patient that you are able to help.
Assist the patient in finding solutions.
Arrange for follow-up (Bober & Varela, 2012).

Figure 17.1 Models for assessment of sexuality.

ASSESSMENT OF SPECIFIC SEXUAL SYMPTOMS

Loss of Libido

Introduction: Loss of libido is extremely common in female cancer survivors; 85% of women on aromatase inhibitors report low libido (Robinson et al., 2017).

Contributing factors: Surgical menopause is more likely to impact negatively on libido than natural menopause (Bıldırcın et al., 2020). Chemotherapy-induced menopause in younger women is also associated with low or absent libido (Cameron et al., 2018; Javadpour et al., 2021). Pain with penetration (dyspareunia) is a contributor to loss of libido as well (Robinson et al., 2017). Other conditions, such as incontinence (Pinheiro Sobreira Bezerra et al., 2020), also have a negative impact on desire.

Assessment: There are no formal measures to assess libido, but the following questions and prompts may be useful:

- What was your previous interest in sex like?
- How has this changed?
- Is this distressing to you?
- What do you think is the cause of this?
- What other factors might be involved?

(*Prompts:* e.g., relationship status/changes, body image, treatment/medication)

Management of low or absent libido:

- *Nonpharmaceutical:* Mindfulness-based meditation has been shown to be effective in improving libido in women with cancer (Jaderek & Lew-Starowicz, 2019). Mindfulness-based sex therapy has also been shown to be effective in treating women with a variety of sexual problems, including low desire and arousal (Brotto et al., 2016; Gunst et al., 2019). For women with loss of libido related to altered body image, cognitive behavioral therapy (CBT), communication training, and sensate focus exercises may be helpful in addressing the psychological and emotional factors that impact on their sexual self-image (ter Kuile et al., 2010). Involvement of the partner in couple's counseling may also be of benefit as a result of improved communication between partners (Regan et al., 2012). Sex therapy or counseling may also be of benefit; discovering the reasons for diminished desire will help identify interventions to improve this aspect of the survivor's sexual experience (Streicher & Simon, 2018). While most sex therapy sessions occur face to face, there is preliminary evidence that an internet-based CBT program improves sexual interest (Stephenson et al., 2021). If the reason for decreased libido is related to pain with sexual touch or penetration (dyspareunia), vaginal lubricants and moisturizers are a first-line treatment.

- *Pharmaceutical:* There has been much interest in a pharmaceutical treatment for low libido in women. The focus has been on the use of androgens (e.g., testosterone; Islam et al., 2019) to increase libido, which have not been approved by the Food and Drug Administration (FDA; Vegunta et al., 2020) due to safety concerns (Jayasena et al., 2019). Two oral medications (flibanserin [Addyi] and bremelanotide [Vyleesi]) have been studied in

Dyspareunia

Introduction: Vulvovaginal atrophy (VVA), one of the symptoms of the genitourinary syndrome of menopause, is common in women after treatment for cancer (Crean-Tate et al., 2020). Loss of elasticity of the tissues as well as loss of lubrication due to changes in vascular function lead to diminished or absent signs of arousal and painful intercourse (Streicher & Simon, 2018). Women describe pain with sexual touch or vaginal penetration, as well as stinging or burning with urination and tenderness when wiping with toilet tissue.

Contributing factors: The use of aromatase inhibitors for prevention of breast cancer recurrence in postmenopausal women is associated with genitourinary syndrome of menopause (Kuehn et al., 2019).

Dyspareunia in turn impacts negatively on libido (Zhu et al., 2019). The impact of these medications on sexual function may lead to discontinuation of therapy (Bowles et al., 2012). Ovarian suppression used in the adjuvant setting for premenopausal women with breast cancer is also associated with genitourinary syndrome of menopause (Bui et al., 2020). Women who are treated with radiation to the pelvis for gynecologic or rectal/anal cancer develop adhesions and shortening of the vagina; stenosis of the vagina will also lead to pain with penetration and pelvic examinations (Summerfield & Leong, 2020). The experience of pain with attempted penetration leads to a cycle of anticipatory pain and a resultant shortening and tightening of the pelvic floor muscles.

Prevalence: Of breast cancer survivors, 42% to 70% report VVA leading to absent arousal and dyspareunia as a result (Biglia et al., 2003). Up to 88% of women who undergo radiation therapy for gynecologic cancer experience vaginal stenosis (Damast et al., 2019).

Assessment:

- The Vaginal Assessment Scale (VAS) and the Vulvar Assessment Scale (VuAS) are validated tools that are completed by the clinician (Eaton et al., 2017) along with a gynecologic exam.

- The Female Sexual Function Index (FSFI; Rosen et al., 2000) is a more complex self-report instrument comprising 19 items that has been validated for use in women with breast cancer (Baser et al., 2012). The FSFI can be downloaded along with the scoring sheet at www.FSFIquestionnaire.com. A shorter version of this tool, the FSFI-6 (Isidori et al., 2010), contains questions about desire, arousal, lubrication, orgasm, satisfaction, and pain.

```
Moisturizers
Lubricants
  • Water-based
  • Silicone-based
Lidocaine
Low-dose local estrogen
Ospemifene
DHEA (Prasterone™)
```

Figure 17.2 Food and Drug Administration-approved management of dyspareunia. DHEA, dehydroepiandrosterone.

■ The Patient-Reported Outcomes Measurement Information System (PROMIS) Sexual Function and Satisfaction Measure v2.0 (SexSF) contains 131 items that measure a wide variety of domains (Narang et al., 2017). Due to its length, it is likely to be too cumbersome for clinical use.

Of note is that these questionnaires do not address distress, an important criterion in the assessment of sexual dysfunction, as well as focus on penetration that may not be applicable to all women. **Management of dyspareunia:** Management of dyspareunia requires a stepped approach.

NONPHARMACEUTICAL MANAGEMENT OF DYSPAREUNIA (FIGURE 17.2)

■ *Moisturizers:* Women are usually advised to start with the use of moisturizers and/or lubricants. It is important to remember that vaginal moisturizers address vaginal dryness only and are not sufficient for penetration. Vaginal moisturizers are designed to rehydrate vaginal tissues and adhere to the vaginal walls; they are used for daily comfort. A variety are available, including over-the-counter vaginal moisturizers, that contain no hormones, with the most effective products containing hyaluronic acid. This ingredient has been shown to be as effective as local estrogen in some women (dos Santos et al., 2021). Because the effects of moisturizers last a few days, they should be used every 2 to 3 days. For women with vulvar dryness, a gel product is preferable to those in suppository form; the gel can be applied externally with a finger. Moisturizers should be used at night so that they can be absorbed fully. Care should be taken to avoid ingredients that contain parabens, glycerin, glycols, nonoxynol-9, or chlorhexidine. Because many women may not be able to read the ingredients of the moisturizers, or the ingredient list may not be clear on the packaging, the healthcare clinician should have a list of recommended products to give to women.

■ *Lubricants:* Lubricants are used for sexual touch and/or penetration and as such provide some comfort to women who experience pain during sexual activity by reducing friction. They should have similar pH and osmolality as vaginal moisturizers, and care should be taken to avoid lubricants that contain irritants (Potter & Panay, 2021), something that is common in lubricants that purport to be warming, cooling, or intensifying. Water-based lubricants are good entry-level products; however, in women treated for cancer, silicone-based lubricants are often more effective. Silicone-based lubricants will have the suffix "-cone" on the list of ingredients. They are freely available at most drugstores or are available online. However, the full list of ingredients may not be printed on the label and so some research may be needed on the product's website to determine exactly what the product contains. Lubricants should be replenished as frequently as necessary during sexual activity; a few drops should be placed on the external genitalia and on the partner's penis or sex toy before penetration. Silicone lubricants should not be used with silicone sex toys as they cause the sex toy to degrade. Hybrid lubricants contain both silicone and ingredients found in water-based lubricants. Any oils (e.g., coconut) should not be used as a lubricant.

- *Pelvic floor physiotherapy:* Pelvic floor physiotherapy has been shown to be an effective but underused intervention in the management of dyspareunia (Berghmans, 2018). A qualified pelvic floor physiotherapist will use a combination of education, manual therapy, pelvic floor muscle exercises with or without biofeedback, as well as home practice to treat women. In one study, 90% of women reported improvement after a 12-week course of treatment (Cyr et al., 2020). Pelvic floor physiotherapy has also been shown to improve pain anxiety and pain catastrophizing in women treated for gynecologic cancer (Cyr et al., 2021). The addition of dilators to this therapy may be of benefit; however, there is no high-level evidence on this (Brennen et al., 2020). The American Board of Physical Therapy Specialties (https://aptaapps.apta.org//APTAPTDirectory/FindAPTDirectory.aspx) has a directory of physiotherapists who specialize in pelvic floor physiotherapy. Not all physiotherapists have been trained in the assessment and management of pelvic floor dysfunction and it is important that a referral be made only to those who have specialty training in these techniques.

- *Dilators:* The use of vaginal dilators is recommended for prevention of vaginal stenosis after radiation therapy to the pelvis. *Stenosis* refers to the shortening and narrowing of the vagina due to the buildup of scar tissue secondary to radiation and loss of estrogen due to medical or surgical menopause (Damast et al., 2019). Women who undergo pelvic radiation are encouraged to use dilators. There are no established guidelines for the initiation or duration of dilator use (Liu et al., 2021), but a consensus opinion suggests that women should use the dilator for 5 to 10 minutes, two to three times a week for an indefinite period

(Matos et al., 2019). It is recommended that women treated with brachytherapy (internal radiation) may need to use dilators for an extended period of time (Stahl et al., 2019). Adherence to the recommended course of treatment with dilators is low, with an average of 50% of women using dilators for 1 year (Haddad et al., 2021). Women report not liking to use dilators as they think the dilator is a sex toy (Cullen et al., 2012) or that it reminds them of their cancer (Bakker et al., 2015). Providing education along with written information improves adherence (Lubotzky et al., 2019).

- *Mindfulness meditation:* Mindfulness meditation is a practice in which purposeful attention to the present moment in a compassionate and nonjudgmental manner is used (Jaderek & Lew-Starowicz, 2019). This practice has shown efficacy in reducing pain with sexual activity in women with gynecologic cancer (Brotto et al., 2008b, 2012). It has also been shown to be helpful in women who experience difficulties with arousal (Brotto, Basson, et al., 2008a; Brotto et al., 2016) and in those with low or absent libido (Brotto & Basson, 2014).

- *Laser and energy-based devices:* Despite significant interest in the use of fractional CO_2 erbium lasers for treatment of the genitourinary syndrome of menopause, there has been limited evidence on their efficacy (Siliquini et al., 2021). Almost all of the studies of these devices are small and observational with short follow-up, if any (Mounir et al., 2021), and there have been no randomized clinical trials to date (Sarmento et al., 2021). Safety outcomes are also underreported (Mension et al., 2022), but cases of scarring, fibrosis, and agglutination of the vaginal walls have been reported (Gordon et al., 2019). In 2018, the FDA released a statement warning against the use of lasers and energy-based devices in treating this condition (FDA, 2018). A limited number of studies have included women with breast cancer (Jha et al., 2019; Quick et al., 2022; Sussman et al., 2019) or gynecologic cancer (Mejia-Gomez et al., 2022). The conclusions reached are that these therapies need large, randomized clinical trials before they can be recommended to women with cancer.

PHARMACEUTICAL MANAGEMENT OF DYSPAREUNIA

- *Lidocaine:* Four percent aqueous lidocaine has been shown to be effective in managing pain at the vaginal introitus (Goetsch et al., 2015). Soaking a gauze pad or cotton ball in the solution and holding it over the area where the pain is most severe for 3 minutes allows for penetration without transfer to the partner. A silicone-based lubricant should be used after application of local lidocaine.

- *Local low-dose estrogen:* If moisturizers and lubricants do not provide relief of pain, local low-dose estrogen can be considered; however, there is controversy regarding the risk of recurrence of hormone-sensitive cancers (Mension et al., 2021). Oncologists are often concerned about this and may refuse to prescribe this therapy (Biglia et al., 2017). In one study of physician behaviors toward treatment of VVA, only 34% of gynecologists and 17% of primary care clinicians felt comfortable prescribing estrogen to women with a history of breast cancer (Kingsberg et al., 2019). However, it has been shown that low-dose (10 mcg) estradiol tablets (Vagifem) or Imvexxy (4 mcg estradiol in a bioadhesive oil) do not increase hormone levels above the postmenopausal range after 1 year of use (Eugster-Hausmann et al., 2010). In women on tamoxifen, the effects of local estrogen may be blocked due to the effects of tamoxifen on estrogen receptors (Cox & Panay, 2019); there is some concern that local estrogen may compromise the effectiveness of aromatase inhibitors. In a meta-analysis of studies on the safety of local estrogen in women on aromatase inhibitors, no systemic absorption of the product was seen and the authors of the meta-analysis concluded that it is safe to prescribe local estrogen to postmenopausal women in this scenario (Pavlović et al., 2019). It is important that the healthcare clinician has a comprehensive discussion with women about the potential risks and benefits so women can make an informed choice on whether to use local estrogen or not.

- *Ospemifene:* A selective estrogen receptor modulator (SERM), ospemifene, has been shown to be effective in treating vulvovaginal dryness with few side effects, with hot flashes being the most common side effect reported (Pingarron et al., 2021), along with a slight increase in urinary tract (Di Donato et al., 2019b). It is an oral agent with a single daily dose of 60 mg (Di Donato et al., 2019a). It is not associated with an increased risk of breast cancer (Pup & Sánchez-Borrego, 2020), and no increased risk of breast cancer recurrence was seen in a matched cohort study (Cai et al., 2020). Adherence and cost are also better than with local estrogen (Faught et al., 2019).

- *Dehydroepiandrosterone (DHEA):* Intravaginal DHEA (Prasterone) 6.5 mg has been shown to be effective in the treatment of genitourinary syndrome of menopause (Simon et al., 2018), with hormone levels within normal postmenopausal levels (Labrie et al., 2016). In women with breast or gynecologic cancer, a rise in blood estrogen levels to within the postmenopausal range has been seen, but not in those taking aromatase inhibitors; improvements were seen in vaginal cytology (Barton et al., 2018). In a systematic review of interventions, DHEA is of greater benefit to sexual function than local estrogen (Febrina et al., 2022).

CHAPTER 17 • SEXUAL DYSFUNCTION IN WOMEN **169**

■ *Intravaginal testosterone:* There is preliminary evidence that the use of intravaginal testosterone (at doses of 150 or 300 mcg) is safe in women with breast cancer who are on endocrine manipulation therapy (Lemke, 2017); however, there is no FDA-approved form of testosterone for women (Karram et al., 2021).

Alterations in Orgasms

Introduction: Low or absent libido or dyspareunia can impact on the woman's ability to achieve orgasms. Altered body image and altered breast sensations may lead to altered orgasm capability. Pelvic floor dysfunction, specifically hypertonic muscles as a result of dyspareunia, may make orgasms more painful.

Contributing factors: One study of women under 35 years of age found that orgasms were affected more frequently than other domains of sexuality (Blouet et al., 2019). Body image changes may also be associated with altered orgasms (van de Grift et al., 2020). Women with colon cancer report a reduction in orgasms following treatment (Milbury et al., 2013). It is important to note that some women may have pretreatment problems with orgasms (Traa et al., 2014) that are exacerbated by cancer treatment.

Assessment of changes to or absence of orgasms: The Bodily Sensations of Orgasm questionnaire (Dubray et al., 2017) is a 22-item questionnaire. While seldom used in clinical practice, it allows for an evaluation of the physical sensations of orgasm. More commonly, questions such as "How have your orgasms changed since . . . " are asked.

Management of orgasmic changes: See Figure 17.3.

Alterations to Body Image

Introduction: Changes to body image after cancer treatment are common and occur in women with a variety of cancers. Most of the research has been done in women with breast cancer because of the role that the breasts play in femininity (Przezdziecki et al., 2013). It is important for women to have a realistic understanding of the esthetic

Reviewing the medications that the woman has been prescribed may identify the contribution of agents such as the selective serotonin reuptake inhibitors (SSRIs) that are known to inhibit orgasms (Lorenz et al., 2016).

Medical devices such as the Eros-Clitoral Therapy Device (https://gesiva.com/product/eros-therapy-kit/), an FDA-approved device that provides gentle suction to the clitoris, may be helpful for some women.

The use of a vibrator may also be useful.

Figure 17.3 Treating the underlying cause of orgasmic changes is the first step. FDA, Food and Drug Administration.

Source: From IsHak, W. W., Bokarius, A., Jeffrey, J. K., Davis, M. C., & Bakhta, Y. (2010). Disorders of orgasm in women: A literature review of etiology and current treatments. *The Journal of Sexual Medicine, 7*(10), 3254–3268. https://doi.org/10.1111/j.1743-6109.2010.01928.x.

outcomes of breast surgery and reconstruction to prevent disappointment (Dikmans et al., 2019). Breast reconstruction following mastectomy may improve body image and sexuality (Zehra et al., 2020; Zhong et al., 2016). Women with rectal or anal cancer also experience changes in sexuality as a result of body image changes (Benedict et al., 2016), and women with cervical cancer report higher sexual distress when they perceive greater physical changes (Bakker et al., 2017).

Prevalence: Of women who underwent surgery for breast cancer, 31% felt disfigured by the surgery and did not want their partner to see their altered body, fearing their reaction (Przezdziecki et al., 2013).

Contributing factors: The presence of lymphedema impacts directly on body image (Alcorso & Sherman, 2016), but also on functionality (Winch et al., 2015). Having to wear a compression garment also has a negative impact on body image and sexuality (Radina et al., 2015).

Assessment: The Body Image Scale (Hopwood et al., 2001) has 10 items and can be used in those with any type of cancer (see Appendix at the end of this chapter).

Management of body image changes: Changes in body image are difficult to treat due to the perception of women about their changed body that may not reflect what others see. CBT may help some women, but better results have come from a program of group therapy accompanied by expressive guided imagery (Esplen et al., 2018).

CASE STUDY

Your patient is a 45-year-old woman with ER+ PR+ HER2/neu negative right-sided breast cancer. She declined immediate reconstruction at the time of her mastectomy. Her scar looks healthy and she has returned to her usual activities with no problems. She states that her relationship is "okay" and she starts to cry.

1.   What further questions should you ask her?

She tells you that her oncologist has prescribed sertraline for her hot flashes but it is not working.

2.   What are the side effects of this medication?

She finally tells you that she is having difficulties achieving orgasm and her partner has become withdrawn.

3.   What advice would you give her after this disclosure?

Loss of Breast Sensuality

Introduction: Gass and colleagues (2017) coined the term *breast sensuality* and reported that breast surgery, including nipple-sparing mastectomy, results in loss of sensation. With 25% of women opting for bilateral mastectomy in recent years (Pesce et al., 2021), the impact on sexuality cannot be ignored. Women who have a lumpectomy appear to retain breast sensation and are more satisfied than those who have more radical surgery.

Prevalence: Only 29.4% of women treated with mastectomy reported that breast touch was pleasurable, suggesting loss of breast sensuality (Gass et al., 2017). Of women treated for breast cancer who are not sexually active, 44% report that their chest/breasts are important for sexuality after surgical treatment, also suggesting loss of breast sensuality (Peifer et al., 2022). Of women who had nipple-sparing mastectomy, 40% report unpleasant breast touch compared with 11% of women who had lumpectomy (Casaubon et al., 2020).

Assessment: Breast-specific sensuality can be assessed by a seven-item questionnaire (Gass et al., 2017) that addresses appearance, the role and importance of the breast in sexuality, frequency of touch/stimulation, importance of the partner seeing the woman's chest without clothing, and changes after mastectomy.

Management of loss of breast sensuality: Counseling interventions are successful in helping women with sexual concerns and are available in individual, group, and internet formats. Inclusion of the woman's partner may enhance the relationship (Reese et al., 2019). While many of the counseling interventions are time-intensive, a two-session intervention for the woman alone showed improvements in sexual satisfaction in women with breast cancer (Abedini et al., 2020). Including the couple in counseling improves communication and relationship functioning and reduces stress (Regan et al., 2012).

GUIDELINES

- **American Society of Clinical Oncology (ASCO)**

  Interventions to Address Sexual Problems in People With Cancer: ASCO Clinical Practice Guideline Adaptation of Cancer Care Ontario Guideline (Carter et al., 2018)

- **National Comprehensive Cancer Network (NCCN)**

  NCCN Guidelines Version 1.2023 Survivorship: Sexual Function (SSF1-SSF-B)

  https://www.nccn.org/professionals/physician_gls/pdf/survivorship.pdf

- **North American Menopause Society (NAMS)**

  "NAMS Position Statement" The 2020 Genitourinary Syndrome of Menopause Position Statement of the North American Menopause Society

  https://www.menopause.org/docs/default-source/default-document-library/2020-gsm-ps.pdf

- **Oncology Nursing Society (ONS)**

    Practice Resources: Sexuality Huddle Card (membership required to access)

- **American College of Obstetricians and Gynecologists**

    Treatment of Urogenital Symptoms in Individuals With a History of Estrogen-Dependent Breast Cancer

    https://www.acog.org/clinical/clinical-guidance/clinical-Consensus/articles/2021/12/Treatment-of-Urogenital-Symptoms-in-Individuals-With-a-History-of-Estrogen-dependent-Breast-Cancer

SUMMARY

Sexual side effects are a cause of distress in women and may impact on relationship satisfaction. While evidence-based interventions are limited, there are certainly enough to encourage advanced practice clinicians to assess for the sexual symptoms/side effects of treatment. While not all interventions are in the scope of practice for nurses, knowing where to refer the patient is an important first step to manage the issue.

A robust set of instructor resources designed to supplement this text is located at http://connect.springerpub.com/content/reference-book/978-0-8261-8524-2. Qualifying Instructors may request access by emailing **textbook@springerpub.com**.

REFERENCES

Abedini, M., Olfati, F., Oveisi, S., Bahrami, N., Astrologo, L., & Chan, Y. H. (2020). Examining the effect of a brief psychoeducation intervention based on self-regulation model on sexual satisfaction for women with breast cancer: A randomized controlled trial. *European Journal of Oncology Nursing*, 47, 101673. https://doi.org/10.1016/j.ejon.2019.101673

Alcorso, J., & Sherman, K. A. (2016). Factors associated with psychological distress in women with breast cancer-related lymphoedema. *Psycho-oncology*, 25(7), 865–872. https://doi.org/10.1002/pon.4021

Annon, J. (1974). *The behavioral treatment of sexual problems*. Enabling Systems.

Bakker, R. M., Kenter, G. G., Creutzberg, C. L., Stiggelbout, A. M., Derks, M., Mingelen, W., Kroon, C. D., Vermeer, W. M., & ter Kuile, M. M. (2017). Sexual distress and associated factors among cervical cancer survivors: A cross-sectional multicenter observational study. *Psycho-oncology*, 26(10), 1470–1477. https://doi.org/10.1002/pon.4317

Bakker, R. M., Vermeer, W. M., Creutzberg, C. L., Mens, J. W. M., Nout, R. A., & ter Kuile, M. M. (2015). Qualitative accounts of patients' determinants of vaginal dilator use after pelvic radiotherapy. *The Journal of Sexual Medicine*, *12*(3), 764–773. https://doi.org/10.1111/jsm.12776

Bartlik, B., Sugarman, A., Seenaraine, S., & Green, S. (2020). FDA-approved (bremelanotide, flibanserin) and off-label medications (testosterone, sildenafil) to enhance sexual desire/function in women. *Online Journal of Complementary and Alternative Medicine*, *4*(1). https://doi.org/10.33552/OJCAM.2020.04.000578

Barton, D. L., Shuster, L. T., Dockter, T., Atherton, P. J., Thielen, J., Birrell, S. N., Sood, R., Griffin, P., Terstriep, S. A., Mattar, B., Lafky, J. M., & Loprinzi, C. L. (2018). Systemic and local effects of vaginal dehydroepiandrosterone (DHEA): NCCTG N10C1 (Alliance). *Supportive Care in Cancer*, *26*(4), 1335–1343. https://doi.org/10.1007/s00520-017-3960-9

Baser, R. E., Li, Y., & Carter, J. (2012). Psychometric validation of the female sexual function index (FSFI) in cancer survivors. *Cancer*, *118*(18), 4606–4618. https://doi.org/10.1002/cncr.26739

Benedict, C., Philip, E. J., Baser, R. E., Carter, J., Schuler, T. A., Jandorf, L., DuHamel, K., & Nelson, C. (2016). Body image and sexual function in women after treatment for anal and rectal cancer. *Psychooncology*, *25*(3), 316–323. https://doi.org/10.1002/pon.3847

Berghmans, B. (2018). Physiotherapy for pelvic pain and female sexual dysfunction: An untapped resource. *International Urogynecology Journal*, *29*(5), 631–638. https://doi.org/10.1007/s00192-017-3536-8

Biglia, N., Bounous, V. E., D'Alonzo, M., Ottino, L., Tuninetti, V., Robba, E., & Perrone, T. (2017). Vaginal atrophy in breast cancer survivors: Attitude and approaches among oncologists. *Clinical Breast Cancer*, *17*(8), 611–617. https://doi.org/10.1016/j.clbc.2017.05.008

Biglia, N., Cozzarella, M., Cacciari, F., Ponzone, R., Roagna, R., Maggiorotto, F., & Sismondi, P. (2003). Menopause after breast cancer: A survey on breast cancer survivors. *Maturitas*, *45*(1), 29–38. https://doi.org/10.1016/S0378-5122(03)00087-2

Bıldırcın, F. D., Özdeş, E. K., Karlı, P., Özdemir, A. Z., & Kökçü, A. (2020). Does type of menopause affect the sex lives of women? *Medical Science Monitor*, *26*, e921811. https://doi.org/10.12659/msm.921811

Blouet, A., Zinger, M., Capitain, O., Landry, S., Bourgeois, H., Seegers, V. T., & Pointreau, Y. (2019). Sexual quality of life evaluation after treatment among women with breast cancer under 35 years old. *Supportive Care in Cancer*, *27*, 879–885.

Bober, S. L., & Varela, V. S. (2012). Sexuality in adult cancer survivors: Challenges and intervention. *Journal of Clinical Oncology*, *30*(30), 3712–3719. https://doi.org/10.1200/jco.2012.41.7915

Bowles, E. J. A., Boudreau, D. M., Chubak, J., Yu, O., Fujii, M., Chestnut, J., & Buist, D. S. M. (2012). Patient-reported discontinuation of endocrine therapy and related adverse effects among women with early-stage breast cancer.

Journal of Oncology Practice, 8(6), e149–e157. https://doi.org/10.1200/jop.2 012.000543

Brennen, R., Lin, K. Y., Denehy, L., & Frawley, H. C. (2020). The effect of pelvic floor muscle interventions on pelvic floor dysfunction after gynecological cancer treatment: A systematic review. *Physical Therapy, 100*(8), 1357–1371. https://doi.org/10.1093/ptj/pzaa081

Brotto, L. A., & Basson, R. (2014). Group mindfulness-based therapy significantly improves sexual desire in women. *Behaviour Research and Therapy, 57,* 43–54. https://doi.org/10.1016/j.brat.2014.04.001

Brotto, L. A., Basson, R., & Luria, M. (2008a). A mindfulness-based group psychoeducational intervention targeting sexual arousal disorder in women. *The Journal of Sexual Medicine, 5*(7), 1646–1659. https://doi.org/10.1111/j.1 743-6109.2008.00850.x

Brotto, L. A., Chivers, M. L., Millman, R. D., & Albert, A. (2016). Mindfulness-based sex therapy improves genital-subjective arousal concordance in women with sexual desire/arousal difficulties. *Archives of Sexual Behavior, 45*(8), 1907–1921. https://doi.org/10.1007/s10508-015-0689-8

Brotto, L. A., Erskine, Y., Carey, M., Ehlen, T., Finlayson, S., Heywood, M., Kwon, J., McAlpine, J., Stuart, G., Thomson, S., & Miller, D. (2012). A brief mindfulness-based cognitive behavioral intervention improves sexual functioning versus wait-list control in women treated for gynecologic cancer. *Gynecologic Oncology, 125*(2), 320–325. https://doi.org/10.1016/j.ygyno.20 12.01.035

Brotto, L. A., Heiman, J., Goff, B., Greer, B., Lentz, G., Swisher, E., Tamimi, H., & Van Blaricom, A. (2008b). A psychoeducational intervention for sexual dysfunction in women with gynecologic cancer. *Archives of Sexual Behavior, 37,* 317–329. https://doi.org/10.1007/s10508-007-9196-x

Bui, K. T., Willson, M. L., Goel, S., Beith, J., & Goodwin, A. (2020). Ovarian suppression for adjuvant treatment of hormone receptor-positive early breast cancer. *Cochrane Database of Systematic Reviews, 3*(3), Cd013538. https://doi.org/10.1002/14651858.Cd013538

Cai, B., Simon, J., Villa, P., Biglia, N., Panay, N., Djumaeva, S., Particco, M., Kanakamedal, H., & Altomare, C. (2020). No increase in incidence or risk of recurrence of breast cancer in ospemifene-treated patients with vulvovaginal atrophy (VVA). *Maturitas, 142,* 38–44. https://doi.org/10.1016/j.maturi tas.2020.06.021

Cameron, K. E., Kole, M. B., Sammel, M. D., Ginsberg, J. P., Gosiengfiao, Y., Mersereau, J. E., Su, H. I., & Gracia, C. R. (2018). Acute menopausal symptoms in young cancer survivors immediately following chemotherapy. *Oncology, 94*(4), 200–206. https://doi.org/10.1159/000485917

Carter, J., Lacchetti, C., Andersen, B. L., Barton, D. L., Bolte, S., Damast, S., Diefenbach, M. A., DuHamel, K., Florendo, J., Ganz, P. A., Goldfarb, S., Hallmeyer, S., Kushner, D. M., & Rowland, J. H. (2018). Interventions to address sexual problems in people with cancer: American society of clinical oncology clinical practice guideline adaptation of cancer care Ontario guideline. *Journal of Clinical Oncology, 36*(5), 492–511. https://doi.org/10.1200/jco.2017.75.8995

Casaubon, J. T., Kuehn, R. B., Pesek, S. E., Raker, C. A., Edmonson, D. A., Stuckey, A., & Gass, J. S. (2020). Breast-specific sensuality and appearance satisfaction: Comparison of breast-conserving surgery and nipple-sparing mastectomy. *Journal of the American College of Surgeons, 230*(6), 990–998. https://doi.org/10.1016/j.jamcollsurg.2020.02.048

Cox, P., & Panay, N. (2019). Vulvovaginal atrophy in women after cancer. *Climacteric, 22*(6), 565–571. https://doi.org/10.1080/13697137.2019.1643180

Crean-Tate, K. K., Faubion, S. S., Pederson, H. J., Vencill, J. A., & Batur, P. (2020). Management of genitourinary syndrome of menopause in female cancer patients: A focus on vaginal hormonal therapy. *American Journal of Obstetrics and Gynecology, 222*(2), 103–113. https://doi.org/10.1016/j.ajog.2019.08.043

Cullen, K., Fergus, K., Dasgupta, T., Fitch, M., Doyle, C., & Adams, L. (2012). From "sex toy" to intrusive imposition: A qualitative examination of women's experiences with vaginal dilator use following treatment for gynecological cancer. *The Journal of Sexual Medicine, 9*(4), 1162–1173. https://doi.org/10.1111/j.1743-6109.2011.02639.x

Cyr, M. P., Dumoulin, C., Bessette, P., Pina, A., Gotlieb, W. H., Lapointe-Milot, K., Mayrand, M.-H., & Morin, M. (2020). Feasibility, acceptability and effects of multimodal pelvic floor physical therapy for gynecological cancer survivors suffering from painful sexual intercourse: A multicenter prospective interventional study. *Gynecologic Oncology, 159*(3), 778–784. https://doi.org/10.1016/j.ygyno.2020.09.001

Cyr, M. P., Dumoulin, C., Bessette, P., Pina, A., Gotlieb, W. H., Lapointe-Milot, K., Mayrand, M.-H., & Morin, M. (2021). A prospective single-arm study evaluating the effects of a multimodal physical therapy intervention on psychosexual outcomes in women with dyspareunia after gynecologic cancer. *The Journal of Sexual Medicine, 18*(5), 946–954. https://doi.org/10.1016/j.jsxm.2021.02.014

Damast, S., Jeffery, D. D., Son, C. H., Hasan, Y., Carter, J., Lindau, S. T., & Jhingran, A. (2019). Literature review of vaginal stenosis and dilator use in radiation oncology. *Practical Radiation Oncology, 9*(6), 479–491. https://doi.org/10.1016/j.prro.2019.07.001

Di Donato, V., Schiavi, M. C., Iacobelli, V., D'Oria, O., Kontopantelis, E., Simoncini, T., Muzii, L., & Benedetti Panici, P. (2019a). Ospemifene for the treatment of vulvar and vaginal atrophy: A meta-analysis of randomized trials. Part I: Evaluation of efficacy. *Maturitas, 121*, 86–92. https://doi.org/10.1016/j.maturitas.2018.11.016

Di Donato, V., Schiavi, M. C., Iacobelli, V., D'Oria, O., Kontopantelis, E., Simoncini, T., Muzii, L., & Benedetti Panici, P. (2019b). Ospemifene for the treatment of vulvar and vaginal atrophy: A meta-analysis of randomized trials. Part II: Evaluation of tolerability and safety. *Maturitas, 121*, 93–100. https://doi.org/10.1016/j.maturitas.2018.11.017

Dikmans, R. E. G., van de Grift, T. C., Bouman, M. B., Pusic, A. L., & Mullender, M. G. (2019). Sexuality, a topic that surgeons should discuss with women before risk-reducing mastectomy and breast reconstruction. *Breast, 43*, 120–122. https://doi.org/10.1016/j.breast.2018.12.003

dos Santos, C. C. M., Uggioni, M. L. R., Colonetti, T., Colonetti, L., Grande, A. J., & Da Rosa, M. I. (2021). Hyaluronic acid in postmenopause vaginal atrophy: A systematic review. *The Journal of Sexual Medicine, 18*(1), 156–166. https://doi.org/10.1016/j.jsxm.2020.10.016

Dubray, S., Gérard, M., Beaulieu-Prévost, D., & Courtois, F. (2017). Validation of a self-report questionnaire assessing the bodily and physiological sensations of orgasm. *The Journal of Sexual Medicine, 14*(2), 255–263. https://doi.org/10.1016/j.jsxm.2016.12.006

Eaton, A. A., Baser, R. E., Seidel, B., Stabile, C., Canty, J. P., Goldfrank, D. J., & Carter, J. (2017). Validation of clinical tools for vaginal and vulvar symptom assessment in cancer patients and survivors. *The Journal of Sexual Medicine, 14*(1), 144–151. https://doi.org/10.1016/j.jsxm.2016.11.317

Esplen, M. J., Wong, J., Warner, E., & Toner, B. (2018). Restoring body image after cancer (ReBIC): Results of a randomized controlled trial. *Journal of Clinical Oncology, 36*(8), 749–756. https://doi.org/10.1200/jco.2017.74.8244

Eugster-Hausmann, M., Waitzinger, J., & Lehnick, D. (2010). Minimized estradiol absorption with ultra-low-dose 10 µg 17β-estradiol vaginal tablets. *Climacteric, 13*(3), 219–227. https://doi.org/10.3109/13697137.2010.483297

Faught, B. M., Soulban, G., Yeaw, J., Maroun, C., Coyle, K., Schaffer, S., & DeKoven, M. (2019). Ospemifene versus local estrogen: Adherence and costs in postmenopausal dyspareunia. *Journal of Comparative Effectiveness Research, 8*(13), 1111–1123. https://doi.org/10.2217/cer-2019-0091

FDA. (2018). Statement from FDA Commissioner Scott Gottlieb, M.D., on efforts to safeguard women's health from deceptive health claims and significant risks related to devices marketed for use in medical procedures for "vaginal rejuvenation". [Press release]

Febrina, F., Triyoga, I. F., White, M., Marino, J. L., & Peate, M. (2022). Efficacy of interventions to manage sexual dysfunction in women with cancer: A systematic review. *Menopause, 29*(5), 609–626. https://doi.org/10.1097/gme.0000000000001953

Gass, J. S., Onstad, M., Pesek, S., Rojas, K., Fogarty, S., Stuckey, A., Raker, C., & Dizon, D. S. (2017). Breast-specific sensuality and sexual function in cancer survivorship: Does surgical modality matter? *Annals of Surgical Oncology, 24*(11), 3133–3140. https://doi.org/10.1245/s10434-017-5905-4

Goetsch, M. F., Lim, J. Y., & Caughey, A. (2015). A practical solution for dyspareunia in breast cancer survivors: A randomized controlled trial. *Journal of*

Clinical Oncology, *33*(30), 3394–3400. https://doi.org/10.1200/JCO.2014.6 0.7366

Gordon, C., Gonzales, S., & Krychman, M. L. (2019). Rethinking the techno vagina: A case series of patient complications following vaginal laser treatment for atrophy. *Menopause*, *26*(4), 423–427. https://doi.org/10.1097/gme .0000000000001293

Gunst, A., Ventus, D., Arver, S., Dhejne, C., Görts-Öberg, K., Zamore-Söderström, E., & Jern, P. (2019). A randomized, waiting-list-controlled study shows that brief, mindfulness-based psychological interventions are effective for treatment of women's low sexual desire. *Journal of Sex Research*, *56*(7), 913–929. https://doi.org/10.1080/00224499.2018.1539463

Haddad, N. C., Soares Brollo, L. C., Pinho Oliveira, M. A., & Bernardo-Filho, M. (2021). Diagnostic methods for vaginal stenosis and compliance to vaginal dilator use: A systematic review. *The Journal of Sexual Medicine*, *18*(3), 493–514. https://doi.org/10.1016/j.jsxm.2020.12.013

Hopwood, P., Fletcher, I., Lee, A., & Al Ghazal, S. (2001). A body image scale for use with cancer patients. *European Journal of Cancer*, *37*(2), 189–197. https://doi.org/10.1016/S0959-8049(00)00353-1

Isidori, A. M., Pozza, C., Esposito, K., Giugliano, D., Morano, S., Vignozzi, L., Corona, G., Lenzi, A., & Jannini, E. A. (2010). Original research—outcomes assessment: Development and validation of a 6-item version of the female sexual function index (FSFI) as a diagnostic tool for female sexual dysfunction. *The Journal of Sexual Medicine*, *7*(3), 1139–1146. https://doi.org/10.1111 /j.1743-6109.2009.01635.x

Islam, R. M., Bell, R. J., Green, S., Page, M. J., & Davis, S. R. (2019). Safety and efficacy of testosterone for women: A systematic review and meta-analysis of randomised controlled trial data. *The Lancet Diabetes & Endocrinology*, *7*(10), 754–766. https://doi.org/10.1016/S2213-8587(19)30189-5

Jaderek, I., & Lew-Starowicz, M. (2019). A systematic review on mindfulness meditation-based interventions for sexual dysfunctions. *The Journal of Sexual Medicine*, *16*(10), 1581–1596. https://doi.org/10.1016/j.jsxm.2019.07.019

Javadpour, S., Sharifi, N., Mosallanezhad, Z., Rasekhjahromi, A., & Jamali, S. (2021). Assessment of premature menopause on the sexual function and quality of life in women. *Gynecological Endocrinology*, *37*(4), 307–311. https://doi.org/10.1080/09513590.2021.1871894

Jayasena, C. N., Alkaabi, F. M., Liebers, C. S., Handley, T., Franks, S., & Dhillo, W. S. (2019). A systematic review of randomized controlled trials investigating the efficacy and safety of testosterone therapy for female sexual dysfunction in postmenopausal women. *Clinical Endocrinology (Oxford)*, *90*(3), 391–414. https://doi.org/10.1111/cen.13906

Jha, S., Wyld, L., & Krishnaswamy, P. H. (2019). The impact of vaginal laser treatment for genitourinary syndrome of menopause in breast cancer survivors: A systematic review and meta-analysis. *Clinical Breast Cancer*, *19*(4), e556–e562. https://doi.org/10.1016/j.clbc.2019.04.007

Jing, L., Zhang, C., Li, W., Jin, F., & Wang, A. (2019). Incidence and severity of sexual dysfunction among women with breast cancer: A meta-analysis based on female sexual function index. *Supportive Care in Cancer*, *27*(4), 1171–1180. https://doi.org/10.1007/s00520-019-04667-7

Karram, M., Glaser, R., Simon, J., & Streicher, L. (2021). Testosterone supplementation in women: When, why, and how. *OBG Management*, *33*(3), 32. https://doi.org/10.12788/obgm.0070

Kingsberg, S. A., Larkin, L., Krychman, M., Parish, S. J., Bernick, B., & Mirkin, S. (2019). WISDOM survey: Attitudes and behaviors of physicians toward vulvar and vaginal atrophy (VVA) treatment in women including those with breast cancer history. *Menopause*, *26*(2), 124–131. https://doi.org/10.1097/gme.0000000000001194

Kuehn, R., Casaubon, J., Raker, C., Edmonson, D., Stuckey, A., & Gass, J. (2019). Sexual dysfunction in survivorship: The impact of menopause and endocrine therapy. *Annals of Surgical Oncology*, *26*(10), 3159–3165. https://doi.org/10.1245/s10434-019-07552-z

Labrie, F., Archer, D. F., Koltun, W., Vachon, A., Young, D., Frenette, L., Portman, D., Montesino, M., Côté, I., Parent, J., Lavoie, L., Beauregard, A., Martel, C., Vaillancourt, M., Balser, J., & Moyneur, É. (2016). Efficacy of intravaginal dehydroepiandrosterone (DHEA) on moderate to severe dyspareunia and vaginal dryness, symptoms of vulvovaginal atrophy, and of the genitourinary syndrome of menopause. *Menopause*, *23*(3), 243–256. https://doi.org/10.1097/GME.0000000000000571

Lemke, E., Madsen, L., & Dains, J. (2017). Vaginal testosterone for management of aromatase inhibitor related sexual dysfunction: An integrative review. *Oncology Nursing Forum*, *44*(3), 296–301.

Liu, M., Juravic, M., Mazza, G., & Krychman, M. L. (2021). Vaginal dilators: Issues and answers. *Sexual Medicine Reviews*, *9*(2), 212–220. https://doi.org/10.1016/j.sxmr.2019.11.005

Lorenz, T., Rullo, J., & Faubion, S. (2016). Antidepressant-induced female sexual dysfunction. *Mayo Clinic Proceedings*, *91*(9), 1280–1286. https://doi.org/10.1016/j.mayocp.2016.04.033

Lubotzky, F. P., Butow, P., Hunt, C., Costa, D. S. J., Laidsaar-Powell, R., Carroll, S., Thompson, S. R., Jackson, M., Tewari, A., Nattress, K., & Juraskova, I. (2019). A psychosexual rehabilitation booklet increases vaginal dilator adherence and knowledge in women undergoing pelvic radiation therapy for gynaecological or anorectal cancer: A randomised controlled trial. *Clinical Oncology: A Journal of the Royal College of Radiologists*, *31*(2), 124–131. https://doi.org/10.1016/j.clon.2018.11.035

Marino, J. L., Saunders, C. M., & Hickey, M. (2017). Sexual inactivity in partnered female cancer survivors. *Maturitas*, *105*, 89–94. https://doi.org/10.1016/j.maturitas.2017.04.020

Matos, S. R. L., Lucas Rocha Cunha, M., Podgaec, S., Weltman, E., Yamazaki Centrone, A. F., & Cintra Nunes Mafra, A. C. (2019). Consensus for vaginal stenosis prevention in patients submitted to pelvic radiotherapy. *PloS One*, *14*(8), e0221054. https://doi.org/10.1371/journal.pone.0221054

Mejia-Gomez, J., Bouteaud, J., Philippopoulos, E., Wolfman, W., & Brezden-Masley, C. (2022). Use of a vaginal CO(2) laser for the management of genitourinary syndrome of menopause in gynecological cancer survivors: A systematic review. *Climacteric*, *25*(3), 228–234. https://doi.org/10.1080/136 97137.2021.1990258

Mension, E., Alonso, I., & Castelo-Branco, C. (2021). Genitourinary syndrome of menopause: Current treatment options in breast cancer survivors—systematic review. *Maturitas*, *143*, 47–58. https://doi.org/10.1016/j.maturit as.2020.08.010

Mension, E., Alonso, I., Tortajada, M., Matas, I., Gómez, S., Ribera, L., Anglès, S., & Castelo-Branco, C. (2022). Vaginal laser therapy for genitourinary syndrome of menopause—systematic review. *Maturitas*, *156*, 37–59. https://do i.org/10.1016/j.maturitas.2021.06.005

Mick, J., Hughes, M., & Cohen, M. (2003). Sexuality and cancer: How oncology nurses can address it BETTER. *Oncology Nursing Forum*, *30*, 152–153.

Milbury, K., Cohen, L., Jenkins, R., Skibber, J. M., & Schover, L. R. (2013). The association between psychosocial and medical factors with long-term sexual dysfunction after treatment for colorectal cancer. *Support Care Cancer*, *21*(3), 793–802. https://doi.org/10.1007/s00520-012-1582-9. Accession Number: 22948439 PMCID: Pmc4437688.

Mounir, D. M., Hernandez, N., & Gonzalez, R. R. (2021). Update: The clinical role of vaginal lasers for the treatment of the genitourinary syndrome of menopause. *Urology*, *151*, 2–7. https://doi.org/10.1016/j.urology.2020. 09.012

Narang, G. L., Pannell, S. C., Laviana, A. A., Huen, K. H. Y., Izard, J., Smith, A. B., & Bergman, J. (2017). Patient-reported outcome measures in urology. *Current Opinion in Urology*, *27*(4), 366–374. https://doi.org/10.1097/mou.0 000000000000412

Pavlović, R. T., Janković, S. M., Milovanović, J. R., Stefanović, S. M., Folić, M. M., Milovanović, O. Z., Mamillapalli, C., & Milosavljević, M. N. (2019). The safety of local hormonal treatment for vulvovaginal atrophy in women with estrogen receptor-positive breast cancer who are on adjuvant aromatase inhibitor therapy: Meta-analysis. *Clinical Breast Cancer*, *19*(6), e731–e740. htt ps://doi.org/10.1016/j.clbc.2019.07.007

Peifer, H. G., Raker, C., Pesek, S., Edmonson, D., Stuckey, A., & Gass, J. S. (2022). Breast-specific sensuality in breast cancer survivors: Sexually active or not. *Annals of Surgical Oncology*, *29*(10), 6225–6233. https://doi.org/10.12 45/s10434-022-12196-7

Pesce, C., Jaffe, J., Kuchta, K., Yao, K., & Sisco, M. (2021). Patient-reported outcomes among women with unilateral breast cancer undergoing breast conservation versus single or double mastectomy. *Breast Cancer Research and Treatment*, *185*(2), 359–369. https://doi.org/10.1007/s10549-020-05964-0

Pettigrew, J. A., & Novick, A. M. (2021). Hypoactive sexual desire disorder in women: Physiology, assessment, diagnosis, and treatment. *Journal of Midwifery & Womens Health, 66*(6), 740–748. https://doi.org/10.1111/jmwh.13283

Pingarron, C., de Lafuente, P., Ierullo, A. M., Poyo Torcal, S., Maroto Díaz, C. J., & Palacios, S. (2021). Ospemifene in clinical practice for vulvo-vaginal atrophy: Results at 3 months of follow-up of use. *Gynecological Endocrinology, 37*(6), 562–566. https://doi.org/10.1080/09513590.2020.1853695

Pinheiro Sobreira Bezerra, L. R., Britto, D. F., Ribeiro Frota, I. P., Lira do Nascimento, S., Morais Brilhante, A. V., Lucena, S. V., & Moura Brasil, D. M. (2020). The impact of urinary incontinence on sexual function: A systematic review. *Sexual Medicine Reviews, 8*(3), 393–402. https://doi.org/10.1016/j.sxmr.2019.06.009

Potter, N., & Panay, N. (2021). Vaginal lubricants and moisturizers: A review into use, efficacy, and safety. *Climacteric, 24*(1), 19–24. https://doi.org/10.1080/13697137.2020.1820478

Przezdziecki, A., Sherman, K. A., Baillie, A., Taylor, A., Foley, E., & Stalgis-Bilinski, K. (2013). My changed body: Breast cancer, body image, distress and self-compassion. *Psychooncology, 22*(8), 1872–1879. https://doi.org/10.1002/pon.3230

Pup, L. D., & Sánchez-Borrego, R. (2020). Ospemifene efficacy and safety data in women with vulvovaginal atrophy. *Gynecological Endocrinology, 36*(7), 569–577. https://doi.org/10.1080/09513590.2020.1757058

Pyke, R. E., & Clayton, A. H. (2019). Lumping, splitting, and treating: Therapies are needed for women with overlapping sexual dysfunctions. *Sexual Medicine Reviews, 7*(4), 551–558. https://doi.org/10.1016/j.sxmr.2019.04.002

Quick, A. M., Hundley, A., Evans, C., Stephens, J. A., Ramaswamy, B., Reinbolt, R. E., Noonan, A. M., Van Deusen, J. B., Wesolowski, R., Stover, D. G., Williams, N. O., Sardesai, S. D., Faubion, S. S., Loprinzi, C. L., & Lustberg, M. B. (2022). Long-term follow-up of fractional CO2 laser therapy for genitourinary syndrome of menopause in breast cancer survivors. *Journal of Clinical Medicine, 11*(3), 774. https://www.mdpi.com/2077-0383/11/3/774

Radina, M. E., Fu, M. R., Horstman, L., & Kang, Y. (2015). Breast cancer-related lymphedema and sexual experiences: A mixed-method comparison study. *Psycho-oncology, 24*(12), 1655–1662. https://doi.org/10.1002/pon.3778

Reese, J. B., Smith, K. C., Handorf, E., Sorice, K., Bober, S. L., Bantug, E. T., Schwartz, S., & Porter, L. S. (2019). A randomized pilot trial of a couple-based intervention addressing sexual concerns for breast cancer survivors. *Journal of Psychosocial Oncology, 37*(2), 242–263. https://doi.org/10.1080/07347332.2018.1510869

Regan, T. W., Lambert, S. D., Girgis, A., Kelly, B., Kayser, K., & Turner, J. (2012). Do couple-based interventions make a difference for couples affected by cancer? A systematic review. *BMC Cancer, 12*, 279. https://doi.org/10.1186/1471-2407-12-279

Robinson, P. J., Bell, R. J., Christakis, M. K., Ivezic, S. R., & Davis, S. R. (2017). Aromatase inhibitors are associated with low sexual desire causing distress and fecal incontinence in women: An observational study. *The Journal of Sexual Medicine, 14*(12), 1566–1574. https://doi.org/10.1016/j.jsxm.2017.09.018

Rosen, R., Brown, C., Heiman, J., Leiblum, S., Meston, C., Shabsigh, R., Ferguson, D., & D'Agostino, R. (2000). The female sexual function index (FSFI): A multidimensional self-report instrument for the assessment of female sexual function. *Journal of Sex & Marital Therapy, 26*(2), 191–208. https://doi.org/10.1080/009262300278597

Sarmento, A. C. A., Lírio, J. F., Medeiros, K. S., Marconi, C., Costa, A. P. F., Crispim, J. C., & Gonçalves, A. K. (2021). Physical methods for the treatment of genitourinary syndrome of menopause: A systematic review. *International Journal of Gynaecology & Obstetrics, 153*(2), 200–219. https://doi.org/10.1002/ijgo.13561

Siliquini, G. P., Bounous, V. E., Novara, L., Giorgi, M., Bert, F., & Biglia, N. (2021). Fractional CO_2 vaginal laser for the genitourinary syndrome of menopause in breast cancer survivors. *The Breast Journal, 27*(5), 448–455. https://doi.org/10.1111/tbj.14211

Simon, J. A., Goldstein, I., Kim, N. N., Davis, S. R., Kellogg-Spadt, S., Lowenstein, L., Pinkerton, J. V., Stuenkel, C. A., Traish, A. M., Archer, D. F., Bachmann, G., Goldstein, A. T., Nappi, R. E., & Vignozzi, L. (2018). The role of androgens in the treatment of genitourinary syndrome of menopause (GSM): International Society for the Study of Women's Sexual Health (ISSWSH) expert consensus panel review. *Menopause, 25*(7), 837–847. https://doi.org/10.1097/gme.0000000000001138

Stabile, C., Goldfarb, S., Baser, R. E., Goldfrank, D. J., Abu-Rustum, N. R., Barakat, R. R., Dickler, M. N., & Carter, J. (2017). Sexual health needs and educational intervention preferences for women with cancer. *Breast Cancer Research and Treatment, 165*(1), 77–84. https://doi.org/10.1007/s10549-017-4305-6

Stahl, J. M., Qian, J. M., Tien, C. J., Carlson, D. J., Chen, Z., Ratner, E. S., Park, H. S., & Damast, S. (2019). Extended duration of dilator use beyond 1 year may reduce vaginal stenosis after intravaginal high-dose-rate brachytherapy. *Supportive Care in Cancer, 27*(4), 1425–1433. https://doi.org/10.1007/s00520-018-4441-5

Stephenson, K. R., Zippan, N., & Brotto, L. A. (2021). Feasibility of a cognitive behavioral online intervention for women with sexual interest/arousal disorder. *Journal of Clinical Psychology, 77*(9), 1877–1893. https://doi.org/10.1002/jclp.23137

Streicher, L., & Simon, J. A. (2018). Sexual function post-breast cancer. *Cancer Treatment and Research, 173*, 167–189. https://doi.org/10.1007/978-3-319-70197-4_11

Summerfield, J., & Leong, A. (2020). Management of radiation therapy-induced vaginal adhesions and stenosis: A New Zealand survey of current practice. *Journal of Medical Radiation Sciences, 67*(2), 128–133. https://doi.org/10.1002/jmrs.386

Sussman, T. A., Kruse, M. L., Thacker, H. L., & Abraham, J. (2019). Managing genitourinary syndrome of menopause in breast cancer survivors receiving endocrine therapy. *Journal of Oncology Practice, 15*(7), 363–370. https://doi.org/10.1200/jop.18.00710

ter Kuile, M. M., Both, S., & van Lankveld, J. J. D. M. (2010). Cognitive behavioral therapy for sexual dysfunctions in women. *Psychiatric Clinics of North America, 33*(3), 595–610. https://doi.org/10.1016/j.psc.2010.04.010

Traa, M. J., de Vries, J., Roukema, J. A., Rutten, H. J., & Den Oudsten, B. L. (2014). The sexual health care needs after colorectal cancer: The view of patients, partners, and health care professionals. *Support Care Cancer, 22*(3), 763–772. https://doi.org/10.1007/s00520-013-2032-z. Accession Number: 24240645.

van de Grift, T. C., Mureau, M. A. M., Negenborn, V. N., Dikmans, R. E. G., Bouman, M. B., & Mullender, M. G. (2020). Predictors of women's sexual outcomes after implant-based breast reconstruction. *Psychooncology, 29*(8), 1272–1279. https://doi.org/10.1002/pon.5415. Accession Number: 32419285 PMCID: PMC7496883.

Vegunta, S., Kling, J., & Kapoor, E. (2020). Androgen therapy in women. *Journal of Women's Health, 29*(1), 57–64. https://doi.org/10.1089/jwh.2018.7494

Wang, L. Y., Pierdomenico, A., Lefkowitz, A., & Brandt, R. (2015). Female sexual health training for oncology providers: New applications. *Sexual Medicine, 3*(3), 189–197. https://doi.org/10.1002/sm2.66

Winch, C., Sherman, K., Koelmeyer, L., Smith, K., Mackie, H., & Boyages, J. (2015). Sexual concerns of women diagnosed with breast cancer-related lymphedema. *Supportive Care in Cancer, 23*(12), 3481–3491. https://doi.org/10.1007/s00520-015-2709-6

Zehra, S., Doyle, F., Barry, M., Walsh, S., & Kell, M. R. (2020). Health-related quality of life following breast reconstruction compared to total mastectomy and breast-conserving surgery among breast cancer survivors: A systematic review and meta-analysis. *Breast Cancer, 27*(4), 534–566. https://doi.org/10.1007/s12282-020-01076-1

Zhong, T., Hu, J., Bagher, S., Vo, A., O'Neill, A. C., Butler, K., Novak, C. B., Hofer, S. O. P., & Metcalfe, K. A. (2016). A comparison of psychological response, body image, sexuality, and quality of life between immediate and delayed autologous tissue breast reconstruction: A prospective long-term outcome study. *Plastic and Reconstructive Surgery, 138*(4), 772–780. https://doi.org/10.1097/prs.0000000000002536

Zhu, Y., Cohen, S. M., Rosenzweig, M. Q., & Bender, C. M. (2019). Symptom map of endocrine therapy for breast cancer: A scoping review. *Cancer Nursing, 42*(5), E19–E30. https://doi.org/10.1097/ncc.0000000000000632

CHAPTER 18

SEXUAL DYSFUNCTION IN MEN

INTRODUCTION

Sexual symptoms are common in men treated for a variety of cancers; however, most of the evidence has been gathered from men with prostate or colorectal cancer. Sexual side effects result from the various treatments that are offered, with surgery producing the worst impact on erections. More rare cancers, such as testicular and penile cancer, have profound effects on both sexual and psychological functions. Sexual symptoms in men include erectile dysfunction (ED), alterations in the occurrence or sensations of orgasm, and loss of libido.

ERECTILE DYSFUNCTION

Introduction

ED causes frustration, depression, and anxiety about sex (Albaugh et al., 2017). Masculinity, self-esteem, and changes to body image are also affected (Bowie et al., 2022). The loss of spontaneity and feelings of shame can be profound (Schantz Laursen, 2017) and may lead to depression (Walker & Santos-Iglesias, 2020). The man's partner is also affected and the relationship may change (Bamidele et al., 2019).

Prevalence

Studies of men with prostate cancer show a high incidence of ED after surgery. Six months after surgery, there was a 95% prevalence of ED in men who had surgery (Neal et al., 2020). Only 43% of younger men see a return to baseline erectile function after surgery (Barocas et al., 2017) and sexual satisfaction remains low for most of them. Radiation therapy has a slightly less deleterious impact on erections (Ávila et al., 2018). The prevalence of ED in men who have radiation therapy is 88% at 6 months (Neal et al., 2020). A newer form of radiation therapy, stereotactic body radiation (SBRT), also causes erectile problems, with 26% to 55% of men reporting ED at 5 years after treatment (Loi et al., 2019). Brachytherapy has the least impact on erections, with men who choose this treatment reporting adequate function 5 years after treatment (Bazinet et al., 2020). After the addition of androgen deprivation to external beam radiation, men report genital shrinkage (42%), pain with orgasm (15%), and decreased skin sensation (27%; Frey et al., 2017). Men who have surgery for rectal cancer experience ED, with 25% of men in one study reporting ED (Li et al., 2021) and 93% of those who had multimodal treatment having ED (Pang et al., 2020). For men with bladder cancer, ED is present in up to 60%, with the prevalence highest among those treated with radical cystectomy and resection of the prostate and seminal vesicles (Kowalkowski et al., 2014; Figure 18.1).

- Thirty-two percent of young men who have had a childhood cancer report at least one problem with sexual functioning (Zebrack et al., 2010).
- Men treated for head and neck cancer report loss of libido and decreased sexual activity (So et al., 2019).
- Allogenic stem cell transplant recipients report profound ED (72%; Zavattaro et al., 2021).
- Graft-versus-host disease causes body image disturbance affecting sexual functioning (Nørskov et al., 2015).

Figure 18.1 Incidence of men reporting sexual problems, erectile dysfunction (ED), after cancer.

Contributing factors

Besides cancer treatment, contributing factors to ED include loss of libido, antidepressants, other medications, and body image issues.

Assessment

Three patient-reported outcome tools are available to measure ED, and all have been validated (Narang et al., 2017; Figure 18.2).

Management

A staged approach to the management of ED is used in clinical practice.

PHARMACEUTICAL MANAGEMENT
- Administration of the oral agents phosphodiesterase 5 Inhibitors (PDE5Is) (Feng et al., 2022) is the first step in the treatment of ED. These medications act by causing smooth muscle relaxation in the vessels supplying the corpora cavernosa in the penis; penile stimulation is required (Mitidieri et al., 2020). While generally well-tolerated, they do have a number of side effects, including facial flushing, nasal congestion, headache,

The IIEF is a 15-item Likert scale frequently used in clinical practice. It evaluates functioning in 5 domains: erectile function, orgasmic function, sexual desire, intercourse satisfaction, and overall satisfaction.

The SHIM is a 5-item Likert scale derived from the IIEF for ease in clinical practice. It measures erectile function and intercourse satisfaction.

The PROMIS SexFS contains 131 items and is cumbersome for use in clinical practice. An advantage of this measure is that it is valid across sexual orientation, age, and partner status.

The QEQ contains 6 items and is not used widely in clinical practice.

Figure 18.2 Patient-reported tools for assessing sexual dysfunction in men. International Index of Erectile Function (IIEF), Sexual health Inventory for Men (SHIM), Patient-Reported Outcomes Management Information System Sexual Function and Satisfaction (PROMIS SexFS), Quality of Erection Questionnaire (QEQ).

dyspepsia, myalgia, and back pain (Burnett et al., 2018). Both vardenafil and sildenafil are available in orodispersible tablets that dissolve quickly. Avanafil may have an advantage over the other medications in this class (Yang et al., 2021). Use of PDE5I has been shown to be effective in men after rectal cancer surgery (Notarnicola et al., 2020).

- The alprostadil suppository that is inserted into the urethra is marginally effective. The most significant side effect is penile or urethral pain, and studies have high attrition due to lack of efficacy (Raina et al., 2007).

- Intracavernosal injection of a combination of prostaglandin E2, phentolamine, and papaverine (commonly called *Trimix*) is a highly effective treatment for ED; rare side effects include priapism (7%), penile curvature (10%), and mild penile pain (Bearelly et al., 2020). A test dose should be provided by a clinician to find a satisfactory response.

- The use of penile implant is usually the last resort in managing ED despite high satisfaction rates (Wang & Levine, 2022). Uptake among men with prostate cancer treated with surgery is low (Tal et al., 2011).

MECHANICAL DEVICES: The penile pump (also called a *vacuum device*) is the most mechanical intervention (Lima et al., 2021). Use of these devices pulls blood into the penis due to the negative pressure exerted on the penis. It is recommended that a constriction device be placed at the base of the penis to trap the blood. Side effects include bruising, numbness, and pain (Lima et al., 2021), as well as the penis feeling cold and loss of spontaneity. There is some evidence that regular use of the pump may mitigate loss of penile length (Lehrfeld & Lee, 2009).

PENILE REHABILITATION: The regular use of oral medications, vacuum devices, and/or intracavernosal injections after radical prostatectomy showed some efficacy in improving erectile function (Padma-Nathan et al., 2008). One meta-analysis suggests that daily use of sildenafil 100 mg or three times a week or tadalafil 20 mg results in a higher likelihood of erectile recovery (Sari Motlagh et al., 2021). It is also suggested that starting sildenafil 100 mg twice a week immediately following removal of the urinary catheter improves erectile recovery (Jo et al., 2018). Adherence to penile rehabilitation protocols is low (55.8%) at 12 months, with lack of improvement to baseline levels of erectile function (Albaugh et al., 2019). Only about a third of men return to the same level of function as they had before surgery (Terrier et al., 2018). Men discontinue the use of these interventions for a variety of reasons, including costs and lack of improvement (Klotz et al., 2005).

MINDFULNESS MEDITATION: An acceptance-based approach to ED for both men and their partners, mindfulness meditation has shown some efficacy (Bossio et al., 2021).

PHYSIOTHERAPY: Pelvic floor muscle therapy with and without the addition of biofeedback and vibratory stimulation has not been shown to be an effective treatment for ED (Feng et al., 2022).

NEW TREATMENTS: New therapies for the management of ED include low-intensity extracorporeal shockwave therapy (Li-ESWT), stem cell therapy, and platelet-rich plasma (Raheem et al., 2020); there is limited evidence on their efficacy in the nononcology scenario. While improvements in International Index of Erectile Function (IIEF) scores have been seen for shockwave therapy (Dong et al., 2019), use of this treatment in men following prostate cancer surgery is not clinically significant (Baccaglini et al., 2020). Herbal supplements do not appear to be useful (Borrelli et al., 2018).

ALTERATIONS IN ORGASMS

Introduction

More intense or painful orgasms are also possible after surgery for prostate cancer (Frey et al., 2014; Nolsøe et al., 2021). Men who have surgery for colorectal cancer also report this issue (Towe et al., 2019). The absence of ejaculation that occurs after surgical removal of the prostate may be confused with anorgasmia in some men.

Prevalence

The inability to achieve orgasm (anorgasmia) occurs in up to 70% of men after radical prostatectomy and changes in orgasm intensity (dysorgasmia) in up to 14% of men (Haney et al., 2018). Radiation therapy is also associated with anorgasmia (Devlin et al., 2019).

Contributing factors

It is theorized that painful orgasms are a result of overactive pelvic floor muscles (Padoa et al., 2021).

Management

No effective treatments have been described (Clavell-Hernández et al., 2018). If painful orgasms are related to hypertonic pelvic floor muscles, pelvic floor physiotherapy may be helpful in this regard.

LOSS OF LIBIDO

Introduction

In men who are not able to achieve or maintain an erection, a reactive loss of libido may occur. However, the major cause of loss of libido is the use of androgen deprivation therapy (ADT) for management of advanced or recurrent prostate cancer. Loss of libido impacts negatively on couple functioning and relationship satisfaction (Collaço et al., 2021).

Prevalence

Men on ADT report worsening sexual function (libido and erections) over time and increased bother with these changes (Donovan et al.,

2018; Fode et al., 2020). Up to 97% of men on ADT are not sexually active. Of men with testicular cancer who are commonly below 34 years of age, more than 20% reported diminished interest in sex, resulting in a decrease in sexual activity (Wortel et al., 2015).

Contributing factors

Two years after cessation of ADT, only 51% of men return to their baseline level of testosterone (Nascimento et al., 2019). Third-generation ADTs such as enzalutamide and abiraterone may cause less sexual dysfunction (Kaplan et al., 2021).

Management of loss of libido due to androgen deprivation therapy: Intermittent therapy, where treatment stops when markers of the disease drop and then is initiated again if signs of progression occur, allows testosterone levels to rise and may allow sexual function to improve (Corona et al., 2021). Education of men and their partners about the effects of ADT on both sexual and relationship functioning and satisfaction is important (Wibowo et al., 2020). Couples should be told that men can still have orgasms despite absent or reduced libido and without erections (Corona et al., 2021), but more intense stimulation is needed. It is also important for couples to mourn what they have lost in order to create a new way of being sexual (Wittmann et al., 2011).

CASE STUDY

Your patient is a 70-year-old man who had a radical prostatectomy 6 months ago for high-risk prostate cancer. He states that he is frustrated with erections that do not last long enough. He has tried "the pills" and says that they don't work and he "can't afford them anyway." He is angry that he wasn't told about this as a side effect before the surgery and he is worried that his "girlfriend" is going to leave him if the situation is not resolved.

1. What additional questions do you want to ask?

2. What next step would you advise him and why?

He calls you 2 weeks later and says that what you suggested has not helped at all. He is even more frustrated and says that if you can't help him, he doesn't know what he is going to do.

3. What is your response to this?

4. What other suggestions can you make?

OTHER SEXUAL SIDE EFFECTS

Penile shrinkage with an average of ½ inch/1 cm loss in length is seen to occur after prostate surgery (El-Khatib et al., 2021; Vasconcelos et al., 2012). Bladder leakage with arousal (Bach et al., 2019) or orgasm (Jimbo et al., 2020) is also known to occur (see Chapter 16 for incontinence).

Ten percent of men develop Peyronie disease (curvature of the penis) after surgery to remove the prostate (Frey et al., 2014).

GUIDELINES

- **American Society of Clinical Oncology (ASCO)**

    Interventions to Address Sexual Problems in People With Cancer: American Society of Clinical Oncology Clinical Practice Guideline Adaptation of Cancer Care Ontario Guideline (Carter et al., 2018)

- **American Urological Association (AUA)**

    Erectile Dysfunction: AUA Guideline 2018

    https://www.auanet.org//guidelines/guidelines/erectile-dysfunction-(ed)-guideline

- **National Comprehensive Cancer Network (NCCN)**

    NCCN Guidelines Version 1.2023 Survivorship: Sexual Function (SSF1–SSF-B)

    https://www.nccn.org/professionals/physician_gls/pdf/survivorship.pdf

- **Oncology Nursing Society (ONS)**

    Practice Resources: Sexuality Huddle Card (membership required to access)

SUMMARY

Sexual dysfunction is common after treatment for cancers affecting men. Oral agents that were developed to treat ED have shown limited effectiveness in this patient population. Loss of libido occurs as a reaction to ED, but also from androgen deprivation therapy (ADT). There is also a psychological factor for men treated for other cancers with sexual impacts and the partner relationship is negatively affected.

A robust set of instructor resources designed to supplement this text is located at http://connect.springerpub.com/content/reference-book/978-0-8261-8524-2.
Qualifying Instructors may request access by emailing **textbook@springerpub.com**.

REFERENCES

Albaugh, J., Adamic, B., Chang, C., Kirwen, N., & Aizen, J. (2019). Adherence and barriers to penile rehabilitation over 2 years following radical prostatectomy. *BMC Urology, 19*(1), 89. https://doi.org/10.1186/s12894-019-0516-y

Albaugh, J. A., Sufrin, N., Lapin, B. R., Petkewicz, J., & Tenfelde, S. (2017). Life after prostate cancer treatment: A mixed methods study of the experiences of men with sexual dysfunction and their partners. *BMC Urology*, *17*(1), 45. https://doi.org/10.1186/s12894-017-0231-5

Ávila, M., Patel, L., López, S., Cortés-Sanabria, L., Garin, O., Pont, À., Ferrer, F., Boladeras, B., Zamora, V., Fosså, S., Storås, A. H., Sanda, M., Serra-Sutton, V., & Ferrer, M. (2018). Patient-reported outcomes after treatment for clinically localized prostate cancer: A systematic review and meta-analysis. *Cancer Treatment Reviews*, *66*, 23–44. https://doi.org/10.1016/j.ctrv.2018.03.005

Baccaglini, W., Linck Pazeto, C., Corrêa Barros, E. A., Timóteo, F., Monteiro, L., Saad Rached, R. Y., Navas, A., & Glina, S. (2020). PS-5–9 Erectile dysfunction after radical prostatectomy: Low-Intensity Extracorporeal Shockwave Therapy (LIESWT) plays a role? *The Journal of Sexual Medicine*, *17*(6), S136. https://doi.org/10.1016/j.jsxm.2020.04.054

Bach, P. V., Salter, C. A., Katz, D., Schofield, E., Nelson, C. J., & Mulhall, J. P. (2019). Arousal incontinence in men following radical prostatectomy: Prevalence, impact and predictors. *The Journal of Sexual Medicine*, *16*(12), 1947–1952. https://doi.org/10.1016/j.jsxm.2019.09.015

Bamidele, O., Lagan, B. M., McGarvey, H., Wittmann, D., & McCaughan, E. (2019). "…It might not have occurred to my husband that this woman, his wife who is taking care of him has some emotional needs as well…": The unheard voices of partners of Black African and Black Caribbean men with prostate cancer. *Supportive Care in Cancer*, *27*(3), 1089–1097. https://doi.org/10.1007/s00520-018-4398-4

Barocas, D. A., Alvarez, J., Resnick, M. J., Koyama, T., Hoffman, K. E., Tyson, M. D., Conwill, R., McCollum, D., Cooperberg, M. R., Goodman, M., Greenfield, S., Hamilton, A. S., Hashibe, M., Kaplan, S. H., Paddock, L. E., Stroup, A. M., Wu, X.-C., & Penson, D. F. (2017). Association between radiation therapy, surgery, or observation for localized prostate cancer and patient-reported outcomes after 3 years. *JAMA*, *317*(11), 1126–1140. https://doi.org/10.1001/jama.2017.1704

Bazinet, A., Zorn, K. C., Taussky, D., Delouya, G., & Liberman, D. (2020). Favorable preservation of erectile function after prostate brachytherapy for localized prostate cancer. *Brachytherapy*, *19*(2), 222–227. https://doi.org/10.1016/j.brachy.2019.11.003

Bearelly, P., Phillips, E. A., Pan, S., O'Brien, K., Asher, K., Martinez, D., & Munarriz, R. (2020). Long-term intracavernosal injection therapy: Treatment efficacy and patient satisfaction. *International Journal of Impotence Research*, *32*(3), 345–351. https://doi.org/10.1038/s41443-019-0186-z

Borrelli, F., Colalto, C., Delfino, D. V., Iriti, M., & Izzo, A. A. (2018). Herbal dietary supplements for erectile dysfunction: A systematic review and meta-analysis. *Drugs*, *78*(6), 643–673. https://doi.org/10.1007/s40265-018-0897-3

Bossio, J. A., Higano, C. S., & Brotto, L. A. (2021). Preliminary development of a mindfulness-based group therapy to expand couples; Sexual intimacy after prostate cancer: A mixed methods approach. *Sexual Medicine*, *9*(2). https://doi.org/10.1016/j.esxm.2020.100310

Bowie, J., Brunckhorst, O., Stewart, R., Dasgupta, P., & Ahmed, K. (2022). Body image, self-esteem, and sense of masculinity in patients with prostate cancer:

A qualitative meta-synthesis. *Journal of Cancer Survivorship, 16*(1), 95–110. https://doi.org/10.1007/s11764-021-01007-9

Burnett, A. L., Nehra, A., Breau, R. H., Culkin, D. J., Faraday, M. M., Hakim, L. S., Heidelbaugh, J., Khera, M., McVary, K. T., Miner, M. M., Nelson, C. J., Sadeghi-Nejad, H., Sefte, A. D., & Shindel, A. W. (2018). Erectile dysfunction: AUA guideline. *The Journal of Urology, 200*(3), 633–641. https://doi.org/10.1016/j.juro.2018.05.004

Carter, J., Lacchetti, C., Andersen, B. L., Barton, D. L., Bolte, S., Damast, S., Diefenbach, M. A., DuHamel, K., Florendo, J., Ganz, P. A., Goldfarb, S., Hallmeyer, S., Kushner, D. M., & Rowland, J. H. (2018). Interventions to address sexual problems in people with cancer: American Society of Clinical Oncology Clinical Practice Guideline Adaptation of Cancer Care Ontario Guideline. *Journal of Clinical Oncology, 36*(5), 492–511. https://doi.org/10.1200/jco.2017.75.8995

Clavell-Hernández, J., Martin, C., & Wang, R. (2018). Orgasmic dysfunction following radical prostatectomy: Review of current literature. *Sexual Medicine Reviews, 6*(1), 124–134. https://doi.org/10.1016/j.sxmr.2017.09.003. Accession Number: 29108976.

Collaço, N., Wagland, R., Alexis, O., Gavin, A., Glaser, A., & Watson, E. K. (2021). The experiences and needs of couples affected by prostate cancer aged 65 and under: A qualitative study. *Journal of Cancer Survivorship, 15*, 358–366.

Corona, G., Filippi, S., Comelio, P., Bianchi, N., Frizza, F., Dicuio, M., Rastrelli, G., Concetti, S., Sforza, A., Vignozzi, L., & Maggi, M. (2021). Sexual function in men undergoing androgen deprivation therapy. *International Journal of Impotence Research, 33*(4), 439–447. https://doi.org/10.1038/s41443-021-00418-7

Devlin, E. J., Whitford, H. S., Denson, L. A., & Potter, A. E. (2019). "Just as I expected": A longitudinal cohort study of the impact of response expectancies on side effect experiences during radiotherapy for prostate cancer. *Journal of Pain and Symptom Management, 57*(2), 273–281.e4. https://doi.org/10.1016/j.jpainsymman.2018.11.002. Accession Number: 30447387.

Dong, L., Chang, D., Zhang, X., Li, J., Yang, F., Tan, K., Yang, Y., Yong, S., & Yu, X. (2019). Effect of low-intensity extracorporeal shock wave on the treatment of erectile dysfunction: A systematic review and meta-analysis. *American Journal of Men's Health, 13*(2), 1557988319846749. https://doi.org/10.1177/1557988319846749

Donovan, K. A., Gonzalez, B. D., Nelson, A. M., Fishman, M. N., Zachariah, B., & Jacobsen, P. B. (2018). Effect of androgen deprivation therapy on sexual function and bother in men with prostate cancer: A controlled comparison. *Psychooncology, 27*(1), 316–324. https://doi.org/10.1002/pon.4463. Accession Number: 28557112 PMCID: PMC5709275.

El-Khatib, F., Huynh, L., Osman, M., Choi, E., Yafi, F., & Ahlering, T. (2021). 158 Penile length shortening following robot-assisted radical prostatectomy: Impacts on erections and sexual bother. *The Journal of Sexual Medicine, 18*(3), S86–S87. https://doi.org/10.1016/j.jsxm.2021.01.013

Feng, D., Tang, C., Liu, S., Yang, Y., Han, P., & Wei, W. (2022). Current management strategy of treating patients with erectile dysfunction after radical prostatectomy: A systematic review and meta-analysis. *International Journal of Impotence Research, 34*(1), 18–36. https://doi.org/10.1038/s41443-020-00364-w

Fode, M., Mosholt, K. S., Nielsen, T. K., Tolouee, S., Giraldi, A., Østergren, P. B., & Azawi, N. (2020). Sexual motivators and endorsement of models describing sexual response of men undergoing androgen deprivation therapy for advanced prostate cancer. *Journal of Sex Medicine, 17*(8), 1538–1543. https://doi.org/10.1016/j.jsxm.2020.04.006. Accession Number: 32448679.

Frey, A., Pedersen, C., Lindberg, H., Bisbjerg, R., Sønksen, J., & Fode, M. (2017). Prevalence and predicting factors for commonly neglected sexual side effects to external-beam radiation therapy for prostate cancer. *The Journal of Sexual Medicine, 14*(4), 558–565. https://doi.org/10.1016/j.jsxm.2017.01.015

Frey, A., Sønksen, J., Jakobsen, H., & Fode, M. (2014). Prevalence and predicting factors for commonly neglected sexual side effects to radical prostatectomies: Results from a cross; Sectional questionnaire; Based study. *The Journal of Sexual Medicine, 11*(9), 2318–2326. https://doi.org/10.1111/jsm.12624

Haney, N. M., Alzweri, L. M., & Hellstrom, W. J. G. (2018). Male orgasmic dysfunction post-radical pelvic surgery. *Sexual Medicine Reviews, 6*(3), 429–437. https://doi.org/10.1016/j.sxmr.2017.12.003. Accession Number: 29396282.

Jimbo, M., Alom, M., Pfeifer, Z. D., Haile, E. S., Stephens, D. A., Gopalakrishna, A., Ziegelmann, M. J., Viers, B. R., Trost, L. W., & Kohler, T. S. (2020). Prevalence and predictors of climacturia and associated patient/partner bother in patients with history of definitive therapy for prostate cancer. *The Journal of Sexual Medicine, 17*(6), 1126–1132. https://doi.org/10.1016/j.jsxm.2020.02.016

Jo, J. K., Jeong, S. J., Oh, J. J., Lee, S. W., Lee, S., Hong, S. K., Byun, S.-S., & Lee, S. E. (2018). Effect of starting penile rehabilitation with sildenafil immediately after robot-assisted laparoscopic radical prostatectomy on erectile function recovery: A prospective randomized trial. *The Journal of Urology, 199*(6), 1600–1606. https://doi.org/10.1016/j.juro.2017.12.060

Kaplan, I., Bubley, G. J., Bhatt, R. S., Taplin, M. E., Dowling, S., Mahoney, & K. (2021). Enzalutamide with radiation therapy for intermediate-risk prostate cancer: A Phase 2 study. *International Journal of Radiation Oncollogy, Biology, Physics, 110*(5), 1416–1422. https://doi.org/10.1016/j.ijrobp.2021.02.027. Accession Number: 33636278.

Klotz, T., Mathers, M., Klotz, R., & Sommer, F. (2005). Why do patients with erectile dysfunction abandon effective therapy with sildenafil (Viagra®)? *International Journal of Impotence Research, 17*(1), 2–4. https://doi.org/10.1038/sj.ijir.3901252

Kowalkowski, M. A., Chandrashekar, A., Amiel, G. E., Lerner, S. P., Wittmann, D. A., Latini, D. M., & Goltz, H. H. (2014). Examining sexual dysfunction in non-muscle-invasive bladder cancer: Results of cross-sectional mixed-methods research. *Sexual Medicine*, 2(3), 141–151. https://doi.org/10.1002/sm2.24; 10.1002/sm2.24

Lehrfeld, T., & Lee, D. I. (2009). The role of vacuum erection devices in penile rehabilitation after radical prostatectomy. *International Journal of Impotence Research*, 21(3), 158–164. https://doi.org/10.1038/ijir.2009.3

Li, K., He, X., Tong, S., & Zheng, Y. (2021). Risk factors for sexual dysfunction after rectal cancer surgery in 948 consecutive patients: A prospective cohort study. *European Journal of Surgical Oncology*, 47(8), 2087–2092. https://doi.org/10.1016/j.ejso.2021.03.251

Lima, T. F. N., Bitran, J., Frech, F. S., & Ramasamy, R. (2021). Prevalence of post-prostatectomy erectile dysfunction and a review of the recommended therapeutic modalities. *International Journal of Impotence Research*, 33(4), 401–409. https://doi.org/10.1038/s41443-020-00374-8

Loi, M., Wortel, R. C., Francolini, G., & Incrocci, L. (2019). Sexual function in patients treated with stereotactic radiotherapy for prostate cancer: A systematic review of the current evidence. *The Journal of Sexual Medicine*, 16(9), 1409–1420. https://doi.org/10.1016/j.jsxm.2019.05.019

Mitidieri, E., Cirino, G., d'Emmanuele di Villa Bianca, R., & Sorrentino, R. (2020). Pharmacology and perspectives in erectile dysfunction in man. *Pharmacology & Therapeutics*, 208, 107493. https://doi.org/10.1016/j.pharmthera.2020.107493

Narang, G. L., Pannell, S. C., Laviana, A. A., Huen, K. H. Y., Izard, J., Smith, A. B., & Bergman, J. (2017). Patient-reported outcome measures in urology. *Current Opinion in Urology*, 27(4), 366–374. https://doi.org/10.1097/mou.0000000000000412

Nascimento, B., Miranda, E. P., Jenkins, L. C., Benfante, N., Schofield, E. A., & Mulhall, J. P. (2019). Testosterone recovery profiles after cessation of androgen deprivation therapy for prostate cancer. *Journal of Sex Medicine*, 16(6), 872–879. https://doi.org/10.1016/j.jsxm.2019.03.273. Accession Number: 31080102 PMCID: PMC7546513.

Neal, D. E., Metcalfe, C., Donovan, J. L., Lane, J. A., Davis, M., Young, G. J., Dutton, S. J., Walsh, E. I., Martin, R. M., Peters, T. J., Turner, E. L., Mason, M., Bryant, R., Bollina, P., Catto, J., Doherty, A., Gillatt, D., Gnanapragasam, V., Holding, P., & Hamdy, F. C. (2020). Ten-year mortality, disease progression, and treatment-related side effects in men with localised prostate cancer from the protect randomised controlled trial according to treatment received. *European Urology*, 77(3), 320–330. https://doi.org/10.1016/j.eururo.2019.10.030

Nolsøe, A. B., Jensen, C. F. S., Østergren, P. B., & Fode, M. (2021). Neglected side effects to curative prostate cancer treatments. *International Journal of Impotence Research*, 33(4), 428–438.

Nørskov, K. H., Schmidt, M., & Jarden, M. (2015). Patients' experience of sexuality 1-year after allogeneic Haematopoietic Stem Cell Transplantation. *European Journal of Oncology Nursing*, 19(4), 419–426. https://doi.org/10.1016/j.ejon.2014.12.005

Notarnicola, M., Celentano, V., Gavriilidis, P., Abdi, B., Beghdadi, N., Sommacale, D., Brunetti, F., Coccolini, F., & de'Angelis, N. (2020). PDE-5i management of erectile dysfunction after rectal surgery: A systematic review focusing on treatment efficacy. *American Journal of Men's Health*, *14*(5), 1557988320969061. https://doi.org/10.1177/1557988320969061

Padma-Nathan, H., McCullough, A. R., Levine, L. A., Lipshultz, L. I., Siegel, R., Montorsi, F., Giuliano, F., Brock, G., & on behalf of the Study Group. (2008). Randomized, double-blind, placebo-controlled study of postoperative nightly sildenafil citrate for the prevention of erectile dysfunction after bilateral nerve-sparing radical prostatectomy. *International Journal of Impotence Research*, *20*(5), 479–486. https://doi.org/10.1038/ijir.2008.33

Padoa, A., McLean, L., Morin, M., & Vandyken, C. (2021). "The overactive pelvic floor (OPF) and sexual dysfunction" Part 1: Pathophysiology of OPF and its impact on the sexual response. *Sexual Medicine Reviews*, *9*(1), 64–75. https://doi.org/10.1016/j.sxmr.2020.02.002. Accession Number: 32238325.

Pang, J. H., Jones, Z., Myers, O. B., & Popek, S. (2020). Long term sexual function following rectal cancer treatment. *The American Journal of Surgery*, *220*(5), 1258–1263. https://doi.org/10.1016/j.amjsurg.2020.06.064

Raheem, O. A., Natale, C., Dick, B., Reddy, A. G., Yousif, A., Khera, M., & Baum, N. (2020). Novel treatments of erectile dysfunction: Review of the current literature. *Sexual Medicine Reviews*, *9*(1), 123–132. https://doi.org/10.1016/j.sxmr.2020.03.005

Raina, R., Pahlajani, G., Agarwal, A., & Zippe, C. D. (2007). The early use of transurethral alprostadil after radical prostatectomy potentially facilitates an earlier return of erectile function and successful sexual activity. *BJU International*, *100*(6), 1317–1321. https://doi.org/10.1111/j.1464-410X.2007.07124.x

Sari Motlagh, R., Abufaraj, M., Yang, L., Mori, K., Pradere, B., Laukhtina, E., Mostafaei, H., Schuettfort, V. M., Quhal, F., Montorsi, F., Amjadi, M., Gratzke, C., & Shariat, S. F. (2021). Penile rehabilitation strategy after nerve sparing radical prostatectomy: A systematic review and network meta-analysis of randomized trials. *Journal of Urology*, *205*(4), 1018–1030. https://doi.org/10.1097/ju.0000000000001584

Schantz Laursen, B. (2017). Sexuality in men after prostate cancer surgery: A qualitative interview study. *Scandinavian Journal of Caring Sciences*, *31*(1), 120–127. https://doi.org/10.1111/scs.12328

So, W. K. W., Wong, C. L., Choi, K. C., Chan, C. W. H., Chan, J. C. Y., Law, B. M. H., Wan, R., Mak, S., Ling, W.-M., Ng, W.-T., & Yu, B. W. L. (2019). A mixed-methods study of unmet supportive care needs among head and neck cancer survivors. *Cancer Nursing*, *42*(1), 67–78. https://doi.org/10.1097/ncc.0000000000000542

Tal, R., Jacks, L. M., Elkin, E., & Mulhall, J. P. (2011). Penile implant utilization following treatment for prostate cancer: Analysis of the SEER-Medicare database. *The Journal of Sexual Medicine*, *8*(6), 1797–1804. https://doi.org/10.1111/j.1743-6109.2011.02240.x

Terrier, J. E., Masterson, M., Mulhall, J. P., & Nelson, C. J. (2018). Decrease in intercourse satisfaction in men who recover erections after radical prostatectomy. *The Journal of Sexual Medicine, 15*(8), 1133–1139. https://doi.org/10.1016/j.jsxm.2018.05.020

Towe, M., Huynh, L. M., El-Khatib, F., Gonzalez, J., Jenkins, L. C., & Yafi, F. A. (2019). A review of male and female sexual function following colorectal surgery. *Sexual Medicine Reviews, 7*(3), 422–429. https://doi.org/10.1016/j.sxmr.2019.04.001. Accession Number: 31147295.

Vasconcelos, J. S., Figueiredo, R. T., Nascimento, F. L., Damiao, R., & da Silva, E. A. (2012). The natural history of penile length after radical prostatectomy: A long-term prospective study. *Urology, 80*(6), 1293–1296. https://doi.org/10.1016/j.urology.2012.07.060

Walker, L. M., & Santos-Iglesias, P. (2020). On the relationship between erectile function and sexual distress in men with prostate cancer. *Archives of Sexual Behavior, 49*(5), 1575–1588. https://doi.org/10.1007/s10508-019-01603-y

Wang, V. M., & Levine, L. A. (2022). Safety and efficacy of inflatable penile prostheses for the treatment of erectile dysfunction: Evidence to date. *Medical Devices (Auckland N.Z), 15*, 27–36. https://doi.org/10.2147/mder.S251364

Wibowo, E., Wassersug, R. J., Robinson, J. W., Santos-Iglesias, P., Matthew, A., McLeod, D. L., & Walker, L. M. (2020). An educational program to help patients manage androgen deprivation therapy side effects: Feasibility, acceptability, and preliminary outcomes. *American Journal of Men's Health, 14*(1), 1557988319898991. https://doi.org/10.1177/1557988319898991

Wittmann, D., Foley, S., & Balon, R. (2011). A biopsychosocial approach to sexual recovery after prostate cancer surgery: The role of grief and mourning. *Journal of Sex & Marital Therapy, 37*(2), 130–144. https://doi.org/10.1080/0092623x.2011.560538

Wortel, R. C., Alemayehu, W. G., & Incrocci, L. (2015). Orchiectomy and radiotherapy for stage I-II testicular seminoma: A prospective evaluation of short-term effects on body image and sexual function. *The Journal of Sexual Medicine, 12*(1), 210–218. https://doi.org/10.1111/jsm.12739; 10.1111/jsm.12739

Yang, J., Jian, Z. Y., & Wang, J. (2021). Phosphodiesterase type-5 inhibitors for erectile dysfunction following nerve-sparing radical prostatectomy: A network meta-analysis. *Medicine (Baltimore), 100*(8), e23778. https://doi.org/10.1097/md.0000000000023778

Zavattaro, M., Felicetti, F., Faraci, D., Scaldaferri, M., Dellacasa, C., Busca, A., Dionisi-Vici, M., Cattel, F., Motta, G., Giaccone, L., Ghigo, E., Arvat, E., Lanfranco, F., Bruno, B., & Brignardello, E. (2021). Impact of allogeneic stem cell transplantation on testicular and sexual function. *Transplantation and Cellular Therapy, 27*(2), 182.e181–182.e188. https://doi.org/10.1016/j.jtct.2020.10.020

Zebrack, B. J., Foley, S., Wittmann, D., & Leonard, M. (2010). Sexual functioning in young adult survivors of childhood cancer. *Psycho-Oncology, 19*(8), 814–822. https://doi.org/10.1002/pon.1641

V

Pulmonary Symptoms

CHAPTER 19

DYSPNEA

INTRODUCTION

Dyspnea is a common symptom in patients with lung cancer, as well as those with other advanced cancers. It is common at the time of diagnosis of lung cancer and also during the last 3 months of life in patients with advanced cancers (Button et al., 2016). Dyspnea is a subjective experience of breathing discomfort that varies in intensity and is often described as breathlessness or air hunger (Parshall et al., 2012). It may not be associated with hypoxia or objective lack of air transfer.

PREVALENCE

The prevalence of dyspnea in those with lung cancer ranges from 45% (Kocher et al., 2015) to 75% (Weingaertner et al., 2014). Of patients with malignant pleural mesothelioma, 73% report dyspnea (Hoon et al., 2021).

CONTRIBUTING FACTORS

Preoperative dyspnea confers a 500% risk of long-term dyspnea; clinically significant depression is also a contributing factor (Feinstein et al., 2010). Preexisting conditions, such as chronic obstructive pulmonary disease (COPD), also contribute to dyspnea (Hashimoto et al., 2014).

ASSESSMENT

It is important to understand the impact of dyspnea on the patient's quality of life, the intensity of the symptom, and the distress it causes. Patients will use different terms to describe what they are experiencing, but there are formal questionnaires that provide an objective assessment. Assessment should include the presence of triggers for dyspnea and potential causes that may be reversed or mitigated. There are a number of assessment tools available, including the following:

- Baseline Dyspnea Index (BDI; Mahler et al., 1984; https://www.thoracic.org/members/assemblies/assemblies/srn/question-aires/bdi-tdi.php)

- Borg Rating of Perceived Exertion (RPE) Scale (Williams, 2017)

- Cancer Dyspnea Scale (Uronis et al., 2012)

- Chronic Respiratory Questionnaire (Williams et al., 2001)

- European Organisation for Research and Treatment of Cancer (EORTC-QLQ-LC29; Koller et al., 2017)

- EORTC-LC13 (Bergman et al., 1994; Koller et al., 2015; https://qol.eortc.org/questionnaire/qlq-lc29/)

- Functional Assessment of Cancer Therapy-Lung (FACT-L V.4; https://www.facit.org/_files/ugd/626819_340039bdea6642e-bab42d309b7b716db.pdf)

- Lung Cancer Symptom Scale (LCSS; Gralla et al., 2016)

- Multidimensional Dyspnea Profile (Meek et al., 2012; Williams et al., 2022)

- Numeric Rating Scale (Gift & Narsavage, 1998)

- Revised Edmonton Symptom Assessment Scale (Watanabe et al., 2011)

- Short-Form Chronic Respiratory Disease Questionnaire (Charalambous & Molassiotis, 2017; Tsai et al., 2008)

- Visual Analog Scale of the Effort to Breathe (VAS$_e$; Mador & Kufel, 1992)

MANAGEMENT

Dyspnea is distressing for both the patient and their caregiver(s). There are a number of interventions, ranging from breathing exercises to palliative care. Referral to the palliative care team provides expert symptom management, as well as psychosocial support, to both the patient and their caregivers, decision-making in complex situations, coordination of care teams, and advance care planning (Hui & Bruera, 2020). Specialist breathlessness services provide expertise in managing dyspnea (Farquhar et al., 2014) but are not widely available as yet.

Nonpharmaceutical Management

A battery-operated hand fan blowing room air on the person's face (specifically the cheek) has been shown to be effective in relieving dyspnea at rest (Barnes-Harris et al., 2019; Swan et al., 2019), as well as for those in the terminal stages of illness (Kako et al., 2018). If the patient is not able to hold the fan, a tabletop fan aimed at the face can be used.

Specialist training that includes breath control, anxiety management, relaxation, and pacing may help patients cope with their dyspnea (Johnson et al., 2015). These techniques may be most helpful in the home setting. Inspiratory muscle training (Molassiotis et al., 2015) or mindful breathing (Tan et al., 2019) may also be suggested. Oxygen by mask (Nava et al., 2013) or nasal prongs delivering 2 to 6 L/min (Hui et al., 2021) can also be provided if the patient is hypoxic.

Acupuncture may also be offered (Minchom et al., 2016).

Pharmaceutical Management

Opioids are the first-line pharmaceutical intervention and should be started at low doses and titrated carefully using whichever route of administration is appropriate to the situation (Barnes et al., 2016). Nebulized opioids may be prescribed if systemic opioids are not appropriate for the individual patient (Boyden et al., 2015).

Benzodiazepines should not be offered as first-line treatment of dyspnea due to the risk of delirium (Mori et al., 2020) and respiratory depression when the patient is on opioids (Dowell et al., 2016).

Short-term systemic corticosteroids may be prescribed to select patients with caution due to their well-known side effects (Mori et al., 2017).

Bronchodilators can be used if bronchospasm exists, but should not exceed the maximum daily doses (Hui et al., 2021).

Palliative Sedation

CASE STUDY

An 87-year-old man is seen in the clinic for routine follow-up after treatment for stage 2a non-small cell lung cancer. He was treated with surgical resection and there is now evidence that his cancer has metastasized. He previously refused adjuvant chemotherapy. His daughter who accompanies him is very concerned because he has become increasingly short of breath. He lives alone and she is worried that there is no one at his home to take care of him.

1. How would you assess his condition?

2. What immediate measures would you suggest?

His daughter wants to know what the plan is for her father. He appears weak and emaciated and he is having difficulty staying awake.

3. What are your next steps?

Over the next 5 days, his condition deteriorates. He appears to be in pain and the opioids that were prescribed do not seem to be effective. The palliative care physician suggests that it may be time for palliative sedation. His daughter is opposed to this and she demands to see the hospital administrator.

4. What can you do to help the situation?

Palliative sedation can be used in patients who are imminently dying and are experiencing pain and suffering, including intractable dyspnea that is unresponsive to other palliative interventions (Kirk & Mahon, 2010). It should be offered after a comprehensive discussion with the patient and their family (Bobb, 2016) and consultation with palliative care specialists. It is not the same as euthanasia or physician-assisted suicide.

GUIDELINES

- **American Society of Clinical Oncology (ASCO)**

    Integration of Palliative Care Into Standard Oncology Care: American Society of Clinical Oncology Clinical Practice Guideline Update (2017; Ferrell et al., 2017)

    Management of Dyspnea in Advanced Cancer: ASCO Guideline (2021; Hui et al., 2021)

- **American Thoracic Society**

    An Official American Thoracic Society Statement: Update on the Mechanisms, Assessment, and Management of Dyspnea (2012; Parshall et al., 2012)

SUMMARY

Dyspnea is a distressing symptom that occurs frequently in patients with lung cancer and at or near the end of life in patients with other cancers. Treatment should start with nonpharmaceutical interventions, and consultation with palliative care specialists is recommended, especially if pharmaceutical interventions are needed.

A robust set of instructor resources designed to supplement this text is located at http://connect.springerpub.com/content/reference-book/978-0-8261-8524-2. Qualifying Instructors may request access by emailing **textbook@springerpub.com**.

REFERENCES

Barnes-Harris, M., Allgar, V., Booth, S., Currow, D., Hart, S., Phillips, J., Swan, F., & Johnson, M. J. (2019). Battery operated fan and chronic breathlessness: Does it help? *BMJ Supportive and Palliative Care, 9*(4), 478–481. https://doi.org/10.1136/bmjspcare-2018-001749

Barnes, H., McDonald, J., Smallwood, N., & Manser, R. (2016). Opioids for the palliation of refractory breathlessness in adults with advanced disease and terminal illness. *Cochrane Database of Systematic Reviews, 3*, CD011008.

Bergman, B., Aaronson, N. K., Ahmedzai, S., Kaasa, S., & Sullivan, M. (1994). The EORTC QLQ-LC13: A modular supplement to the EORTC core quality of life questionnaire (QLQ-C30) for use in lung cancer clinical trials. *European Journal of Cancer, 30*(5), 635–642. https://doi.org/10.1016/0959-8049(94)90535-5

Bobb, B. (2016). A review of palliative sedation. *Nursing Clinics of North America*, *51*(3), 449–457. https://doi.org/10.1016/j.cnur.2016.05.008

Boyden, J. Y., Connor, S. R., Otolorin, L., Nathan, S. D., Fine, P. G., Davis, M. S., & Muir, J. C. (2015). Nebulized medications for the treatment of dyspnea: A literature review. *Journal of Aerosol Medicine and Pulmonary Drug Delivery*, *28*(1), 1–19.

Button, E., Chan, R., Chambers, S., Butler, J., & Yates, P. (2016). Signs, symptoms, and characteristics associated with end of life in people with a hematologic malignancy: A review of the literature. *Oncology Nursing Forum*, *43*(5), E178–E187. https://doi.org/10.1188/16.Onf.E178-e187

Charalambous, A., & Molassiotis, A. (2017). Preliminary validation and reliability of the Short Form Chronic Respiratory Disease Questionnaire in a lung cancer population. *European Journal of Cancer Care (England)*, *26*(1), e12418. https://doi.org/10.1111/ecc.12418

Dowell, D., Haegerich, T. M., & Chou, R. (2016). CDC guideline for prescribing opioids for chronic pain—United States, 2016. *JAMA*, *315*(15), 1624–1645.

Farquhar, M. C., Prevost, A. T., McCrone, P., Brafman-Price, B., Bentley, A., Higginson, I. J., Todd, C., & Booth, S. (2014). Is a specialist breathlessness service more effective and cost-effective for patients with advanced cancer and their carers than standard care? Findings of a mixed-method randomised controlled trial. *BMC Medicine*, *12*, 194. https://doi.org/10.1186/s12916-014-0194-2

Feinstein, M. B., Krebs, P., Coups, E. J., Park, B. J., Steingart, R. M., Burkhalter, J., Logue, A., Ostroff, J. S., & Ostroff, J. S. (2010). Current dyspnea among long-term survivors of early-stage non-small cell lung cancer. *Journal of Thoracic Oncology*, *5*(8), 1221–1226. https://doi.org/10.1097/JTO.0b013e3181df61c8

Ferrell, B. R., Temel, J. S., Temin, S., Alesi, E. R., Balboni, T. A., Basch, E. M., Firn, J. I., Paice, J. A., Peppercorn, J. M., Phillips, T., Stovall, E. L., Zimmermann, C., & Smith, T. J. (2017). Integration of palliative care into standard oncology care: American Society of Clinical Oncology Clinical Practice Guideline Update. *Journal of Clinical Oncology*, *35*(1), 96–112. https://doi.org/10.1200/jco.2016.70.1474

Gift, A. G., & Narsavage, G. (1998). Validity of the numeric rating scale as a measure of dyspnea. *American Journal of Critical Care*, *7*(3), 200–204.

Gralla, R. J., Spigel, D. R., Bennett, B., Taylor, F., Penrod, J. R., DeRosa, M., Dastani, H., Orsini, L. S., & Reck, M. (2016). Lung Cancer Symptom Scale (LCSS) as a marker of treatment (tx) benefit with nivolumab (nivo) vs docetaxel (doc) in patients (pts) with advanced (adv) non-squamous (NSQ) NSCLC from CheckMate 057. *Journal of Clinical Oncology*, *34*(15 Suppl), 9031–9031. https://doi.org/10.1200/JCO.2016.34.15_suppl.9031

Hashimoto, N., Matsuzaki, A., Okada, Y., Imai, N., Iwano, S., Wakai, K., Imaizumi, K., Yokoi, K., & Hasegawa, Y. (2014). Clinical impact of prevalence and severity of COPD on the decision-making process for therapeutic management of lung cancer patients. *BMC Pulmonary Medicine, 14*(1), 1–9. https://doi.org/10.1186/1471-2466-14-14

Hoon, S. N., Lawrie, I., Qi, C., Rahman, N., Maskell, N., Forbes, K., Gerry, S., Monterosso, L., Chauhan, A., & Brims, F. J. H. (2021). Symptom burden and unmet needs in malignant pleural mesothelioma: Exploratory analyses from the RESPECT-Meso Study. *Journal of Palliative Care, 36*(2), 113–120. https://doi.org/10.1177/0825859720948975

Hui, D., Bohlke, K., Bao, T., Campbell, T. C., Coyne, P. J., Currow, D. C., Gupta, A., Leiser, A. L., Mori, M., Nava, S., Reinke, L. F., Roeland, E. J., Seigel, C., Walsh, D., & Campbell, M. L. (2021). Management of dyspnea in advanced cancer: ASCO Guideline. *Journal of Clinical Oncology, 39*(12), 1389–1411. https://doi.org/10.1200/jco.20.03465

Hui, D., & Bruera, E. (2020). Models of palliative care delivery for patients with cancer. *Journal of Clinical Oncology, 38*(9), 852.

Hui, D., Mahler, D. A., Larsson, L., Wu, J., Thomas, S., Harrison, C. A., Hess, K., Lopez-Mattei, J., Thompson, K., Gomez, D., Jeter, M., Lin, S., Basen-Engquist, K., & Bruera, E. (2021). High-flow nasal cannula therapy for exertional dyspnea in patients with cancer: A pilot randomized clinical trial. *Oncologist, 26*(8), e1470–e1479. https://doi.org/10.1002/onco.13624

Johnson, M. J., Kanaan, M., Richardson, G., Nabb, S., Torgerson, D., English, A., Barton, R., & Booth, S. (2015). A randomised controlled trial of three or one breathing technique training sessions for breathlessness in people with malignant lung disease. *BMC Medicine, 13*, 213. https://doi.org/10.1186/s12916-015-0453-x

Kako, J., Morita, T., Yamaguchi, T., Kobayashi, M., Sekimoto, A., Kinoshita, H., Ogawa, A., Zenda, S., Uchitomi, Y., Inoguchi, H., & Matsushima, E. (2018). Fan therapy is effective in relieving dyspnea in patients with terminally ill cancer: A parallel-arm, randomized controlled trial. *Journal of Pain and Symptom Management, 56*(4), 493–500. https://doi.org/10.1016/j.jpainsymman.2018.07.001

Kirk, T. W., & Mahon, M. M. (2010). National Hospice and Palliative Care Organization (NHPCO) position statement and commentary on the use of palliative sedation in imminently dying terminally ill patients. *Journal of Pain and Symptom Management, 39*(5), 914–923.

Kocher, F., Hilbe, W., Seeber, A., Pircher, A., Schmid, T., Greil, R., Auberger, J., Nevinny-Stickel, M., Sterlacci, W., Tzankov, A., Jamnig, H., Kohler, K., Zabernigg, A., Frötscher, J., Oberaigner, W., & Fiegl, M. (2015). Longitudinal analysis of 2293 NSCLC patients: A comprehensive study from the TYROL registry. *Lung Cancer, 87*(2), 193–200. https://doi.org/10.1016/j.lungcan.2014.12.006

Koller, M., Hjermstad, M. J., Tomaszewski, K. A., Tomaszewska, I. M., Hornslien, K., Harle, A., Arraras, J. I., Morag, O., Pompili, C., Ioannidis, G., Georgiou, M., Navarra, C., Chie, W.-C., Johnson, C. D., Himpel, A., Schulz, C., Bohrer, T., Janssens, A., Kuliś, D., & Bottomley, A. (2017). An international study to revise the EORTC questionnaire for assessing quality of life in lung cancer patients. *Annals of Oncology, 28*(11), 2874–2881. https://doi.org/10.1093/annonc/mdx453

Koller, M., Warncke, S., Hjermstad, M. J., Arraras, J., Pompili, C., Harle, A., Johnson, C. D., Chie, W.-C., Schulz, C., Zeman, F., van Meerbeeck, J. P., Kuliś, D., Bottomley, A., & European Organisation for Research and Treatment of Cancer (EORTC) Quality of Life Group and the EORTC Lung Cancer Group. (2015). Use of the lung cancer–specific Quality of Life Questionnaire EORTC QLQ-LC13 in clinical trials: A systematic review of the literature 20 years after its development . *Cancer, 121*(24), 4300–4323. https://doi.org/10.1002/cncr.29682

Mador, M. J., & Kufel, T. J. (1992). Reproducibility of visual analog scale measurements of dyspnea in patients with chronic obstructive pulmonary disease. *American Review of Respiratory Disease, 146*(1), 82–87.

Mahler, D. A., Weinberg, D. H., Wells, C. K., & Feinstein, A. R. (1984). The measurement of dyspnea: Contents, interobserver agreement, and physiologic correlates of two new clinical indexes. *Chest, 85*(6), 751–758.

Meek, P. M., Banzett, R., Parsall, M. B., Gracely, R. H., Schwartzstein, R. M., & Lansing, R. (2012). Reliability and validity of the multidimensional dyspnea profile. *Chest, 141*(6), 1546–1553. https://doi.org/10.1378/chest.11-1087

Minchom, A., Punwani, R., Filshie, J., Bhosle, J., Nimako, K., Myerson, J., Gunapala, R., Popat, S., & O'Brien, M. E. (2016). A randomised study comparing the effectiveness of acupuncture or morphine versus the combination for the relief of dyspnoea in patients with advanced non-small cell lung cancer and mesothelioma. *European Journal of Cancer, 61*, 102–110. https://doi.org/10.1016/j.ejca.2016.03.078

Molassiotis, A., Charalambous, A., Taylor, P., Stamataki, Z., & Summers, Y. (2015). The effect of resistance inspiratory muscle training in the management of breathlessness in patients with thoracic malignancies: A feasibility randomised trial. *Supportive Care in Cancer, 23*(6), 1637–1645. https://doi.org/10.1007/s00520-014-2511-x

Mori, M., Morita, T., Matsuda, Y., Yamada, H., Kaneishi, K., Matsumoto, Y., Matsuo, N., Odagiri, T., Aruga, E., Watanabe, H., Tatara, R., Sakurai, H., Kimura, A., Katayama, H., Suga, A., Nishi, T., Shirado, A. N., Watanabe, T., Kuchiba, A. … Watanabe, H. (2020). How successful are we in relieving terminal dyspnea in cancer patients? A real-world multicenter prospective observational study. *Supportive Care in Cancer, 28*(7), 3051–3060.

Mori, M., Shirado, A. N., Morita, T., Okamoto, K., Matsuda, Y., Matsumoto, Y., Yamada, H., Sakurai, H., Aruga, E., Kaneishi, K., Watanabe, H., Yamaguchi, T., Odagiri, T., Hiramoto, S., Kohara, H., Matsuo, N., Katayama, H., Nishi, T., Matsui, T., & Kaneishi, K. (2017). Predictors of response to corticosteroids for dyspnea in advanced cancer patients: A preliminary multicenter prospective observational study. *Supportive Care in Cancer, 25*(4), 1169–1181.

Nava, S., Ferrer, M., Esquinas, A., Scala, R., Groff, P., Cosentini, R., Guido, D., Lin, C.-H., Cuomo, A. M., & Grassi, M. (2013). Palliative use of non-invasive ventilation in end-of-life patients with solid tumours: A randomised feasibility trial. *Lancet Oncology, 14*(3), 219–227. https://doi.org/10.1016/s1 470-2045(13)70009-3

Parshall, M. B., Schwartzstein, R. M., Adams, L., Banzett, R. B., Manning, H. L., Bourbeau, J., Calverley, P. M., Gift, A. G., Harver, A., Lareau, S. C., Mahler, D. A., & Meek, P. M. (2012). An official American Thoracic Society statement: Update on the mechanisms, assessment, and management of dyspnea. *American Journal of Respiratory and Critical Care Medicine, 185*(4), 435–452. https://doi.org/10.1164/rccm.201111-2042ST

Swan, F., Newey, A., Bland, M., Allgar, V., Booth, S., Bausewein, C., Yorke, J., & Johnson, M. (2019). Airflow relieves chronic breathlessness in people with advanced disease: An exploratory systematic review and meta-analyses. *Palliative Medicine, 33*(6), 618–633. https://doi.org/10.1177/0269216319 835393

Tan, S. B., Liam, C. K., Pang, Y. K., Leh-Ching Ng, D., Wong, T. S., Wei-Shen Khoo, K., Ooi, C.-Y., & Chai, C. S. (2019). The effect of 20-minute mindful breathing on the rapid reduction of dyspnea at rest in patients with lung diseases: A randomized controlled trial. *Journal of Pain and Symptom Management, 57*(4), 802–808. https://doi.org/10.1016/j.jpainsymman.2019. 01.009

Tsai, C.-L., Hodder, R. V., Page, J. H., Cydulka, R. K., Rowe, B. H., & Camargo, C. A. (2008). The short-form chronic respiratory disease questionnaire was a valid, reliable, and responsive quality-of-life instrument in acute exacerbations of chronic obstructive pulmonary disease. *Journal of Clinical Epidemiology, 61*(5), 489–497. https://doi.org/10.1016/j.jclinepi.2007.07.003

Uronis, H. E., Shelby, R. A., Currow, D. C., Ahmedzai, S. H., Bosworth, H. B., Coan, A., & Abernethy, A. P. (2012). Assessment of the psychometric properties of an English version of the cancer dyspnea scale in people with advanced lung cancer. *Journal of Pain and Symptom Management, 44*(5), 741–749. https://doi.org/10.1016/j.jpainsymman.2011.10.027

Watanabe, S. M., Nekolaichuk, C., Beaumont, C., Johnson, L., Myers, J., & Strasser, F. (2011). A multicenter study comparing two numerical versions of the Edmonton Symptom Assessment system in palliative care patients. *Journal of Pain and Symptom Management, 41*(2), 456–468. https://doi.org/10. 1016/j.jpainsymman.2010.04.020

Weingaertner, V., Scheve, C., Gerdes, V., Schwarz-Eywill, M., Prenzel, R., Bausewein, C., Higginson, I. J., Voltz, R., Herich, L., & Simon, S. T. (2014). Breathlessness, functional status, distress, and palliative care needs over time in patients with advanced chronic obstructive pulmonary disease or lung cancer: A cohort study. *Journal of Pain and Symptom Management, 48*(4), 569–581.e561. https://doi.org/10.1016/j.jpainsymman.2013.11.011

Williams, J. E., Singh, S. J., Sewell, L., Guyatt, G. H., & Morgan, M. D. (2001). Development of a self-reported Chronic Respiratory Questionnaire (CRQ-SR). *Thorax, 56*(12), 954–959. https://doi.org/10.1136/thorax. 56.12.954

Williams, M. T., Lewthwaite, H., Paquet, C., Johnston, K., Olsson, M., Belo, L. F., Pitta, F., Morelot-Panzini, C., & Ekström, M. (2022). Dyspnoea-12 and multidimensional dyspnea profile: Systematic review of use and properties. *Journal of Pain and Symptom Management, 63*(1), e75–e87. https://doi.org/10.1016/j.jpainsymman.2021.06.023

Williams, N. (2017). The Borg Rating of Perceived Exertion (RPE) scale. *Occupational Medicine, 67*(5), 404–405. https://doi.org/10.1093/occmed/kqx063

CHAPTER 20

HEMOPTYSIS

INTRODUCTION

Hemoptysis occurs in patients with lung cancer and may be fatal. Pulmonary cancer is the most frequent cause of this, comprising 19% of all cases (Mondoni et al., 2018). It is thought to occur when cavitation of the tumor leads to a fistula between the airway and bronchial circulation (Oskan et al., 2017). The location of squamous cell lung cancer is most often central in the chest and is thus more likely to invade the large blood vessels. *Life-threatening hemoptysis* is defined as approximately 150 mL of blood in a 24-hour period (quantifiable by patients as roughly a half cup of blood in 24 hours) or bleeding at a rate of ≥100 mL/hr (Ibrahim, 2008).

PREVALENCE

Nonlife-threatening hemoptysis occurs in 7% to 10% of patients with lung cancer at diagnosis, and 20% of patients with lung cancer will experience hemoptysis intermittently (Cahill & Ingbar, 1994).

Life-threatening hemoptysis occurs in approximately 2% of patients (Mondoni et al., 2018).

CONTRIBUTING FACTORS

Radiation-induced necrosis, cancer therapies that cause cavitation such as bevacizumab, and brachytherapy are risk factors for hemoptysis (Oskan et al., 2017), but there is some debate about these factors (Hellmann et al., 2013).

ASSESSMENT

If the patient is not experiencing life-threatening hemoptysis or their breathing is not compromised, evaluate the frequency, severity, and location of the source of the bleeding. Laboratory studies (hematocrit and hemoglobin), chest x-ray (Thirumaran et al., 2009), and CT of the chest with intravenous (IV) contrast (American College of Radiology [ACR] Appropriateness Criteria® Hemoptysis [2019]) should be ordered.

CASE STUDY

A 45-year-old man with known lung cancer reports at his regular visit that he has been coughing blood.

1. What do you need to consider in this case?
2. What investigations should you order?

All investigations are essentially normal.

3. What should you advise him?

MANAGEMENT

Bronchoscopy is recommended for nonlife-threatening hemoptysis to identify the source of the bleeding. If there is a visible lesion, referral to the appropriate specialist for control of bleeding should be made (Simoff et al., 2013). For patients with large volume of bleeding, emergency procedures including endotracheal intubation should be initiated (Simoff et al., 2013).

GUIDELINES

- **American College of Chest Physicians**

    American College of Chest Physicians Evidence-Based Clinical Practice Guidelines: Symptom Management in Patients With Lung Cancer Diagnosis and Management of Lung Cancer, Third Edition (2013; Simoff et al., 2013)

- **American College of Radiology (ACR)**

    ACR Appropriateness Criteria® Hemoptysis (2019)

    https://acsearch.acr.org/docs/69449/Narrative/

SUMMARY

Hemoptysis is not an uncommon symptom in patients with lung cancer and is usually self-limiting and not life-threatening. However, large volumes of blood may be expectorated in some cases and this is an emergency.

A robust set of instructor resources designed to supplement this text is located at http://connect.springerpub.com/content/reference-book/978-0-8261-8524-2.
Qualifying Instructors may request access by emailing **textbook@springerpub.com**.

REFERENCES

Cahill, B. C., & Ingbar, D. H. (1994). Massive hemoptysis. Assessment and management. *Clinics in Chest Medicine, 15*(1), 147–167.

Hellmann, M. D., Chaft, J. E., Rusch, V., Ginsberg, M. S., Finley, D. J., Kris, M. G., Price, K. A. R., Azzoli, C. G., Fury, M. G., Riely, G. J., Krug, L. M., Downey, R. J., Bains, M. S., Sima, C. S., Rizk, N., Travis, W. D., Rizvi, N., & Paik, P. K. (2013). Risk of hemoptysis in patients with resected squamous cell and other high-risk lung cancers treated with adjuvant bevacizumab. *Cancer Chemotherapy and Pharmacology, 72*(2), 453–461. https://doi.org/10.1007/s0 0280-013-2219-5

Ibrahim, W. H. (2008). Massive haemoptysis: the definition should be revised. *European Respiratory Journal, 32*(4), 1131–1132. https://doi.org/10.1183/090 31936.00080108

Mondoni, M., Carlucci, P., Job, S., Parazzini, E. M., Cipolla, G., Pagani, M., Tursi, F., Negri, L., Fois, A., Canu, S., Arcadu, A., Pirina, P., Bonifazi, M., Gasparini, S., Marani, S., Comel, A. C., Ravenna, F., Dore, S., Alfano, F., & Sotgiu, G. (2018). Observational, multicentre study on the epidemiology of haemoptysis. *European Respiratory Journal, 51*(1). https://doi.org/10.1183/13 993003.01813-2017

Oskan, F., Becker, G., & Bleif, M. (2017). Specific toxicity after stereotactic body radiation therapy to the central chest: A comprehensive review. *Strahlentherapie und Onkologie, 193*(3), 173–184. https://doi.org/10.1007/s0 0066-016-1063-z

Simoff, M. J., Lally, B., Slade, M. G., Goldberg, W. G., Lee, P., Michaud, G. C., Wahidi, M. M., & Chawla, M. (2013). Symptom management in patients with lung cancer: Diagnosis and management of lung cancer: American College of Chest Physicians evidence-based clinical practice guidelines. *Chest, 143*(5), e455S–e497S. https://doi.org/10.1378/chest.12-2366

Thirumaran, M., Sundar, R., Sutcliffe, I. M., & Currie, D. C. (2009). Is investigation of patients with haemoptysis and normal chest radiograph justified? *Thorax, 64*(10), 854–856. https://doi.org/10.1136/thx.2008.108795

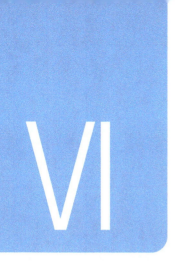

Neurologic Symptoms

CHAPTER 21

HEARING LOSS

INTRODUCTION

Some of the most widely used chemotherapy agents (cisplatin, carboplatin, and oxaliplatin) cause hearing impairment and/or tinnitus. Used in the treatment of solid tumors, such as ovarian, cervical, testicular, non-small cell lung, bladder, and head and neck, these side effects impact negatively on quality of life, including the development of depression, anxiety, and social anxiety. An estimated 500,000 people are diagnosed with these cancers each year and are eligible for treatment with these agents, causing a significant burden due to ototoxicity (Siegel et al., 2022). Hearing loss usually occurs at higher frequencies initially and may be permanent (Rybak, 2007). The impact on the inner ear also leads to poor balance and a risk of falls (Phillips et al., 2023). These symptoms can occur at any time during treatment and can affect one or both ears. Radiation therapy to the head also causes hearing loss due to damage to structures such as the temporal bones, the cochlea, the middle ear, and the Eustachian tube (Lambert et al., 2016).

PREVALENCE

Up to 36% of adults treated with these agents will experience changes in auditory function (tinnitus, pain, and hearing loss), with greater severity with cumulative exposure to the chemotherapy agents (Karasawa & Steyger, 2015). A higher prevalence of tinnitus (60.5%) and hearing loss (56.4%) has been reported in men with testicular cancer (Sanchez et al., 2023), and these symptoms were associated with fatigue, cognitive dysfunction, and depression. Up to 67% of patients treated with radiation for head and neck cancer have hearing loss, with permanent loss at 6 months after treatment (Lambert et al., 2016).

CONTRIBUTING FACTORS

Platinum-based chemotherapy and radiation to the head are contributing factors to these symptoms.

CASE STUDY

Your patient is a 74-year-old man with stage 2 non-small cell lung cancer who will start chemotherapy with cisplatin. He will have radiation after completion of chemotherapy. You notice that he seems to not understand what you have told him.

1. What might be causing this?
2. What else should be considered?

He declines further testing but his daughter who is with him tries to convince him to follow your suggestions.

3. What can you do if he refuses a hearing test?

His score on the patient self-report test suggests that he has moderate hearing loss. He continues to deny this.

4. What are your next steps?

ASSESSMENT

The Revised Hearing Handicap Inventory (RHHI) contains 18 items (Cassarly et al., 2020) that are scored from 0 (no) to 2 (sometimes) and 4 (yes), with a cutoff score of ≥6. A screening version (RHHI-S) contains 10 items with the same scoring and cutoff point (Figure 21.1).

Does a hearing problem cause you difficulty when listening to TV or radio?
Does a hearing problem cause you difficulty when attending a party?
Does a hearing problem cause you to feel frustrated when talking to members of your family?
Does a hearing problem cause you to feel left out when you are with a group of people?
Does a hearing problem cause you difficulty when visiting friends, relatives, or neighbors?
Do you feel handicapped by a hearing problem?
Do you feel that any difficulty with your hearing limits or hampers your personal or social life?
Does a hearing problem cause you to feel uncomfortable when talking to friends?
Does a hearing problem cause you to avoid groups of people?
Does a hearing problem cause you to visit friends, relatives, or neighbors less often than you would like?

Figure 21.1 Revised Hearing Handicap Inventory and Screening.

Source: From Cassarly, C., Matthews, L. J., Simpson, A. N., & Dubno, J. R. (2020). The Revised Hearing Handicap Inventory and Screening tool based on psychometric reevaluation of the hearing handicap inventories for the elderly and adults. *Ear and Hearing, 41*(1), 95–105. https://doi.org/10.1097/aud.0000000000000746.

The Common Terminology Criteria for Adverse Events (CTCAE) provides criteria to assess both hearing loss and tinnitus (www.ctep. cancer.gov/protocoldevelopment/electronic_applications/docs/ ctcae_v5_quick_reference_8.5x11.pdf).

Grading of hearing impairment is presented in Boxes 21.1, and 21.2. Grading for tinnitus is presented in Box 21.3.

Hearing Impairment for Patients on a Monitoring Program

Box 21.1 Hearing Impairment Grading for Patients on a Monitoring Program

Grade 1	Threshold shift of 15–25 dB averaged at two contiguous test frequencies in at least one ear
Grade 2	Threshold shift of >25 dB averaged at two contiguous test frequencies in at least one ear
Grade 3	Threshold shift of >25 dB averaged at three contiguous test frequencies in at least one ear (intervention indicated)
Grade 4	Profound bilateral hearing loss >80 dB

Hearing Impairment for Patients <u>Not</u> on a Monitoring Program

Box 21.2 Hearing Impairment Grading for Patients <u>Not</u> on a Monitoring Program

Grade 1	Subjective change in hearing in the absence of documented hearing loss
Grade 2	Hearing loss with hearing aid or intervention not indicated; limiting instrumental ADL
Grade 3	Hearing loss with hearing aid or intervention indicated; limiting self-care ADL

ADL, activities of daily living.

Tinnitus

Box 21.3 Tinnitus Grading

Grade 1	Mild symptoms; intervention not indicated
Grade 2	Moderate symptoms; limiting instrumental ADL
Grade 3	Severe symptoms; limiting self-care ADL

ADL, activities of daily living.

The Tinnitus Primary Function Questionnaire (TPFQ; Tyler et al., 2014) can be used to assess tinnitus and its impact in four domains (Figure 21.2). Scores on the TPFQ range from 0 (completely disagree)

Concentration

- I feel like my tinnitus makes it difficult for me to concentrate on some tasks.
- I have difficulty focusing my attention on some important tasks because of tinnitus.
- My inability to think about something undisturbed is one of the worst effects of my tinnitus.

Emotion

- My emotional peace is one of the worst effects of my tinnitus.
- I am depressed because of my tinnitus.
- I am anxious because of my tinnitus.

Hearing

- My tinnitus masks some speech sounds.
- In addition to my hearing loss, my tinnitus interferes with my understanding of speech.
- One of the worst things about my tinnitus is its effect on my speech understanding, over and above any effect of my hearing loss.

Sleep

- I am tired during the day because my tinnitus has disrupted my sleep.
- I lie awake at night because of my tinnitus.
- When I wake up in the night, my tinnitus makes it difficult to get back to sleep.

Figure 21.2 The Tinnitus Primary Function Questionnaire.

Source: From Tyler, R., Ji, H., Perreau, A., Witt, S., Noble, W., & Barros Coelho, C. (2014). Development and validation of the tinnitus primary function questionnaire. *American Journal of Audiology, 23*, 260–272. https://doi.org/10.1044/2014_AJA-13-0014.

to 100 (completely agree). The higher the score, the greater the impact of tinnitus on activities of daily living. There are a number of other measures for tinnitus that can be accessed on the American Tinnitus Association's website (www.ata.org). Adherence to ototoxicity monitoring is poor due in part to lack of data regarding its importance for rehabilitation and quality of life (Santucci et al., 2021).

MANAGEMENT

Prevention is the core mitigation strategy at the present time; there are no Food and Drug Administration (FDA)-approved pharmaceutical agents for the treatment of hearing loss in this population (Chattaraj et al., 2023). A baseline evaluation of hearing for all patients prescribed platinum-based therapy should be conducted using both behavioral and objective measures (Durrant et al., 2009). There is concern that some patients may not be able to accurately assess their hearing during treatment. The U.S. Department of Veterans Affairs has proposed a comprehensive ototoxicity monitoring program for its members (COMP-VA; Konrad-Martin et al., 2014), which includes a pretreatment risk assessment, screening for early hearing changes, screening for outer hair cell dysfunction, follow-up testing, screening and referral for tinnitus, and patient and clinician education about rehabilitation. When hearing loss and/or tinnitus are identified, referral to an audiologist or auditory clinic is recommended (Clemens et al., 2019). It is important to minimize further damage to hearing loss; if hearing loss is permanent, amplification devices, assisted hearing devices, or cochlear implants, in addition to communication strategies, can be considered (Ganesan et al., 2018).

GUIDELINES

- **American Academy of Audiology**

    American Academy of Audiology Position Statement and Clinical Practice Guidelines: Ototoxicity Monitoring (Durrant et al., 2009)

- **American Speech-Language-Hearing Association**

    American Speech-Language-Hearing Association Audiologic Management of Individuals Receiving Cochleotoxic Drug Therapy

    www.asha.org/policy/gl1994-00003/

SUMMARY

Ototoxicity refers to auditory changes caused by platinum-based chemotherapy and/or radiation to the head that exposes the structures responsible for hearing. These changes are experienced as hearing loss that may be permanent and/or tinnitus that impact on social functioning, sleep, and mental health.

A robust set of instructor resources designed to supplement this text is located at http://connect.springerpub.com/content/reference-book/978-0-8261-8524-2. Qualifying Instructors may request access by emailing **textbook@springerpub.com**.

REFERENCES

Cassarly, C., Matthews, L. J., Simpson, A. N., & Dubno, J. R. (2020). The revised hearing handicap inventory and screening tool based on psychometric reevaluation of the hearing handicap inventories for the elderly and adults. *Ear and Hearing*, 41(1), 95–105. https://doi.org/10.1097/aud.0000000000000746

Chattaraj, A., Syed, M. P., Low, C. A., & Owonikoko, T. K. (2023). Cisplatin-induced ototoxicity: A concise review of the burden, prevention, and interception strategies. *JCO Oncology Practice*, 19(5), 278–283. https://doi.org/10.1200/op.22.00710

Clemens, E., van, den Heuvel-Eibrink, M. M., Mulder, R. L., Kremer, L. C. M., Hudson, M. M., Skinner, R., Constine, L. S., Bass, J. K., Kuehni, C. E., Langer, T., van Dalen, E. C., Bardi, E., Bonne, N.-X., Brock, P. R., Brooks, B., Carleton, B., Caron, E., Chang, K. W., Johnston, K., & Landier, W. (2019). Recommendations for ototoxicity surveillance for childhood, adolescent, and young adult cancer survivors: A report from the international late effects of childhood cancer guideline harmonization group in collaboration with the PanCare consortium. *Lancet Oncol, 20*(1), e29–e41. https://doi.org/10.1016/s1470-2045(18)30858-1

Durrant, J., Campbell, K., Fausti, S., Guthrie, O., Jacobson, G., Lonsbury-Martin, B., & Poling, G. (2009). *American Academy of Audiology position statement and clinical practice guidelines: Ototoxicity monitoring.* American Academ y of Audiology.

Ganesan, P., Schmiedge, J., Manchaiah, V., Swapna, S., Dhandayutham, S., & Kothandaraman, P. P. (2018). Ototoxicity: A challenge in diagnosis and treatment. *Journal of Audiology & Otology, 22*(2), 59–68. https://doi.org/10.7874/jao.2017.00360

Karasawa, T., & Steyger, P. S. (2015). An integrated view of cisplatin-induced nephrotoxicity and ototoxicity. *Toxicology Letters, 237*(3), 219–227. https://doi.org/10.1016/j.toxlet.2015.06.012

Konrad-Martin, D., Reavis, K. M., McMillan, G., Helt, W. J., & Dille, M. (2014). Proposed comprehensive ototoxicity monitoring program for VA healthcare (COMP-VA). *Journal of Rehabilitation Research and Development, 51*(1), 81.

Lambert, E. M., Gunn, G. B., & Gidley, P. W. (2016). Effects of radiation on the temporal bone in patients with head and neck cancer. *Head & Neck, 38*(9), 1428–1435. https://doi.org/10.1002/hed.24267

Phillips, O. R., Baguley, D. M., Pearson, S. E., & Akeroyd, M. A. (2023). The long-term impacts of hearing loss, tinnitus and poor balance on the quality of life of people living with and beyond cancer after platinum-based chemotherapy: A literature review. *Journal of Cancer Survivorship, 17*(1), 40–58. https://doi.org/10.1007/s11764-022-01314-9

Rybak, L. P. (2007). Mechanisms of cisplatin ototoxicity and progress in otoprotection. *Current Opinion in Otolaryngology & Head and Neck Surgery, 15*(5), 364–369.

Sanchez, V. A., Shuey, M. M., Jr, P. C. D., Monahan, P. O., Fosså, S. D., Sesso, H. D., Dolan, M. E., Einhorn, L. H., Vaughn, D. J., Martin, N. E., Feldman, D. R., Kroenke, K., Fung, C., Frisina, R. D., & Travis, L. B. (2023). Patient-reported functional impairment due to hearing loss and tinnitus after cisplatin-based chemotherapy. *Journal of Clinical Oncology, 41*(12), 2211–2226. https://doi.org/10.1200/jco.22.01456

Santucci, N. M., Garber, B., Ivory, R., Kuhn, M. A., Stephen, M., & Aizenberg, D. (2021). Insight into the current practice of ototoxicity monitoring during cisplatin therapy. *Journal of Otolaryngology-Head & Neck Surgery, 50*(1), 19. https://doi.org/10.1186/s40463-021-00506-0

Siegel, R. L., Miller, K. D., Fuchs, H. E., & Jemal, A. (2022). Cancer statistics, 2022. *CA: A Cancer Journal for Clinicians, 72*(1), 7–33.

Tyler, R., Ji, H., Perreau, A., Witt, S., Noble, W., & Barros Coelho, C. (2014). Development and validation of the tinnitus primary function questionnaire. *American Journal of Audiology, 23*, 260–272. https://doi.org/10.1044/2014_AJA-13-0014

CHAPTER 22

PERIPHERAL NEUROPATHY

INTRODUCTION

Chemotherapy-induced peripheral neuropathy (CIPN) is a common side effect of specific chemotherapy agents that is dose-dependent, cumulative, and has a negative impact on quality of life. CIPN predominately affects the sensory nerves in a glove-and-stocking distribution (Emery et al., 2022) and usually improves over time; however, for some patients, it can become chronic. Patients report numbness, tingling, and pain which may alter gait and balance (Campbell & Skubic, 2018). Oxaliplatin and paclitaxel cause acute neuropathy (cold sensitivity, throat discomfort especially when swallowing cold liquids, muscle cramps), usually peaking 2 to 3 days after infusion. Paclitaxel causes a pain syndrome that is felt in the trunk and hips, also peaking 2 to 3 days after each dose (Loprinzi et al., 2020). Both docetaxel (Bandos et al., 2017) and oxaliplatin (Briani et al., 2014) are associated with long-term peripheral neuropathy.

PREVALENCE

CIPN occurs in up to 70% of patients (Pachman et al., 2011). In most patients, there is a gradual decline in symptoms, but it is estimated that 30% of patients will still have symptoms at 6 months after chemotherapy treatment (Seretny et al., 2014).

CONTRIBUTING FACTORS

The agents with the greatest risk of developing CIPN are platinum agents (cisplatin and oxaliplatin), taxanes (paclitaxel, docetaxel), vinca alkaloids (vincristine), and bortezomib. Dose and duration of treatment, combination with other neurotoxic agents, and cumulative dose are responsible for the degree of nerve damage. Comorbidities that affect the nerves such as diabetes also impact on the development of this condition (Pachman et al., 2011). Environmental factors such as cold temperatures may also contribute (Pulvers & Marx, 2017).

ASSESSMENT

There are a number of instruments to assess CIPN, but most have been used with single cancer populations; there is no single tool to measure this condition in the general oncology population (Curcio, 2016; Figure 22.1).

Other measures include the following:

- Chemotherapy-Induced Peripheral Neuropathy Assessment Tool (CIPNAT; Tofthagen et al., 2011)

- Scale for Chemotherapy-Induced Long-Term Neurotoxicity Scale (SCIN; Oldenburg et al., 2006)

- European Organisation for Research and Treatment of Cancer Quality of Life Questionnaire-Chemotherapy Induced Peripheral Neuropathy20 Questionnaire (Lavoie Smith et al., 2013)

- Patient Neurotoxicity Questionnaire (Shimozuma et al., 2009)

- Functional Assessment of Cancer Therapy-Taxane (FACT-Taxane; Cella et al., 2003)

The grade of peripheral neuropathy is assessed by the National Cancer Institute Common Terminology Criteria for Adverse Events (NCI CTCAE; Box 22.1; https://ctep.cancer.gov/protocoldevelopment/electronic_applications/docs/CTCAE_v5_Quick_Reference_8.5x11.pdf).

The Functional Assessment of Cancer Therapy/Gynecologic Oncology Group–Neurotoxicity (FACT/GOG-Ntx-4)

This 4-item patient-report measure assesses numbness or tingling and discomfort in hands and feet over the past 7 weeks.

(Calhoun et al., 2003; Cheng et al., 2020)

Reduced Total Neuropathy Score (TNSr)

TNSr includes clinical assessment of sensory symptoms, pin and vibration sensibility, motor strength, and deep tendon reflexes as well as reduction in sural nerve sensory action potential and peroneal nerve compound muscle action potential.

(Cavaletti et al., 2007)

Total Neuropathy Score (TNSc; clinical examination).

This tool includes clinical assessment of sensory symptoms, pin and vibration sensibility, motor strength, and deep tendon reflexes but EXCLUDES assessment of reduction in sural nerve sensory action potential and peroneal nerve compound muscle action potential.

(Cavaletti et al., 2006)

Figure 22.1 Recommended tools to assess chemotherapy-induced peripheral neuropathy.

CHAPTER 22 • PERIPHERAL NEUROPATHY **221**

Box 22.1 Grade of Peripheral Neuropathy Assessed by the National Cancer Institute Common Terminology Criteria for Adverse Events

Grade 1	Asymptomatic
Grade 2	Moderate symptoms that limit instrumental activities of daily living
Grade 3	Severe symptoms limiting self-care activities of daily living
Grade 4	Life-threatening consequences with urgent interventions indicated

There are a number of measures to assess balance and gait (Abbenhardt et al., 2013), including sensor-based measures such as body-worn sensors and gaming systems.

MANAGEMENT

The risk from the type of chemotherapy prescribed should be assessed in patients with comorbidities that predispose to CIPN. An automated symptom monitoring system that prompts engagement with a nurse clinician has been shown to reduce the prevalence, severity, and distress associated with CIPN (Kolb et al., 2018).

- *Pharmaceutical management:* Small studies suggest that duloxetine may help those treated with cisplatin rather than taxanes, while venlafaxine may be helpful to those treated with oxaliplatin. There is limited evidence on the use of gabapentin or pregabalin. Amitriptyline may be helpful in treating CIPN (Jordan et al., 2020).

- *Nonpharmaceutical management:* There is limited evidence about commonly suggested interventions to treat CIPN, including acupuncture, cryotherapy, compression therapy, exercise, or ganglioside-monosialic acid (GM-1; Loprinzi et al., 2020).

- *Self-management strategies:* Avoidance of extreme temperatures and tight clothing and shoes, caution when handling sharp objects, and paying attention to good foot and hand care are all important to discuss with the patient and their caregivers (Jordan et al., 2020). Patients will often modify their activities of daily living by managing their environment and asking their family and friends for help (Speck et al., 2012). Getting enough sleep may be helpful in improving CIPN symptoms (Stevinson et al., 2009).

CASE STUDY

Your patient is a 62-year-old woman with breast cancer. She is about to start chemotherapy and asks you what she can expect

(continued)

CASE STUDY (*CONTINUED*)

about the side effects. She mentions that her sister was treated a number of years ago and she had bad peripheral neuropathy and she would like to avoid this side effect.

1. What advice should you give her?

After a discussion with her oncologist, she consents to a regimen that is known to cause chemotherapy-induced peripheral neuropathy (CIPN). When you see her after her first dose, she states that the symptoms have started and she is having a hard time taking care of her family.

2. What questions should you ask her?

3. Based on her response, what advice can you give her?

GUIDELINES

- **American Society of Clinical Oncology (ASCO)**

  ASCO Prevention and Management of Chemotherapy-Induced Peripheral Neuropathy in Survivors of Adult Cancers (2020)

  https://old-prod.asco.org/practice-patients/guidelines/patient-and-survivor-care#/9541

- **European Society for Medical Oncology (ESMO), European Oncology Nursing Society (EONS), and European Association of Neuro-Oncology (EANO)**

  Systemic Anticancer Therapy-Induced Peripheral and Central Neurotoxicity: ESMO–EONS–EANO Clinical Practice Guidelines for Diagnosis, Prevention, Treatment, and Follow-Up (2020; Jordan et al., 2020)

- **Oncology Nursing Society (ONS)**

  Oncology Nursing Society (2014). Putting Evidence Into Practice (PEP Guidelines; Aiello-Laws et al., 2009)

  https://www-ons-org.uml.idm.oclc.org/practice-resources/pep

SUMMARY

CIPN is a common adverse event with few interventions. The agents causing this are commonly used to treat breast, gynecologic, and colorectal cancers. The condition negatively affects quality of life and activities of daily living.

A robust set of instructor resources designed to supplement this text is located at http://connect.springerpub.com/content/reference-book/978-0-8261-8524-2.
Qualifying Instructors may request access by emailing **textbook@springerpub.com**.

REFERENCES

Abbenhardt, C., McTiernan, A., Alfano, C. M., Wener, M. H., Campbell, K. L., Duggan, C., Foster-Schubert, K. E., Kong, A., Toriola, A. T., Potter, J. D., Mason, C., Xiao, L., Blackburn, G. L., ,., Bain, C., & Ulrich, C. M. (2013). Effects of individual and combined dietary weight loss and exercise interventions in postmenopausal women on adiponectin and leptin levels. *Journal of Internal Medicine, 274*(2), 163–175. https://doi.org/10.1111/joim.12062

Aiello-Laws, L., Janice Reynolds, R., Nancy Deizer, M., & Mary Peterson, R. (2009). Putting evidence into practice: What are the pharmacologic interventions for nociceptive and neuropathic cancer pain in adults? *Clinical Journal of Oncology Nursing, 13*(6), 649.

Bandos, H., Melnikow, J., Rivera, D. R., Swain, S. M., Sturtz, K., Fehrenbacher, L., Wade, J. L., Brufsky, A. M., Julian, T. B., Margolese, R. G., McCarron, E. C., & Ganz, P. A. (2017). Long-term Peripheral neuropathy in breast cancer patients treated with adjuvant chemotherapy: NRG Oncology/NSABP B-30. *JNCI: Journal of the National Cancer Institute, 110*(2), djx162. https://doi.org/10.1093/jnci/djx162

Briani, C., Argyriou, A. A., Izquierdo, C., Velasco, R., Campagnolo, M., Alberti, P., Frigeni, B., Cacciavillani, M., Bergamo, F., Cortinovis, D., Cazzaniga, M., Bruna, J., Cavaletti, G., & Kalofonos, H. P. (2014). Long-term course of oxaliplatin-induced polyneuropathy: A prospective 2-year follow-up study. *Journal of the Peripheral Nervous System, 19*(4), 299–306. https://doi.org/10.1111/jns.12097

Calhoun, E. A., Welshman, E. E., Chang, C. H., Lurain, J. R., Fishman, D. A., Hunt, T. L., & Cella, D. (2003). Psychometric evaluation of the Functional Assessment of Cancer Therapy/Gynecologic Oncology Group—Neurotoxicity (Fact/GOG-Ntx) questionnaire for patients receiving systemic chemotherapy. *International Journal of Gynecologic Cancer, 13*(6), 741. https://doi.org/10.1136/ijgc-00009577-200311000-00003

Campbell, G., & Skubic, M. A. (2018). Balance and gait impairment: Sensor-based assessment for patients with peripheral neuropathy. *Clinical Journal of Oncology Nursing, 22*(3), 316–325. https://doi.org/10.1188/18.Cjon.316-325

Cavaletti, G., Frigeni, B., Lanzani, F., Piatti, M., Rota, S., Briani, C., Zara, G., Plasmati, R., Pastorelli, F., Caraceni, A., Pace, A., Manicone, M., Lissoni, A., Colombo, N., Bianchi, G., & Zanna, C. (2007). The Total Neuropathy Score as an assessment tool for grading the course of chemotherapy-induced peripheral neurotoxicity: Comparison with the National Cancer Institute-Common Toxicity Scale. *Journal of the Peripheral Nervous System, 12*(3), 210–215. https://doi.org/10.1111/j.1529-8027.2007.00141.x

Cavaletti, G., Jann, S., Pace, A., Plasmati, R., Siciliano, G., Briani, C., Cocito, D., Padua, L., Ghiglione, E., Manicone, M., & Giussani, G. (2006). Multicenter assessment of the Total Neuropathy Score for chemotherapy-induced peripheral neurotoxicity. *Journal of the Peripheral Nervous System, 11*(2), 135–141. https://doi.org/10.1111/j.1085-9489.2006.00078.x

Cella, D., Peterman, A., Hudgens, S., Webster, K., & Socinski, M. A. (2003). Measuring the side effects of taxane therapy in oncology. *Cancer, 98*(4), 822–831. https://doi.org/10.1002/cncr.11578

Cheng, H. L., Lopez, V., Lam, S. C., Leung, A. K. T., Li, Y. C., Wong, K. H., Kie Au, J. S., Sundar, R., Chan, A., De Ng, T. R., Ping Suen, L. K., Chan, C. W., Yorke, J., & Molassiotis, A. (2020). Psychometric testing of the Functional Assessment of Cancer Therapy/Gynecologic Oncology Group—Neurotoxicity (FACT/GOG-Ntx) subscale in a longitudinal study of cancer patients treated with chemotherapy. *Health Qual Life Outcomes, 18*(1), 246. https://doi.org/10.1186/s12955-020-01493-y

Curcio, K. R. (2016). Instruments for assessing chemotherapy-induced peripheral neuropathy: A review of the literature. *Clinical Journal of Oncology Nursing, 20*(2), 144–151. https://doi.org/10.1188/16.Cjon.20-01ap

Emery, J., Butow, P., Lai-Kwon, J., Nekhlyudov, L., Rynderman, M., & Jefford, M. (2022). Management of common clinical problems experienced by survivors of cancer. *Lancet, 399*(10334), 1537–1550. https://doi.org/10.1016/s0140-6736(22)00242-2

Jordan, B., Margulies, A., Cardoso, F., Cavaletti, G., Haugnes, H. S., Jahn, P., Le Rhun, E., Preusser, M., Scotté, F., Taphoorn, M. J. B., & Jordan, K. (2020). Systemic anticancer therapy-induced peripheral and central neurotoxicity: ESMO-EONS-EANO Clinical Practice Guidelines for diagnosis, prevention, treatment and follow-up. *Annals of Oncology, 31*(10), 1306–1319. https://doi.org/10.1016/j.annonc.2020.07.003

Kolb, N. A., Smith, A. G., Singleton, J. R., Beck, S. L., Howard, D., Dittus, K., Karafiath, S., & Mooney, K. (2018). Chemotherapy-related neuropathic symptom management: A randomized trial of an automated symptom-monitoring system paired with nurse practitioner follow-up. *Supportive Care in Cancer, 26*(5), 1607–1615. https://doi.org/10.1007/s00520-017-3970-7

Lavoie Smith, E. M., Barton, D. L., Qin, R., Steen, P. D., Aaronson, N. K., & Loprinzi, C. L. (2013). Assessing patient-reported peripheral neuropathy: The reliability and validity of the European Organization for Research and Treatment of Cancer QLQ-CIPN20 Questionnaire. *Quality of Life Research, 22*(10), 2787–2799. https://doi.org/10.1007/s11136-013-0379-8

Loprinzi, C. L., Lacchetti, C., Bleeker, J., Cavaletti, G., Chauhan, C., Hertz, D. L., Kelley, M. R., Lavino, A., Lustberg, M. B., Paice, J. A., Schneider, B. P., Lavoie Smith, E. M., Smith, M. L., Smith, T. J., Wagner-Johnston, N., & Hershman, D. L. (2020). Prevention and management of chemotherapy-induced peripheral neuropathy in survivors of adult cancers: ASCO

Guideline update. *Journal of Clinical Oncology, 38*(28), 3325–3348. https://doi.org/10.1200/jco.20.01399

Oldenburg, J., Fosså, S. D., & Dahl, A. A. (2006). Scale for Chemotherapy-induced Long-term Neurotoxicity (SCIN): Psychometrics, validation, and findings in a sample of testicular cancer survivors. *Quality of Life Research, 15*(5), 791–800. https://doi.org/10.1007/s11136-005-5370-6

Pachman, D. R., Barton, D. L., Watson, J. C., & Loprinzi, C. L. (2011). Chemotherapy-induced peripheral neuropathy: Prevention and treatment. *Clinical Pharmacology & Therapeutics, 90*(3), 377–387. https://doi.org/10.1038/clpt.2011.115

Pulvers, J. N., & Marx, G. (2017). Factors associated with the development and severity of oxaliplatin-induced peripheral neuropathy: A systematic review. *Asia Pacific Journal of Clinical Oncology, 13*(6), 345–355. https://doi.org/10.1111/ajco.12694

Seretny, M., Currie, G. L., Sena, E. S., Ramnarine, S., Grant, R., MacLeod, M. R., Colvin, L. A., & Fallon, M. (2014). Incidence, prevalence, and predictors of chemotherapy-induced peripheral neuropathy: A systematic review and meta-analysis. *PAIN®, 155*(12), 2461–2470. https://doi.org/10.1016/j.pain.2014.09.020

Shimozuma, K., Ohashi, Y., Takeuchi, A., Aranishi, T., Morita, S., Kuroi, K., Ohsumi, S., Makino, H., Mukai, H., Katsumata, N., Sunada, Y., Watanabe, T., & Hausheer, F. H. (2009). Feasibility and validity of the Patient Neurotoxicity Questionnaire during taxane chemotherapy in a phase III randomized trial in patients with breast cancer: N-SAS BC 02. *Supportive Care in Cancer, 17*(12), 1483. https://doi.org/10.1007/s00520-009-0613-7

Speck, R. M., DeMichele, A., Farrar, J. T., Hennessy, S., Mao, J. J., Stineman, M. G., & Barg, F. K. (2012). Scope of symptoms and self-management strategies for chemotherapy-induced peripheral neuropathy in breast cancer patients. *Supportive Care in Cancer, 20*(10), 2433–2439.

Stevinson, C., Steed, H., Faught, W., Tonkin, K., Vallance, J. K., Ladha, A. B., Schepansky, A., Capstick, V., & Courneya, K. S. (2009). Physical activity in ovarian cancer survivors: Associations with fatigue, sleep, and psychosocial functioning. *International Journal of Gynecologic Cancer, 19*(1), 73. https://doi.org/10.1111/IGC.0b013e31819902ec

Tofthagen, C. S., McMillan, S. C., & Kip, K. E. (2011). Development and psychometric evaluation of the chemotherapy-induced peripheral neuropathy assessment tool. *Cancer Nursing, 34*(4), E10–E20. https://journals.lww.com/cancernursingonline/Fulltext/2011/07000/Development_and_Psychometric_Evaluation_of_the.13.aspx

CHAPTER 23

COGNITIVE DYSFUNCTION

INTRODUCTION

Commonly referred to as *chemo brain* or *brain fog*, cognitive changes are among the most feared side effects of cancer treatment that have a negative impact on quality of life and may persist for years. Much of the research on this symptom has been conducted in women with breast cancer; however, cognitive changes are not exclusive to patients with breast cancer. Cognitive changes include memory deficits, poor attention and concentration, difficulty with language, and changes in executive functioning (Oldacres et al., 2023). It is suggested that these changes are associated with frontoparietal hyperactivation during tasks involving working memory (Sousa et al., 2020).

The four common domains of cognitive effects of chemotherapy for breast, colorectal, and prostate cancer are executive function, memory, verbal memory, and recall. Women with breast cancer experience more changes than patients with colorectal or prostate cancer (McDougall et al., 2014); however, most of the research on cognitive changes has been conducted in the breast cancer population. Older women with breast cancer may experience an accelerated decline in cognitive functioning (Coughlin et al., 2019) and these cognitive changes are predictive of poor overall survival (Magnuson et al., 2019). Lower cognitive function may lead to a slightly increased risk of cancer-specific mortality (Rostamian et al., 2022). African American women have reported not knowing about this due to lack of information from oncology care clinicians (Husain et al., 2019). The result of this may be fear of changes with no explanation as to the reason.

PREVALENCE

Up to 70% of people treated with chemotherapy for non-central nervous system (CNS) cancers report this symptom (Bray et al., 2018). The prevalence in patients with brain tumors is higher, with up to 90% experiencing changes in at least one domain of cognitive function (Bergo et al., 2016). The greatest impact on cognitive functioning occurs in those with gliomas, with cognitive changes that may be lifelong (Allen & Loughan, 2018).

CONTRIBUTING FACTORS

A major contributing factor is treatment with chemotherapy. Women who have been treated with cyclophosphamide, 5-fluorouracil, and methotrexate report cognitive changes during or soon after chemotherapy treatment (Bray et al., 2018).

There are a number of other factors that contribute to cognitive changes, including symptom burden (e.g., pain, fatigue), emotional distress, and comorbidities. Older age, lower cognitive reserve, being postmenopausal, endocrine manipulation therapies for women with breast cancer, depression, and anxiety are known contributing factors (Henneghan, 2016). Frailty and low cognitive reserve in older patients are markers of negative changes to cognition (Mandelblatt et al., 2013). Radiation therapy for brain tumors is a known factor in the development of cognitive changes (Jacob et al., 2018).

ASSESSMENT

There is a significant difference between self-perceived and objective measures of cancer-related cognitive impairment, due in part to the psychological characteristics of the individual (Bellens et al., 2022). There is no standardized testing for cognitive changes, but the following assessment tools may be used to objectively measure cognitive change. Caution is advised as these tools do not have the sensitivity for the more gradual decline in cognition that is more typical for cancer survivors (National Comprehensive Cancer Network [NCCN] Guidelines; https://www.nccn.org/professionals/physician_gls/pdf/survivorship.pdf).

- The Mini-Mental State Examination (MMSE; www.psychdb.com/cognitive-testing/mmse) is frequently used to assess cognitive functioning in older adults. It contains 11 questions in five areas of cognitive function (orientation, registration, attention and calculation, recall, and language).

- The Montreal Cognitive Assessment (MOCA; https://mocacognition.com) is a rapid assessment of the following domains with 30 questions: short-term memory, visuospatial abilities; executive function; attention, concentration, and working memory; language; and orientation. A training and certification program is necessary before administering and scoring the test.

There is one cancer-specific questionnaire that is available; however, there are no established cut-points for diagnosis (Dyk et al., 2019).

- The Functional Assessment of Cancer Therapy-Cognitive Function (https://www.facit.org/measures/FACT-Cog) is a 37-item

CHAPTER 23 • COGNITIVE DYSFUNCTION

questionnaire that measures chemotherapy-induced cognitive changes in the following domains: perceived cognitive impairments, impact of perceived cognitive impairments on quality of life, comments from others, and perceived cognitive abilities.

Patients should also be screened for potentially reversible conditions such as depression, fatigue, sleep disturbance, and delirium (Oh, 2017).

CASE STUDY

A 53-year-old woman with HER2/neu negative breast cancer tells you that she is increasingly forgetful and she is terrified that this is an early sign of Alzheimer.

1. What can you tell her?

2. What should you do to assess this?

She is reassured with the information but says that she wants to do something about this.

3. What evidence-based suggestions can you make?

MANAGEMENT

- *Pharmaceutical management:* There is limited evidence to support the use of agents such as donepezil, methylphenidate, and modafinil in mitigating the cognitive changes associated with radiation to the brain (Kirkman et al., 2022), as well as chemotherapy-associated cognitive dysfunction (Kohli et al., 2009; Lundorff et al., 2009; Sood et al., 2006).

- *Nonpharmaceutical management:* Treating modifiable factors associated with cognitive changes is the first step in helping those affected. These include improving sleep quality, reducing stress, and encouraging social support (Henneghan, 2016), as well as treating the underlying depression, anxiety, and distress (Atkins & Zimmer, 2023; Figure 23.1).

Computer-Based Training
Focuses on retraining a cognitive skill through practice and computer tasks
Strategy Training
Includes cognitive behavioral therapy aimed at retraining lost cognitive abilities and learning compensatory behaviors through psychoeducation, stress reduction, and peer support

Figure 23.1 Cognitive rehabilitation.

The evidence to support exercise as a method to mitigate cognitive changes is limited (Campbell et al., 2020); however, upon self-report, women with breast cancer have stated that they experienced improvements in executive function when participating in physical activity (Ren et al., 2022). Computer-based cognitive training has shown effectiveness in breast cancer survivors in the domains of processing speed and executive function (Bail & Meneses, 2016) and has positive effects on anxiety, depression, and fatigue (Bray et al., 2017). Strategy training using psychoeducation methods such as the Insight (Bray et al., 2017) and the Cancer and Living Meaningfully (CALM; Ding et al., 2020) programs has shown improvement in cognitive symptoms. Mindfulness-based stress reduction may be helpful in women with breast cancer who report altered cognitive function (Melis et al., 2023; Zhang et al., 2019). Cognitive therapy in a group setting has shown improvement in memory in patients with early-stage gliomas (Piil et al., 2016), but unfortunately interventions are rarely offered to patients with brain tumors due to their poor prognosis (Bergo et al., 2016). There is preliminary evidence that immersive virtual reality may have positive effects on cognition (Zeng et al., 2022).

GUIDELINES

- **National Comprehensive Cancer Network (NCCN)**

    NCCN Guidelines Version 1.2023 Survivorship: Cognitive Function

    https://www.nccn.org/professionals/physician_gls/pdf/survivorship.pdf

- **International Cognition and Cancer Task Force**

    International Cognition and Cancer Task Force Recommendations to Harmonize Studies of Cognitive Function in Patients With Cancer (Wefel et al., 2011)

SUMMARY

Cognitive changes due to cancer treatment are a distressing symptom that impacts on quality of life, employment, and social functioning. Self-reported changes are greater than those measured objectively, but this should not mean that interventions are not offered for perceived changes. Pharmaceutical interventions are limited, but cognitive training, psychoeducation, and mindfulness-based stress reduction show efficacy and promise.

A robust set of instructor resources designed to supplement this text is located at http://connect.springerpub.com/content/reference-book/978-0-8261-8524-2.
Qualifying Instructors may request access by emailing **textbook@springerpub.com**.

REFERENCES

Allen, D. H., & Loughan, A. R. (2018). Impact of cognitive impairment in patients with Gliomas. *Seminars in Oncology Nursing, 34*(5), 528–546. https://doi.org/10.1016/j.soncn.2018.10.010

Atkins, S. L. P., & Zimmer, A. S. (2023). Neurologic complications of breast cancer. *Cancer, 129*(4), 505–520. https://doi.org/ 10.1002/cncr.34518

Bail, J., & Meneses, K. (2016). Computer-based cognitive training for chemotherapy-related cognitive impairment in breast cancer survivors. *Clinical Journal of Oncology Nursing, 20*(5), 504–509. https://doi.org/10.1188/16.Cjon.504-509

Bellens, A., Roelant, E., Sabbe, B., Peeters, M., & van Dam, P. A. (2022). Evaluation of a new online cognitive assessment tool in breast cancer survivors with cognitive impairment: A prospective cohort study. *Supportive Care in Cancer, 30*(1), 21–31. https://doi.org/10.1007/s00520-021-06397-1

Bergo, E., Lombardi, G., Pambuku, A., Della Puppa, A., Bellu, L., D'Avella, D., & Zagonel, V. (2016). Cognitive rehabilitation in patients with gliomas and other brain tumors: State of the art. *Biomed Research International, 2016,* 3041824. https://doi.org/10.1155/2016/3041824

Bray, V. J., Dhillon, H. M., Bell, M. L., Kabourakis, M., Fiero, M. H., Yip, D., Boyle, F., Price, M. A., & Vardy, J. L. (2017). Evaluation of a web-based cognitive rehabilitation program in cancer survivors reporting cognitive symptoms after chemotherapy. *Journal of Clinical Oncology, 35*(2), 217–225. https://doi.org/10.1200/JCO.2016.67.8201

Bray, V. J., Dhillon, H. M., & Vardy, J. L. (2018). Systematic review of self-reported cognitive function in cancer patients following chemotherapy treatment. *Journal of Cancer Survivorship, 12*(4), 537–559. https://doi.org/1 0.1007/s11764-018-0692-x

Campbell, K. L., Zadravec, K., Bland, K. A., Chesley, E., Wolf, F., & Janelsins, M. C. (2020). The effect of exercise on cancer-related cognitive impairment and applications for physical therapy: Systematic review of randomized controlled trials. *Physical Therapy, 100*(3), 523–542. https://doi.org/10.1093/ptj/pzz090

Coughlin, S. S., Paxton, R. J., Moore, N., Stewart, J. L., & Anglin, J. (2019). Survivorship issues in older breast cancer survivors. *Breast Cancer Res Treat, 174*(1), 47–53. https://doi.org/10.1007/s10549-018-05078-8

Ding, K., Zhang, X., Zhao, J., Zuo, H., Bi, Z., & Cheng, H. (2020). Managing cancer and living meaningfully (CALM) intervention on chemotherapy-related cognitive impairment in breast cancer survivors. *Integrative Cancer Therapies, 19,* 153473542093845–1534735420938450. https://doi.org/10.1177/1534735420938450

Dyk, K. V., Crespi, C. M., Petersen, L., & Ganz, P. A. (2019). Identifying cancer-related cognitive impairment using the FACT-Cog perceived cognitive impairment. *JNCI Cancer Spectrum, 4*(1), pkz099. https://doi.org/10.1093/jncics/pkz099

Henneghan, A. (2016). Modifiable factors and cognitive dysfunction in breast cancer survivors: A mixed-method systematic review. *Supportive Care in Cancer*, *24*(1), 481–497. https://doi.org/10.1007/s00520-015-2927-y

Husain, M., Nolan, T. S., Foy, K., Reinbolt, R., Grenade, C., & Lustberg, M. (2019). An overview of the unique challenges facing African-American breast cancer survivors. *Supportive Care in Cancer*, *27*(3), 729–743. https://doi.org/10.1007/s00520-018-4545-y

Jacob, J., Durand, T., Feuvret, L., Mazeron, J. J., Delattre, J. Y., Hoang-Xuan, K., Psimaras, D., Douzane, H., Ribeiro, M., Capelle, L., Carpentier, A., Ricard, D., & Maingon, P. (2018). Cognitive impairment and morphological changes after radiation therapy in brain tumors: A review. *Radiotherapy and Oncology*, *128*(2), 221–228. https://doi.org/10.1016/j.radonc.2018.05.027

Kirkman, M. A., Day, J., Gehring, K., Zienius, K., Grosshans, D., Taphoorn, M., Li, J., & Brown, P. D. (2022). Interventions for preventing and ameliorating cognitive deficits in adults treated with cranial irradiation. *Cochrane Database of Systematic Reviews*, *11*. https://doi.org/10.1002/14651858.CD011335.pub3

Kohli, S., Fisher, S. G., Tra, Y., Adams, M. J., Mapstone, M. E., Wesnes, K. A., Roscoe, J. A., & Morrow, G. R. (2009). The effect of modafinil on cognitive function in breast cancer survivors. *Cancer*, *115*(12), 2605–2616. https://doi.org/10.1002/cncr.24287

Lundorff, L. E., Jønsson, B. H., & Sjøgren, P. (2009). Modafinil for attentional and psychomotor dysfunction in advanced cancer: A double-blind, randomised, cross-over trial. *Palliative Medicine*, *23*(8), 731–738. https://doi.org/10.1177/0269216309106872

Magnuson, A., Sattar, S., Nightingale, G., Saracino, R., Skonecki, E., & Trevino, K. M. (2019). A practical guide to geriatric syndromes in older adults with cancer: A focus on falls, cognition, polypharmacy, and depression. *American Society of Clinical Oncology Educational Book*, *39*, e96–e109. https://doi.org/10.1200/edbk_237641

Mandelblatt, J. S., Hurria, A., McDonald, B. C., Saykin, A. J., Stern, R. A., VanMeter, J. W., VanMeter, J. W., McGuckin, M., Traina, T., Denduluri, N., Turner, S., Howard, D., Jacobsen, P. B., & Ahles, T. (2013). Cognitive effects of cancer and its treatments at the intersection of aging: What do we know; what do we need to know? *Seminars in Oncology*, *40*(6), 709–725. https://doi.org/10.1053/j.seminoncol.2013.09.006

McDougall, G. J., Jr., Oliver, J. S., & Scogin, F. (2014). Memory and cancer: A review of the literature. *Archives of Psychiatric Nursing*, *28*(3), 180–186. https://doi.org/10.1016/j.apnu.2013.12.005

Melis, M., Schroyen, G., Leenaerts, N., Smeets, A., Sunaert, S., Van der Gucht, K., & Deprez, S. (2023). The impact of mindfulness on cancer-related cognitive impairment in breast cancer survivors with cognitive complaints. *Cancer*, *129*, 1105–1116. https://doi.org/10.1002/cncr.34640

Oh, P. J. (2017). Predictors of cognitive decline in people with cancer undergoing chemotherapy. *European Journal of Oncology Nursing, 27*, 53–59. https://doi.org/10.1016/j.ejon.2016.12.007

Oldacres, L., Hegarty, J., O'Regan, P., Murphy-Coakley, N. M., & Saab, M. M. (2023). Interventions promoting cognitive function in patients experiencing cancer related cognitive impairment: A systematic review. *Psycho-oncology, 32*, 214–228. https://doi.org/10.1002/pon.6073

Piil, K., Juhler, M., Jakobsen, J., & Jarden, M. (2016). Controlled rehabilitative and supportive care intervention trials in patients with high-grade gliomas and their caregivers: A systematic review. *BMJ Supportive & Palliative Care, 6*(1), 27–34. https://doi.org/10.1136/bmjspcare-2013-000593

Ren, X., Wang, X., Sun, J., Hui, Z., Lei, S., Wang, C., & Wang, M. (2022). Effects of physical exercise on cognitive function of breast cancer survivors receiving chemotherapy: A systematic review of randomized controlled trials. *Breast, 63*, 113–122. https://doi.org/10.1016/j.breast.2022.03.014

Rostamian, S., le Cessie, S., Marijt, K. A., Jukema, J. W., Mooijaart, S. P., van Buchem, M. A., van Hall, T., Gussekloo, J., & Trompet, S. (2022). Association of cognitive function with increased risk of cancer death and all-cause mortality: Longitudinal analysis, systematic review, and meta-analysis of prospective observational studies. *PLOS ONE, 17*(1), e0261826. https://doi.org/10.1371/journal.pone.0261826

Sood, A., Barton, D. L., & Loprinzi, C. L. (2006). Use of methylphenidate in patients with cancer. *American Journal of Hospice and Palliative Medicine, 23*(1), 35–40. https://doi.org/10.1177/104990910602300106

Sousa, H., Almeida, S., Bessa, J., & Pereira, M. G. (2020). The developmental trajectory of cancer-related cognitive impairment in breast cancer patients: A systematic review of longitudinal neuroimaging studies. *Neuropsychology Review, 30*(3), 287–309. https://doi.org/10.1007/s11065-020-09441-9

Wefel, J. S., Vardy, J., Ahles, T., & Schagen, S. B. (2011). International Cognition and Cancer Task Force recommendations to harmonise studies of cognitive function in patients with cancer. *The Lancet Oncology, 12*(7), 703–708. https://doi.org/10.1016/S1470-2045(10)70294-1

Zeng, Y., Zeng, L., Cheng, A. S. K., Wei, X., Wang, B., Jiang, J., & Zhou, J. (2022). The use of immersive virtual reality for cancer-related cognitive impairment assessment and rehabilitation: A clinical feasibility study. *Asia-Pacific Journal of Oncology Nursing, 9*(12), 100079. https://doi.org/10.1016/j.apjon.2022.100079

Zhang, Q., Zhao, H., & Zheng, Y. (2019). Effectiveness of mindfulness-based stress reduction (MBSR) on symptom variables and health-related quality of life in breast cancer patients—a systematic review and meta-analysis. *Supportive Care in Cancer, 27*(3), 771–781. https://doi.org/10.1007/s00520-018-4570-x

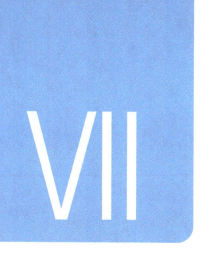

Cutaneous Symptoms

CHAPTER 24

SKIN AND NAIL CHANGES

INTRODUCTION

Traditional chemotherapy targets rapidly dividing cancer cells, as well as other organs/systems that contain rapidly dividing cells. The largest of these is the skin and mucus membranes (see Chapter 8 for mucositis), as well as the hair (see Chapter 7 for alopecia) and nails.

SKIN TOXICITIES

The most common cutaneous side effect is toxic erythema of chemotherapy (TEC; also known as *palmar-plantar erythrodysesthesia*), which presents mainly on the hands and feet (hand–foot syndrome; Shi et al., 2016), but also in the axillae and groin. The symptoms of TEC include painful edema and redness in the affected areas. Capecitabine is known to cause patients to lose their fingerprints, and while this side effect is usually temporary, it can pose a problem in situations where fingerprint identification is necessary (van Doorn et al., 2017).

Novel agents that target specific signaling pathways are noted to cause cutaneous toxicities, mainly a papulopustular rash (also known as *acneiform rash*) but also vitiligo (Mineiro Dos Santos Garrett et al., 2021), that differ from those of traditional chemotherapy agents. Hand–foot skin reaction (HFSR) occurs with the use of multikinase inhibitors and affects mainly areas on the feet that are prone to friction from shoes. Symptoms include painful blisters that are sharply demarcated, red, and edematous, and over time become swollen and painful calluses (Segaert et al., 2009).

Prevalence

Cutaneous side effects are common and impact negatively on quality of life (Hirayama et al., 2020); this may result in limiting or ceasing treatment (Figure 24.1).

SECTION VII • CUTANEOUS SYMPTOMS

Hand–foot syndrome	Up to 77%
Hand–foot skin reaction	Up to 30%
Papulopustular rash	Up to 90%

Figure 24.1 Prevalence of common skin side effects.

Contributing Factors

The frequency of skin reactions is dependent on the type of chemotherapy agent used and the dose prescribed.

- *Nontargeted chemotherapy agents* include fluorouracil, taxanes, vinca alkaloids, platinum agents, anthracyclines, and topoisomerase inhibitors.

- *Targeted chemotherapy agents* include epidermal growth factor receptor (EGFR) inhibitors, multikinase inhibitors, BRAF inhibitors, cytotoxic T-lymphocyte associated protein 4 (CTLA-4), and programmed cell death protein 1 (PD-1) inhibitors.

Assessment

Assessment includes physical examination of the affected areas, noting the extent of body surface involvement, presence of inflammation, size of any lesions, and signs of infection. The subjective experience of the patient is important: impact of the symptoms on activities of daily living and quality of life (Figure 24.2).

The Multinational Association of Supportive Care in Cancer (MASCC) EGFR Inhibitor Skin Toxicity Tool can be used in patients treated with EGFR agents (https://mascc.org/resources/assessment-tools/mascc-egfr-inhibitor-skin-toxicity-tool-mestt).

Grade 1	Minimal skin changes without pain
Grade 2	Skin changes with pain that limit instrumental activities of daily living
Grade 3	Severe skin changes with pain, limiting self-care activities of daily living

Figure 24.2 Grading of toxic erythema of chemotherapy and hand–foot skin reaction.

Source: From https://ctep.cancer.gov/protocoldevelopment/electronic_applications/docs/ctcae_v5_quick_reference_5x7.pdf.

CASE STUDY

A 36-year-old African American woman with triple-negative breast cancer presents to you 6 weeks after the start of neoadjuvant chemotherapy. She is very concerned about a change in the color

(continued)

CASE STUDY (*CONTINUED*)

of her thumb nail on her right hand. She thinks she may have melanoma.

1. What would you assess?

2. What can you tell her?

She remains anxious despite your explanation and asks for a biopsy. The pathology comes back as melanosis, a benign form of hyperpigmentation.

3. How would your management change as a result of this?

Management

PREVENTION: Prevention of TEC includes patient education on avoiding friction, avoiding heat, using emollients without excessive rubbing, and reporting any skin erosion that may become infected (Kwakman et al., 2020). The use of a 10% urea-based cream has been shown to be effective in preventing both hand–foot syndrome and HFSR (Pandy et al., 2022). These strategies also apply to the prevention of HFSR (Manchen et al., 2011).

TREATMENT: Drug interruption or decreasing the dose of chemotherapy is the main treatment for TEC as well as HFSR. Other treatments that may help reduce suffering from this side effect include topical steroids, urea-based creams, and analgesia including topical lidocaine (Manchen et al., 2011; Salzmann et al., 2019). There is limited evidence in support of regional cooling or celecoxib, the latter due to adverse effects (Pandy et al., 2022).

RADIATION-INDUCED CUTANEOUS TOXICITY

Radiation recall dermatitis (RRD) is an inflammatory skin reaction in the radiated skin area after administration of a variety of chemotherapy agents, including docetaxel (Strouthos et al., 2016) and gemcitabine most commonly (Bhangoo et al., 2022). Concurrent chemoradiation therapy may cause more skin toxicities than chemotherapy alone or in sequential chemotherapy (Lüftner et al., 2018). Local treatment of the affected area with Mepitel Film (Morgan, 2014) or a hyaluronic gel (Presta et al., 2019) has shown to be effective in reducing pain from this skin reaction. Treatment with corticosteroids may be required (Bhangoo et al., 2022).

NAIL CHANGES

Changes to the nails occur commonly, and while usually cosmetic and temporary the changes cause pain and impact on activities of daily living. The risk of experiencing nail changes is related to the number of chemotherapy cycles and cumulative dose (Hong et al., 2007). The most common changes to the nails are pigmentation changes; the color change is often to red-brown or black (melanonychia) and appears in bands on the nails. The fingernails are more commonly affected than the toenails (Mittal et al., 2022). The *nail matrix* may be affected, resulting in changes in the *nail plate*, resulting in Beau's lines (depressed bands on the nail plate), separation of the nail plate from the nail matrix (onychomadesis or onycholysis), fragile nails, and Mees' lines (leukonychia) appearing as white lines or bands on the nail plate. Damage to the *nail bed* results in Muehrcke lines (similar in appearance to Mees' lines) and onycholysis. See Figures 24.3 through 24.5 for examples.

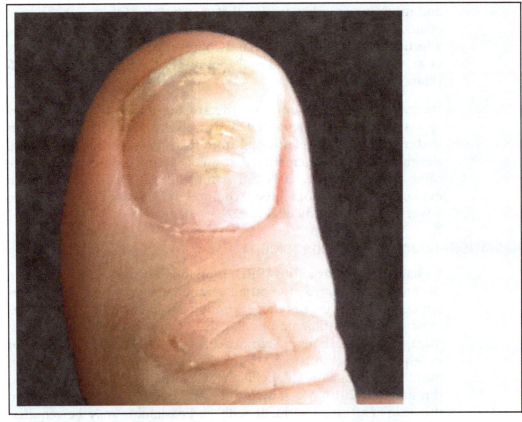

Figure 24.3 Beau's lines. Depicted on the image is an example of Beau's lines on the middle fingernail of the left hand.

Source: https://en.wikipedia.org/wiki/Beau%27s_lines.

CHAPTER 24 • SKIN AND NAIL CHANGES **241**

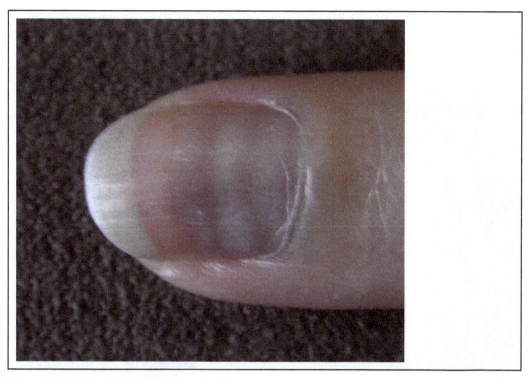

Figure 24.4 Mees' lines. Depicted on the image is an example of Mees' lines resulting from chemotherapy.
Source: https://commons.wikimedia.org/wiki/File:Mees%27_lines.jpg.

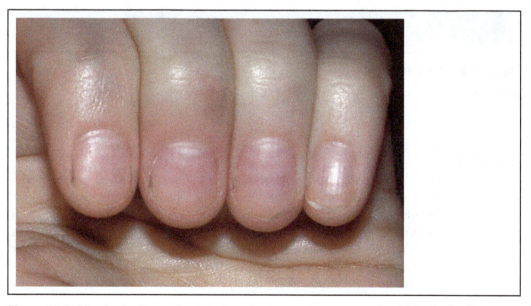

Figure 24.5 Muehrcke lines. Depicted on the image is an example of Muehrcke lines.
Source: https://commons.wikimedia.org/wiki/File:Muehrcke%27s_lines.JPG.

Damage to the nail fold can result in paronychia or periungual pyogenic granuloma, a proliferation of capillaries in the nail fold that can bleed (Zawar et al., 2019; Figure 24.6).

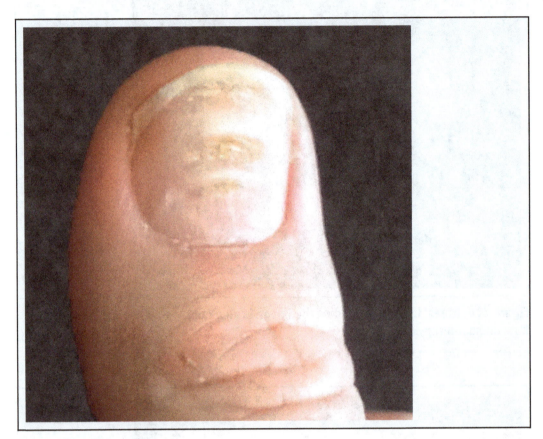

Figure 24.6 Mild paronychia.
Source: https://commons.wikimedia.org/wiki/File:Paronychia.jpg.

Prevalence

There is limited reporting on the prevalence of nail changes associated with traditional and novel agents. These changes usually occur months after treatment and may not be reported to oncology care clinicians. In women with breast or gynecologic cancers, 23.1% report nail changes or nail loss (Hackbarth et al., 2008). Other studies report a range of 5% to 44% in women with all stages of breast cancer treated with taxanes (Minisini et al., 2003).

Contributing Factors

The type of chemotherapy agent used is responsible for nail changes. Chemotherapy-associated nail changes are presented in Figure 24.7.

Nail matrix Melanonychia	Cyclophosphamide, doxorubicin, taxanes, capecitabine, cisplatin, busulfan, bleomycin
Leukonychia	Doxorubicin, cyclophosphamide, vincristine
Beau's lines	Almost all cytotoxic medications
Nail bed Onycholysis	Capecitabine, etoposide, doxorubicin, taxanes, targeted therapies (anti-EGFR and MEK inhibitors)
Nail fold Paronychia	Anti-EGFR and MEK inhibitors, mTOR inhibitors, capecitabine, doxorubicin

Figure 24.7 Chemotherapy-associated nail changes. EGFR, epidermal growth factor receptor; mTOR, mammalian target of rapamycin.

Source: From Mittal, S., Khunger, N., & Kataria, S. P. (2022). Nail changes with chemotherapeutic agents and targeted therapies. *Indian Dermatology Online Journal, 13*(1), 13–22. https://doi.org/10.4103/idoj.IDOJ_801_20.

Assessment

The National Cancer Institute (NCI) Common Terminology Criteria for Adverse Events (CTCAE) presents a limited grading scale for nail changes associated with chemotherapy (Robert et al., 2015; Figure 24.8).

An alternative grading scale (Lacouture et al., 2010) specific to the changes associated with EGFR inhibitors includes patient-reported health quality of life impacts.

Management

Prevention plays a role in mitigating these changes. Prevention includes avoiding trauma and pressure to the nails from manicures or nail biting, avoiding harsh chemicals such as nail polish removers and hardeners,

	Grade 1	Grade 2	Grade 3
Paronychia	Nail fold edema or erythema; disruption of the cuticle	Local intervention needed; oral intervention indicated; associated with discharge or nail plate separation; limiting instrumental ADL	IV antibiotic indicated or surgical intervention; limiting self-care ADL
Nail discoloration	Asymptomatic; clinical or diagnostic observations only; intervention not indicated	–	–
Nail loss	Asymptomatic separation of the nail bed from the nail plate or nail loss	Symptomatic separation of the nail bed from the nail plate or nail loss; limiting instrumental ADL	–
Nail ridging	Asymptomatic; clinical or diagnostic observations only; intervention not indicated	–	–

Figure 24.8 Grading scale for nail changes.

wearing socks and comfortable shoes, using vinyl gloves when washing the dishes, using an emollient cream daily, and regularly trimming the nails. The use of frozen gloves during treatment with taxanes has been shown to reduce nail toxicity (Marks et al., 2018; Robert et al., 2015). It is important that patients are educated about these changes and to expect improvement over the months following the end of treatment. For patients who experience paronychia, topical corticosteroids or oral tetracyclines may be prescribed if severe (Mittal et al., 2022).

GUIDELINES

- **European Society for Medical Oncology (ESMO)**

    Prevention and Management of Dermatological Toxicities Related to Anticancer Agents: ESMO Clinical Practice Guidelines (Lacouture et al., 2021)

- **Oncology Nursing Society (ONS)**

    Skin Toxicity Clinical Summary of the ONS Guidelines™ for Cancer Treatment-Related Skin Toxicity (Wiley et al., 2020)

SUMMARY

Skin and nail toxicities are common after administration of both traditional and novel agents for cancer. The changes are mostly cosmetic and resolve in months after cessation of treatment; however, they may also cause functional impairment, affecting quality of life and activities of daily living. Patient education about these changes is important, and prevention remains the mainstay of treatment.

A robust set of instructor resources designed to supplement this text is located at http://connect.springerpub.com/content/reference-book/978-0-8261-8524-2. Qualifying Instructors may request access by emailing **textbook@springerpub.com**.

REFERENCES

Bhangoo, R. S., Cheng, T. W., Petersen, M. M., Thorpe, C. S., DeWees, T. A., Anderson, J. D., Vargas, C. E., Patel, S. H., Halyard, M. Y., Schild, S. E., & Wong, W. W. (2022). Radiation recall dermatitis: A review of the literature. *Semin Oncol, 49*(2), 152–159. https://doi.org/10.1053/j.seminoncol.2022.04.001

Hackbarth, M., Haas, N., Fotopoulou, C., Lichtenegger, W., & Sehouli, J. (2008). Chemotherapy-induced dermatological toxicity: Frequencies and impact on quality of life in women's cancers. Results of a prospective study. *Supportive Care in Cancer, 16*(3), 267–273. https://doi.org/10.1007/s00520-007-0318-8

Hirayama, K., Su, Y., Chiba, M., Izutsu, M., & Yuki, M. (2020). Relationships between quality of life and skin toxicities of epidermal growth factor receptor inhibitors in cancer patients: A literature review. *Japan Journal of Nursing Science, 17*(3), e12321. https://doi.org/10.1111/jjns.12321

Hong, J., Park, S. H., Choi, S. J., Lee, S. H., Lee, K. C., Lee, J. I., Kyung, S. Y., An, C. H., Lee, S. P., Park, J. W., Jeong, S. H., Nam, E., Bang, S.-M., Cho, E. K., Shin, D. B., & Lee, J. H. (2007). Nail toxicity after treatment with docetaxel: A prospective analysis in patients with advanced non-small cell lung cancer. *Japanese Journal of Clinical Oncology, 37*(6), 424–428. https://doi.org/10.1093/jjco/hym042

Kwakman, J. J. M., Elshot, Y. S., Punt, C. J. A., & Koopman, M. (2020). Management of cytotoxic chemotherapy-induced hand-foot syndrome. *Oncology Reviews, 14*(1), 442. https://doi.org/10.4081/oncol.2020.442

Lacouture, M. E., Maitland, M. L., Segaert, S., Setser, A., Baran, R., Fox, L. P., Epstein, J. B., Barasch, A., Einhorn, L., Wagner, L., West, D. P., Rapoport, B. L., Kris, M. G., Basch, E., Eaby, B., Kurtin, S., Olsen, E. A., Chen, A., Dancey, J. E., & Trotti, A. (2010). A proposed EGFR inhibitor dermatologic adverse event-specific grading scale from the MASCC skin toxicity study group. *Supportive Care in Cancer, 18,* 509–522.

Lacouture, M. E., Sibaud, V., Gerber, P. A., van den Hurk, C., Fernández-Peñas, P., Santini, D., Jahn, F., & Jordan, K. (2021). Prevention and management of dermatological toxicities related to anticancer agents: ESMO Clinical Practice Guidelines☆. *Annals of Oncology, 32*(2), 157–170. https://doi.org/10.1016/j.annonc.2020.11.005

Lüftner, D., Dell'Acqua, V., Selle, F., Khalil, A., Leonardi, M. C., De La Torre Tomás, A., Shenouda, G., Romero Fernandez, J., Orecchia, R., Moyal, D., & Seité, S. (2018). Evaluation of supportive and barrier-protective skin care products in the daily prevention and treatment of cutaneous toxicity during systemic chemotherapy. *OncoTargets and Therapy, 11,* 5865–5872. https://doi.org/10.2147/ott.S155438

Manchen, E., Robert, C., & Porta, C. (2011). Management of tyrosine kinase inhibitor-induced hand-foot skin reaction: Viewpoints from the medical oncologist, dermatologist, and oncology nurse. *Journal of Supportive Oncology, 9*(1), 13–23. https://doi.org/10.1016/j.suponc.2010.12.007

Marks, D. H., Qureshi, A., & Friedman, A. (2018). Evaluation of prevention interventions for taxane-induced dermatologic adverse events: A systematic review. *JAMA Dermatology, 154*(12), 1465–1472. https://doi.org/10.1001/jamadermatol.2018.3465

Mineiro Dos Santos Garrett, N. F., Carvalho da Costa, A. C., Barros Ferreira, E., Damiani, G., Diniz Dos Reis, P. E., & Inocêncio Vasques, C. (2021). Prevalence of dermatological toxicities in patients with melanoma undergoing immunotherapy: Systematic review and meta-analysis. *PloS One, 16*(8), e0255716. https://doi.org/10.1371/journal.pone.0255716

Minisini, A. M., Tosti, A., Sobrero, A. F., Mansutti, M., Piraccini, B. M., Sacco, C., & Puglisi, F. (2003). Taxane-induced nail changes: Incidence, clinical presentation and outcome. *Annals of Oncology, 14*(2), 333–337. https://doi.org/10.1093/annonc/mdg050

Mittal, S., Khunger, N., & Kataria, S. P. (2022). Nail changes with chemotherapeutic agents and targeted therapies. *Indian Dermatology Online Journal, 13*(1), 13–22. https://doi.org/10.4103/idoj.IDOJ_801_20

Morgan, K. (2014). Radiotherapy-induced skin reactions: prevention and cure. *British Journal of Nursing, 23*(16), S24, s26–32. https://doi.org/10.12968/bjon.2014.23.Sup16.S24

Pandy, J. G. P., Franco, P. I. G., & Li, R. K. (2022). Prophylactic strategies for hand-foot syndrome/skin reaction associated with systemic cancer treatment: A meta-analysis of randomized controlled trials. *Supportive Care in Cancer, 30*(11), 8655–8666. https://doi.org/10.1007/s00520-022-07175-3

Presta, G., Puliatti, A., Bonetti, L., Tolotti, A., Sari, D., & Valcarenghi, D. (2019). Effectiveness of hyaluronic acid gel (Jalosome soothing gel) for the treatment of radiodermatitis in a patient receiving head and neck radiotherapy associated with cetuximab: A case report and review. *International Wound Journal, 16*(6), 1433–1439. https://doi.org/10.1111/iwj.13210

Robert, C., Sibaud, V., Mateus, C., Verschoore, M., Charles, C., Lanoy, E., & Baran, R. (2015). Nail toxicities induced by systemic anticancer treatments. *Lancet Oncology, 16*(4), e181–189. https://doi.org/10.1016/s1470-2045(14)71133-7

Salzmann, M., Marmé, F., & Hassel, J. C. (2019). Prophylaxis and management of skin toxicities. *Breast Care, 14*(2), 72–77. https://doi.org/10.1159/000497232

Segaert, S., Chiritescu, G., Lemmens, L., Dumon, K., Van Cutsem, E., & Tejpar, S. (2009). Skin toxicities of targeted therapies. *European Journal of Cancer, 45*(Suppl. 1), 295–308. https://doi.org/10.1016/s0959-8049(09)70044-9

Shi, V. J., Levy, L. L., & Choi, J. N. (2016). Cutaneous manifestations of non-targeted and targeted chemotherapies. *Seminars in Oncology, 43*(3), 419–425. https://doi.org/10.1053/j.seminoncol.2016.02.018

Strouthos, I., Tselis, N., & Zamboglou, N. (2016). Docetaxel-induced radiation recall dermatitis: A case report and literature review. *Strahlentherapie und Onkologie, 192*(10), 730–736. https://doi.org/10.1007/s00066-016-0984-x

van Doorn, L., Veelenturf, S., Binkhorst, L., Bins, S., & Mathijssen, R. (2017). Capecitabine and the risk of fingerprint loss. *JAMA Oncology, 3*(1), 122–123. https://doi.org/10.1001/jamaoncol.2016.2638

Wiley, K., Ebanks, J. G. L., Shelton, G., Strelo, J., & Ciccolini, K. (2020). Skin toxicity: Clinical summary of the ONS guidelines™ for cancer treatment-related skin toxicity. *Clinical Journal of Oncology Nursing, 24*(5), 561–565. https://doi.org/10.1188/20.CJON.561-565

Zawar, V., Bondarde, S., Pawar, M., & Sankalecha, S. (2019). Nail changes due to chemotherapy: A prospective observational study of 129 patients. *Journal of the European Academy of Dermatology and Venereology, 33*(7), 1398–1404. https://doi.org/10.1111/jdv.15508

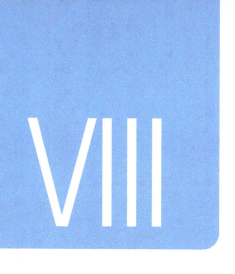

Psychosocial Symptoms

CHAPTER 25

ANXIETY

INTRODUCTION

Anxiety, often but not always coupled with depression, is a common symptom among individuals along the disease trajectory, beginning even before the time of diagnosis. The diagnosis of a life-threatening illness is characterized by uncertainty and fear of pain, suffering, disability, and death (Traeger et al., 2012). Fear of recurrence of the cancer in those currently on treatment and after treatment is a well-described manifestation of anxiety, and death anxiety is common in those with advanced cancer near or at the end of life. Other anxiety disorders seen in cancer survivors include agoraphobia, panic disorder, social anxiety disorder, obsessive-compulsive disorder, and posttraumatic stress disorder (Traeger et al., 2012). These are thought to be reactivation of a preexisting disorder due to the stress of the cancer diagnosis or treatment (Kangas et al., 2005).

PREVALENCE

Anxiety tends to fluctuate at key points over the course of the disease. It is common for symptoms to increase before and after tests or scans; this is described by patients as "scanxiety" (Figure 25.1).

Prostate cancer	23% (S. Watts et al., 2015)
Gynecologic cancer	19%–27.09% (Watts, Prescott et al., 2015)
Breast cancer	17.9%–33.3% (Maass et al., 2015)
Colorectal cancer	1.0%–47.2% (Peng et al., 2019)

Figure 25.1 Prevalence of anxiety for four common cancers.

Overall, women experience more anxiety than men (24% vs. 12.9%), and older patients experience less anxiety than their younger counterparts (Linden et al., 2012).

CONTRIBUTING FACTORS

A wide range of contributing factors play a role in anxiety, and chief among them is a preexisting history of anxiety or trauma (Traeger et al., 2012). Other contributing factors include the following:

- *psychosocial:* social isolation, caregiving responsibilities
- *cancer-related fears:* treatments, uncertainty, suffering, pain, fatigue, dyspnea, insomnia, depression
- *treatment-related factors:* medication side effects, cardiac and respiratory symptoms

ASSESSMENT

It is recommended that all patients with cancer are screened for anxiety on a regular basis, starting at diagnosis and at transition points in the disease trajectory (Andersen et al., 2014). The seven-item Generalized Anxiety Disorder (GAD-7) is recommended due to ease of use, with a score of ≥5 indicative of mild anxiety and scores of 10 and 15 suggestive of moderate and severe anxiety, respectively. Assessment of risk of self-harm or harm to others should be conducted if moderate to severe anxiety is present or if mild anxiety worsens. An urgent referral to a mental health professional should follow (Andersen et al., 2014; Figure 25.2).

The Seven-Item Generalized Anxiety Disorder (GAD-7; Spitzer et al., 2006)	7 items
Generalized Anxiety Disorder Questionnaire (GAD-Q-IV; Newman et al., 2002)	9 items
Beck Anxiety Inventory (BAI; Beck et al., 1993)	21 items
Hospital Anxiety and Depression Scale (HADS; Zigmond & Snaith, 1983)	14 items

Figure 25.2 Self-report measures of anxiety.

MANAGEMENT

Nonpharmaceutical Management

The updated American Society of Clinical Oncology (ASCO) guidelines on the management of anxiety and depression (Andersen et al., 2023) recommend psychosocial interventions for *moderate* symptoms of anxiety (see Chapter 26 for depression). Examples of these are cognitive behavioral therapy (CBT), behavioral activation (BA), structured physical activity, and exercise. These can be used in individual or group therapy. For those with *severe* anxiety, individual therapy with CBT, BA, and mindfulness-based stress reduction (MBSR) is recommended. A range of psychosocial interventions, including music therapy, stress management, and yoga, are recommended to reduce anxiety (Lyman et al., 2018). Coping skills training may be more effective in younger patients (Buffart et al., 2020). Hypnosis (progressive muscle relaxation or rhythmic breathing) has been shown to reduce anxiety in women with breast cancer (Roberts et al., 2017; Sine et al., 2022). Mindfulness-based interventions show efficacy in women with breast cancer (Zhang et al., 2019) as well as in patients with advanced cancer (Zimmermann et al., 2018). Exercise has shown positive effects on anxiety in women with breast cancer (Singh et al., 2018). Prehabilitation, with a focus on preparing patients for the stress associated with cancer treatment, has been shown to reduce anxiety in young to midlife patients (Scriney et al., 2022).

Pharmaceutical Management

The latest guidelines from the ASCO (Andersen et al., 2023) do not provide details on pharmaceutical treatment of anxiety. Referral to a mental health specialist for pharmaceutical management may be warranted (see National Comprehensive Cancer Network [NCCN] Guidelines). Selective serotonin reuptake inhibitors (SSRIs) may be helpful in reducing anxiety; benzodiazepines may be used to treat acute anxiety in the weeks before the SSRI takes effect.

CASE STUDY

Your patient is a 29-year-old woman with metastatic breast cancer. She recently finished chemotherapy treatment and tells you that she is not sleeping despite being deeply fatigued. She has two young children, and even though she has good family support she is feeling overwhelmed.

1. What questions should you ask her?

She denies feeling depressed, but you can see that she is experiencing stress. She says she wants a break from treatment.

2. What can you suggest that may be helpful?

FEAR OF CANCER RECURRENCE

Fear that the cancer will progress or recur may be present up to 5 or more years in cancer survivors (Sharpe et al., 2018). This fear is characterized by preoccupation with thoughts about progression or recurrence, unhelpful coping strategies, impaired daily functioning, inability to plan for the future, and clinically significant distress (Lebel et al., 2016). Fear of recurrence has been reported in 30% of women with gynecologic cancer (Mell et al., 2022) and as high as 99% of women with cancer in general (Koch et al., 2014). Contributing factors include distress, anxiety, and hopelessness. Fear of recurrence may be associated with death anxiety, although the relationship between the two is not clear (Sharpe et al., 2018).

Assessment

The *Cancer Worry Scale* (Custers et al., 2014) is an eight-item Likert scale that assesses the frequency of worry that the cancer will recur, the impact of these worries on mood and daily activities, and worry about family members getting cancer.

Nonpharmaceutical Management

Psychosocial interventions including CBT, mindfulness-based programs, psychoeducation, and communication training have shown efficacy in reducing fear of recurrence (Chen et al., 2018).

DEATH ANXIETY

Death anxiety is said to occur when death in the future is recognized by the patient. It is related to past and future regret and how the person imagines their death (Soleimani et al., 2020). Individual, social, and cultural factors influence death anxiety (Peters et al., 2013). Women with breast cancer have higher death anxiety than people with other cancers, and those who are married have higher death anxiety than single individuals (Soleimani et al., 2020). The overall prevalence is as high as 80% (Grossman et al., 2018).

There are several tools to assess death anxiety. These include the following:

- *Death and Dying Distress Scale (DADDS):* This scale (Lo et al., 2011) is a 15-item Likert scale that addresses feelings of distress over the previous 2 weeks. Questions include regret about not having achieved their goals, not having talked to their loved ones, being a burden to others, and the impact of the death on their family.

- *Templer's Death Anxiety Scale (T-DAS):* T-DAS is a 15-item scale with possible yes/no responses to questions related to the severity of death anxiety (Templer, 1970).

- *Revised Death Anxiety Scale (RDAS):* The RDAS contains 25 items. It may be too cumbersome for clinical use in individuals near the end of life (Thorson & Powell, 1992).

- *Death Anxiety Questionnaire (DAQ):* A 15-item scale, this questionnaire assesses worries about the process of death and dying (Conte et al., 1982).

Psychosocial interventions that focus on meaning, dignity, spiritual well-being, and relationships have been shown to be useful in managing death anxiety (Grossman et al., 2018).

GUIDELINES

- **American Society of Clinical Oncology (ASCO)**

    Management of Anxiety and Depression in Adult Survivors of Cancer: ASCO Guideline Update (2023; Andersen et al., 2023)

    Screening, Assessment, and Care of Anxiety and Depressive Symptoms in Adults With Cancer: An American Society of Clinical Oncology Guideline Adaptation (2014; Andersen et al., 2014)

- **Canadian Association of Psychosocial Oncology**

    Pan-Canadian Practice Guideline: Screening, Assessment and Management of Psychosocial Distress, Depression and Anxiety in Adults With Cancer Version 2 (2015)

    https://capo.ca/resources/Documents/36APAN~1.PDF

- **National Comprehensive Cancer Network (NCCN)**

    NCCN Version 1.2023 Survivorship: Anxiety, Depression, Trauma, and Distress

    https://www.nccn.org/professionals/physician_gls/pdf/survivorship.pdf

SUMMARY

Anxiety, fear of cancer recurrence, and death anxiety are conditions affecting a sizeable proportion of individuals across the cancer trajectory. While pharmaceutical management with SSRIs or anxiolytics may be offered, psychosocial interventions that have proven efficacy with minimal to no adverse effects are available.

 A robust set of instructor resources designed to supplement this text is located at http://connect.springerpub.com/content/reference-book/978-0-8261-8524-2. Qualifying Instructors may request access by emailing **textbook@springerpub.com**.

REFERENCES

Andersen, B., DeRubeis, R., Berman, B., Gruman, J., Champion, V., Massie, M., Holland, J. C., Partridge, A. H., Bak, K., Somerfield, M. R., & Rowland, J. (2014). Screening, assessment, and care of anxiety and depressive symptoms in adults with cancer: An American Society of Clinical Oncology guideline adaptation. *Journal of Clinical Oncology*, 32(15), 1605–1619. https://doi.org/10.1200/JCO.2013.52.4611

Andersen, B. L., Lacchetti, C., Ashing, K., Berek, J. S., Berman, B. S., Bolte, S., Dizon, D. S., Given, B., Nekhlyudov, L., Pirl, W., Stanton, A. L., & Rowland, J. H. (2023). Management of anxiety and depression in adult survivors of cancer: ASCO guideline update. *Journal of Clinical Oncology, 14*(18), 3426–3453. https://doi.org/10.1200/jco.23.00293

Beck, A. T., Epstein, N., Brown, G., & Steer, R. (1993). Beck anxiety inventory. *Journal of Consulting and Clinical Psychology, 56*, 893–897. https://doi.org/10.1037/0022-006X.56.6.893

Buffart, L. M., Schreurs, M. A. C., Abrahams, H. J. G., Kalter, J., Aaronson, N. K., Jacobsen, P. B., Newton, R. U., Courneya, K. S., Armes, J., Arving, C., Braamse, A. M., Brandberg, Y., Dekker, J., Ferguson, R. J., Gielissen, M. F., Glimelius, B., Goedendorp, M. M., Graves, K. D., Heiney, S.P., & Verdonck-de Leeuw, I. M. (2020). Effects and moderators of coping skills training on symptoms of depression and anxiety in patients with cancer: Aggregate data and individual patient data meta-analyses. *Clinical Psychology Review, 80*, 101882. https://doi.org/10.1016/j.cpr.2020.101882

Chen, D., Sun, W., Liu, N., Wang, J., Zhao, J., Zhang, Y., Liu, J., & Zhang, W. (2018). Fear of cancer recurrence: A systematic review of randomized, controlled trials. *Oncology Nursing Forum, 45*(6), 703–712. https://doi.org/10.1188/18.Onf.703-712

Conte, H. R., Weiner, M. B., & Plutchik, R. (1982). Measuring death anxiety: Conceptual, psychometric, and factor-analytic aspects. *Journal of Personality and Social Psychology, 43*(4), 775. https://doi.org/10.1037//0022-3514.43.4.775

Custers, J. A. E., van den Berg, S. W., van Laarhoven, H. W. M., Bleiker, E. M. A., Gielissen, M. F. M., & Prins, J. B. (2014). The cancer worry scale: Detecting fear of recurrence in breast cancer survivors. *Cancer Nursing, 37*(1), E44–E50. https://doi.org/10.1097/NCC.0b013e3182813a17

Grossman, C. H., Brooker, J., Michael, N., & Kissane, D. (2018). Death anxiety interventions in patients with advanced cancer: A systematic review. *Palliative Medicine, 32*(1), 172–184. https://doi.org/10.1177/0269216317722123

Kangas, M., Henry, J. L., & Bryant, R. A. (2005). The course of psychological disorders in the 1st year after cancer diagnosis. *Journal of Consulting and Clinical Psychology, 73*(4), 763. https://doi.org/10.1037/0022-006X.73.4.763

Koch, L., Bertram, H., Eberle, A., Holleczek, B., Schmid-Höpfner, S., Waldmann, A., Zeissig, S. R., Brenner, H., & Arndt, V. (2014). Fear of recurrence in long-term breast cancer survivors—Still an issue. Results on prevalence, determinants, and the association with quality of life and depression from the cancer survivorship—A multi-regional population-based study. *Psycho-Oncology, 23*(5), 547–554. https://doi.org/10.1002/pon.3452

Lebel, S., Ozakinci, G., Humphris, G., Mutsaers, B., Thewes, B., Prins, J., Dinkel, A., & Butow, P. (2016). From normal response to clinical problem: Definition and clinical features of fear of cancer recurrence. *Supportive Care in Cancer, 24*, 3265–3268. https://doi.org/10.1007/s00520-016-3272-5

Linden, W., Vodermaier, A., MacKenzie, R., & Greig, D. (2012). Anxiety and depression after cancer diagnosis: prevalence rates by cancer type, gender, and age. *Journal of Affective Disorders, 141*(2–3), 343–351. https://doi.org/10.1016/j.jad.2012.03.025

Lo, C., Hales, S., Zimmermann, C., Gagliese, L., Rydall, A., & Rodin, G. (2011). Measuring death-related anxiety in advanced cancer: Preliminary psychometrics of the death and dying distress scale. *Journal of Pediatric Hematology/Oncology, 33*(Suppl. 2), S140–S145. https://doi.org/10.1097/MPH.0b013e318230e1fd

Lyman, G. H., Greenlee, H., Bohlke, K., Bao, T., DeMichele, A. M., Deng, G. E., Fouladbakhsh, J. M., Gil, B., Hershman, D. L., Mansfield, S., Mussallem, D. M., Mustian, K. M., Price, E., Rafte, S., & Cohen, L. (2018). Integrative therapies during and after breast cancer treatment: ASCO endorsement of the SIO clinical practice guideline. *Journal of Clinical Oncology, 36*(25), 2647–2655. https://doi.org/10.1200/jco.2018.79.2721

Maass, S. W., Roorda, C., Berendsen, A. J., Verhaak, P. F., & de Bock, G. H. (2015). The prevalence of long-term symptoms of depression and anxiety after breast cancer treatment: A systematic review. *Maturitas, 82*(1), 100–108. https://doi.org/10.1016/j.maturitas.2015.04.010

Mell, C. A., Jewett, P. I., Teoh, D., Vogel, R. I., & Everson-Rose, S. A. (2022). Psychosocial predictors of fear of cancer recurrence in a cohort of gynecologic cancer survivors. *Psycho-oncology, 31*(12), 2141–2148. https://doi.org/https://doi.org/10.1002/pon.6055

Newman, M. G., Zuellig, A. R., Kachin, K. E., Constantino, M. J., Przeworski, A., Erickson, T., & Cashman-McGrath, L. (2002). Preliminary reliability and validity of the Generalized Anxiety Disorder Questionnaire-IV: A revised self-report diagnostic measure of generalized anxiety disorder. *Behavior Therapy, 33*(2), 215–233. https://doi.org/10.1016/S0005-7894(02)80026-0

Peng, Y. N., Huang, M. L., & Kao, C. H. (2019). Prevalence of depression and anxiety in colorectal cancer patients: A literature review. *International Journal of Environmental Research and Public Health, 16*(3), 411. https://doi.org/10.3390/ijerph16030411

Peters, L., Cant, R., Payne, S., O'Connor, M., Mcdermott, F., Hood, K., Morphet, J., & Shimoinaba, K. (2013). How death anxiety impacts nurses' caring for patients at the end of life: A review of literature. *Open Nursing Journal, 7*, 14. https://doi.org/10.2174/1874434601307010014

Roberts, R. L., Na, H., Yek, M. H., & Elkins, G. (2017). Hypnosis for hot flashes and associated symptoms in women with breast cancer. *American Journal of Clinical Hypnosis, 60*(2), 123–136. https://doi.org/10.1080/00029157.2017.1334622

Scriney, A., Russell, A., Loughney, L., Gallagher, P., & Boran, L. (2022). The impact of prehabilitation interventions on affective and functional outcomes for young to midlife adult cancer patients: A systematic review. *Psychooncology, 31*(12), 2050–2062. https://doi.org/10.1002/pon.6029

Sharpe, L., Curran, L., Butow, P., & Thewes, B. (2018). Fear of cancer recurrence and death anxiety. *Psychooncology, 27*(11), 2559–2565. https://doi.org/10.1002/pon.4783

Sine, H., Achbani, A., & Filali, K. (2022). The effect of hypnosis on the intensity of pain and anxiety in cancer patients: A systematic review of controlled experimental trials. *Cancer Investigation, 40*(3), 235–253. https://doi.org/10.1080/07357907.2021.1998520

Singh, B., Spence, R. R., Steele, M. L., Sandler, C. X., Peake, J. M., & Hayes, S. C. (2018). A systematic review and meta-analysis of the safety, feasibility, and effect of exercise in women with stage II+ breast cancer. *Archives of Physical Medicine and Rehabilitation, 99*(12), 2621–2636. https://doi.org/10.1016/j.apmr.2018.03.026

Soleimani, M. A., Bahrami, N., Allen, K. A., & Alimoradi, Z. (2020). Death anxiety in patients with cancer: A systematic review and meta-analysis. *European Journal of Oncology Nursing, 48*, 101803. https://doi.org/10.1016/j.ejon.2020.101803

Spitzer, R. L., Kroenke, K., Williams, J. B., & Löwe, B. (2006). A brief measure for assessing generalized anxiety disorder: The GAD-7. *Archives of Internal Medicine, 166*(10), 1092–1097.

Templer, D. I. (1970). The construction and validation of a death anxiety scale. *The Journal of General Psychology, 82*(2), 165–177. https://doi.org/10.1080/00221309.1970.9920634

Thorson, J. A., & Powell, F. C. (1992). A revised death anxiety scale. *Death Studies, 16*(6), 507–521. https://doi.org/10.1080/07481189208252595

Traeger, L., Greer, J. A., Fernandez-Robles, C., Temel, J. S., & Pirl, W. F. (2012). Evidence-based treatment of anxiety in patients with cancer. *Journal of Clinical Oncology, 30*(11), 1197–1205. https://doi.org/10.1200/jco.2011.39.5632

Watts, S., Leydon, G., Eyles, C., Moore, C. M., Richardson, A., Birch, B., Prescott, P., Powell, C., & Lewith, G. (2015). A quantitative analysis of the prevalence of clinical depression and anxiety in patients with prostate cancer undergoing active surveillance. *BMJ Open, 5*(5), e006674. https://doi.org/10.1136/bmjopen-2014-006674

Watts, S., Prescott, P., Mason, J., McLeod, N., & Lewith, G. (2015). Depression and anxiety in ovarian cancer: a systematic review and meta-analysis of prevalence rates. *BMJ Open, 5*(11), e007618. https://doi.org/10.1136/bmjopen-2015-007618

Zhang, Q., Zhao, H., & Zheng, Y. (2019). Effectiveness of mindfulness-based stress reduction (MBSR) on symptom variables and health-related quality of life in breast cancer patients-a systematic review and meta-analysis. *Supportive Care in Cancer, 27*(3), 771–781. https://doi.org/10.1007/s00520-018-4570-x

Zigmond, A. S., & Snaith, R. P. (1983). The hospital anxiety and depression scale. *Acta Psychiatrica Scandinavica, 67*. https://doi.org/10.1111/j.1600-0447.1983.tb09716.x

Zimmermann, F. F., Burrell, B., & Jordan, J. (2018). The acceptability and potential benefits of mindfulness-based interventions in improving psychological well-being for adults with advanced cancer: A systematic review. *Complementary Therapies in Clinical Practice, 30*, 68–78. https://doi.org/10.1016/j.ctcp.2017

CHAPTER 26

DEPRESSION

INTRODUCTION

Depression and anxiety are common among cancer survivors and may persist for 3 months or more after cancer treatment (Burgess et al., 2005). This chapter will describe the prevalence, contributing factors, assessment, and management of depression, while anxiety is described in Chapter 25. Younger women with breast cancer experience high levels of depression around the time of diagnosis and during treatment, and the depression may worsen for those with existing mental illness (Fernandes-Taylor et al., 2015). For older patients (60 years and older), depression is the most common symptom and is associated with disability, morbidity, and mortality (Parpa et al., 2015). Depression is associated with all-cause and cancer-specific mortality; anxiety is associated with all-cause mortality (Wang et al., 2020).

PREVALENCE

Depression usually starts at diagnosis and continues through the treatment phase(s), and for some through the years of survivorship. For many, anxiety begins when symptoms first occur and continues in the years after treatment is over as a fear of recurrence (Figure 26.1).

Low-income ethnic minority patients are less likely to be diagnosed and treated for depression (Ell et al., 2005). African American women with breast cancer experience high levels of depression that may go unrecognized and undertreated (Sheppard et al., 2013). African American men with prostate cancer, however, appear to experience less depression than their White counterparts (Nelson et al., 2010).

CONTRIBUTING FACTORS

The type of cancer a patient has been diagnosed with is a well-established factor contributing to depression, with pancreatic and lung cancers a significant predictor of depression. Women are more likely than men to experience depression (Linden et al., 2012). Metastases and

Pancreatic cancer: 33%–50% (Massie, 2004)
Oropharyngeal cancer: 22%–57% (Massie, 2004)
Gynecologic cancer: 12.7%–25.3% (Watts, Prescott et al., 2015)
Prostate cancer: 12.5% (S. Watts et al., 2015)
Lung cancer: 11%–44% (Massie, 2004)
Colorectal cancer: 1.6%–57% (Peng et al., 2019)
Breast cancer: 0.4%–66.1% (Maass et al., 2015)

Figure 26.1 Prevalence of depression.

pain also contribute to depression (Smith, 2015), as do certain medications used to treat cancer, such as glucocorticoids, interferon-alpha, vincristine, vinblastine, procarbazine, and cytokine-releasing regimens (Miller et al., 2008; Raison & Miller, 2003; Torres et al., 2013). Living alone, not having a partner, and poor social support also contribute to the development of depression (Zhao et al., 2014).

ASSESSMENT

Patients may present with fatigue, weight change (either increased or decreased), loss of appetite, or poor cognition, all of which may be ascribed to the cancer itself or to the treatment and so healthcare clinicians may not consider depression (Smith, 2015; Figure 26.2).

Major depression can be identified by dysphoria, anhedonia, feeling of being worthless or guilty, having impaired concentration, difficulty making decisions, and displaying suicidal ideation and suicidal behavior. It is very important to screen for past and current suicidal ideation and behavior. There are two questionnaires that are used clinically to screen patients, the Patient Health Questionnaire (PHQ)-2, containing two questions, and the PHQ-9, containing nine questions (Thekkumpurath et al., 2011). It is suggested that all patients be

Depressed mood (dysphoria)
Loss of interest or pleasure (anhedonia)
Change in appetite
Sleep disturbance
Loss of energy
Neurocognitive dysfunction
Psychomotor agitation or slowing

Figure 26.2 Symptoms of depression.

> Over the past 2 weeks, how often* have you been bothered by any of the following:
>
> Little interest or pleasure in doing things
> Feeling down, depressed, or hopeless
>
> *Frequency: not at all, several days, more than half the days, nearly every day
>   0   1   2   3
>
> Cutoff point for depression: ≥2

Figure 26.3 Patient Health Questionnaire (PHQ)-2.

Source: From Mitchell, A. J. (2008). Are one or two simple questions sufficient to detect depression in cancer and palliative care? A Bayesian meta-analysis. *British Journal of Cancer, 98*(12), 1934–1943. https://doi.org/10.1038/sj.bjc.6604396.

regularly asked the first two questions of the PHQ-9 (these are the same as the two questions of the PHQ-2) to screen for low mood and anhedonia (Figure 26.3).

For patients who endorse either or both, they should then be screened with the full PHQ-9. The cutoff score for the PHQ-9 in the cancer population is ≥8 (Andersen et al., 2014).

Alternatives include the following:

- Hospital Anxiety and Depression Scale (HADS), with two sub-scales, seven items for depression and seven for anxiety

- Beck Depression Inventory-Fast Screen, with seven items for patients with medical conditions

- Center for Epidemiologic Studies Depression Scale (CES-D), with a 5- or 10-item version (Smarr & Keefer, 2011)

CASE STUDY

You receive a call from a patient's spouse. The patient, a man in his 60s, was recently diagnosed with high-risk prostate cancer; he is due to have surgery to remove his prostate next week. The patient's spouse says he is sleeping 18 hours a day and she is concerned about him.

1. What might be happening in this situation?

The patient calls you back a couple of hours later.

2. What would you use to assess his mental status?

He scores within the range for depression but says that he is not going to take any pills.

3. What else can you suggest?

MANAGEMENT

The American Society of Clinical Oncology (ASCO) recommends the following management strategies:

- Anyone with cancer and those who are identified caregivers should be provided with information about depression and should be offered resources as appropriate.

- A stepped-care approach should be used, selecting the most effective and less resource-intense intervention, depending on symptom severity.

- For patients who are also anxious, treatment for depression takes precedence, or a combination of cognitive behavioral therapies (CBTs) addressing both issues can be used.

- For those who have moderate symptoms of depression, recommendations include individual or group therapy with CBT, behavioral activation (BA), structured physical activity and exercise, mindfulness-based stress reduction (MBSR), and other psychosocial interventions that are evidence-based such as relaxation or problem-solving.

- For those with severe symptoms, individual therapy with CBT, BA, and MBSR should be offered.

- Assessment after 8 weeks of these interventions and a change of intervention or addition of another intervention (including a pharmaceutical agent) should be considered.

- For those without access to the psychosocial interventions discussed above or for those who prefer pharmaceutical management or who do not improve after psychosocial interventions, pharmaceutical treatments can be offered (Andersen et al., 2023).

The evidence supporting psychosocial interventions is presented in the following:

- Mindfulness-based meditation is effective in reducing depression (Chang et al., 2021; Zhang et al., 2019) and ruminative thinking (Mao et al., 2023).

- CBT has been shown to be effective in women with breast cancer (Jassim et al., 2015) and in patients with colorectal cancer (Hoon et al., 2013).

- Physical exercise is effective in managing depression in patients with hematologic cancer (Knips et al., 2019), women with breast cancer (Singh et al., 2018), and those with lung cancer (Yang et al., 2020).

- Psychoeducation by phone is helpful in reducing depression in a variety of cancer populations (Champarnaud et al., 2020; Chen et al., 2018).

- Mind–body interventions, such as yoga, are helpful (Danhauer et al., 2017; Hsueh et al., 2021).

- Music therapy improves depression (Li et al., 2020).

- Bibliotherapy (self-help workbooks, novels, audiobooks) is helpful for patients with depression and also increases coping skills (Malibiran et al., 2018).

- Spirituality and interventions that focus on creating meaning and purpose may be appropriate for some patients and may reduce depression (Xing et al., 2018).

Pharmaceutical interventions

The latest guidelines from the ASCO (Andersen et al., 2023) do not provide details on the pharmaceutical treatment of depression; however, the previous guidelines (Andersen et al., 2014) do and are presented as follows:

- Patients with moderate to severe depression may benefit from antidepressants; the choice of medication depends on the side effects, how tolerable these are to the individual patient, and the potential for drug interactions (Andersen et al., 2014).

- There is limited evidence on the choice of one medication over another (Andersen et al., 2014).

- All patients should be educated about potential side effects of these medications, as well as when to inform the oncology team of worsening symptoms.

Antidepressants

- Serotonin–norepinephrine reuptake inhibitors (duloxetine) may also help with neuropathic pain and duloxetine is suggested to be more effective than venlafaxine (Farshchian et al., 2018).

- Selective serotonin reuptake inhibitors (fluoxetine and desipramine; Fisch et al., 2003) may be effective.

- Tricyclic antidepressants have the advantage of being sedating; this may be helpful to patients who experience agitation, but they have side effects (dry mouth, urinary retention, constipation, nausea, blurred vision, and tachycardia) that may prove intolerable (Anderson et al., 2008).

- Trazadone is a serotonin modulator that is sedating and may be helpful to patients with sleep disturbance (Mendelson, 2005).

- Psychostimulants (methylphenidate) may be prescribed as an alternative; at high doses, they have significant side effects (Fernandez et al, 1987).

GUIDELINES

- **American Society of Clinical Oncology (ASCO)**

    Management of Anxiety and Depression in Adult Survivors of Cancer: ASCO Guideline Update (2023; Andersen et al., 2023)

    ASCO Screening, Assessment, and Care of Anxiety and Depressive Symptoms in Adults With Cancer: An American Society of Clinical Oncology Guideline Adaptation (2014; Andersen et al., 2014)

- **National Comprehensive Cancer Network (NCCN)**

    National Comprehensive Cancer Network Version 1.2023. Survivorship: Anxiety, Depression, Trauma, and Distress

    https://www.nccn.org/professionals/physician_gls/pdf/survivorship.pdf

- **Oncology Nursing Society (ONS)**

    ONS—Putting Evidence Into Practice: Evidence-Based Interventions for Depression (Fulcher et al., 2008)

SUMMARY

Depression is a common issue in individuals with cancer; it often occurs with anxiety and treatment is similar for both. Screening for depression is important in this population and should occur regularly. Mild depression can be treated with supportive care, while moderate depression responds to many psychosocial interventions.

A robust set of instructor resources designed to supplement this text is located at http://connect.springerpub.com/content/reference-book/978-0-8261-8524-2. Qualifying Instructors may request access by emailing **textbook@springerpub.com**.

REFERENCES

Andersen, B., DeRubeis, R., Berman, B., Gruman, J., Champion, V., Massie, M., Holland, J. C., Partridge, A. H., Bak, K., Somerfield, M. R., & Rowland, J. (2014). & American Society of Clinical Oncology. Screening, assessment, and care of anxiety and depressive symptoms in adults with cancer: An American society of clinical oncology guideline adaptation. *Journal of Clinical Oncology*, 32(15), 1605–1619. https://doi.org/10.1200/JCO.2013.52.4611

Andersen, B. L., Lacchetti, C., Ashing, K., Berek, J. S., Berman, B. S., Bolte, S., Dizon, D. S., Given, B., Nekhlyudov, L., Pirl, W., Stanton, A. L., & Rowland,

J. H. (2023). Management of anxiety and depression in adult survivors of cancer: ASCO guideline update. *Journal of Clinical Oncology, 41*(18), 3426–3453. https://doi.org/10.1200/jco.23.00293

Anderson, I. M., Ferrier, I. N., Baldwin, R. C., Cowen, P. J., Howard, L., Lewis, G., Matthews, K., McAllister-Williams, R. H., Peveler, R. C., Scott, J., & Tylee, A. (2008). Evidence-based guidelines for treating depressive disorders with antidepressants: A revision of the 2000 British association for psychopharmacology guidelines. *Journal of Psychopharmacology, 22*(4), 343–396. https://doi.org/10.1177/0269881107088441

Burgess, C., Cornelius, V., Love, S., Graham, J., Richards, M., & Ramirez, A. (2005). Depression and anxiety in women with early breast cancer: Five year observational cohort study. *British Medical Journal, 330*(7493), 702. https://doi.org/10.1136/bmj.38343.670868.D3

Champarnaud, M., Villars, H., Girard, P., Brechemier, D., Balardy, L., & Nourhashémi, F. (2020). Effectiveness of therapeutic patient education interventions for older adults with cancer: A systematic review. *The Journal of Nutrition, Health and Aging, 24*(7), 772–782. https://doi.org/10.1007/s12603-020-1395-3

Chang, Y. C., Yeh, T. L., Chang, Y. M., & Hu, W. Y. (2021). Short-term effects of randomized mindfulness-based intervention in female breast cancer survivors: A systematic review and meta-analysis. *Cancer Nursing, 44*(6), E703–e714. https://doi.org/10.1097/ncc.0000000000000889

Chen, Y. Y., Guan, B. S., Li, Z. K., & Li, X. Y. (2018). Effect of telehealth intervention on breast cancer patients' quality of life and psychological outcomes: A meta-analysis. *Journal of Telemedicine and Telecare, 24*(3), 157–167. https://doi.org/10.1177/1357633x16686777

Danhauer, S. C., Addington, E. L., Sohl, S. J., Chaoul, A., & Cohen, L. (2017). Review of yoga therapy during cancer treatment. *Supportive Care in Cancer, 25*(4), 1357–1372. https://doi.org/10.1007/s00520-016-3556-9

Ell, K., Sanchez, K., Vourlekis, B., Lee, P. J., Dwight-Johnson, M., & Lagomasino, I., Muderspach, L., & Russell, C. (2005). Depression, correlates of depression, and receipt of depression care among low-income women with breast or gynecologic cancer. *Journal of Clinical Oncology, 23*(13), 3052–3060. https://doi.org/ 10.1200/jco.2005.08.041

Farshchian, N., Alavi, A., Heydarheydari, S., & Moradian, N. (2018). Comparative study of the effects of venlafaxine and duloxetine on chemotherapy-induced peripheral neuropathy. *Cancer Chemotherapy and Pharmacology, 82*(5), 787–793. https://doi.org/10.1007/s00280-018-3664-y

Fernandes-Taylor, S., Adesoye, T., & Bloom, J. R. (2015). Managing psychosocial issues faced by young women with breast cancer at the time of diagnosis and during active treatment. *Current Opinion in Supportive and Palliative Care, 9*(3), 279–284. https://doi.org/10.1097/spc.0000000000000161

Fernandez, F., Adams, F., Holmes, V. F., Levy, J. K., & Neidhart, M. (1987). Methylphenidate for depressive disorders in cancer patients. An alternative to standard antidepressants. *Psychosomatics, 28*(9), 455–461. https://doi.org/10.1016/s0033-3182(87)72476-1

Fisch, M. J., Loehrer, P. J., Kristeller, J., Passik, S., Jung, S. H., Shen, J., Arquette, M. A., Brames, M. J., & Einhorn, L. H. (2003). Fluoxetine versus placebo in advanced cancer outpatients: A double-blinded trial of the Hoosier oncology group. *Journal of Clinical Oncology, 21*(10), 1937–1943. https://doi.org/10.1200/jco.2003.08.025

Fulcher, C. D., Badger, T., Gunter, A. K., Marrs, J. A., & Reese, J. M. (2008). Putting evidence into practice: Interventions for depression. *Clinical Journal of Oncology Nursing, 12*(1), 131–140. https://doi.org/10.1188/08.CJON.131-140

Hoon, L. S., Chi Sally, C. W., & Hong-Gu, H. (2013). Effect of psychosocial interventions on outcomes of patients with colorectal cancer: A review of the literature. *European Journal of Oncology Nursing, 17*(6), 883–891. https://doi.org/10.1016/j.ejon.2013.05.001

Hsueh, E. J., Loh, E. W., Lin, J. J., & Tam, K. W. (2021). Effects of yoga on improving quality of life in patients with breast cancer: A meta-analysis of randomized controlled trials. *Breast Cancer, 28*(2), 264–276. https://doi.org/10.1007/s12282-020-01209-6

Jassim, G. A., Whitford, D. L., Hickey, A., & Carter, B. (2015). Psychological interventions for women with non-metastatic breast cancer. *Cochrane Database of Systematic Reviews, 5.* https://doi.org/10.1002/14651858.CD008729.pub2

Knips, L., Bergenthal, N., Streckmann, F., Monsef, I., Elter, T., & Skoetz, N. (2019). Aerobic physical exercise for adult patients with haematological malignancies. *Cochrane Database of Systematic Reviews, 1*(1), Cd009075. https://doi.org/10.1002/14651858.CD009075.pub3

Li, Y., Xing, X., Shi, X., Yan, P., Chen, Y., Li, M., Zhang, W., Li, X., & Yang, K. (2020). The effectiveness of music therapy for patients with cancer: A systematic review and meta-analysis. *Journal of advanced nursing, 76*(5), 1111–1123. https://doi.org/10.1111/jan.14313

Linden, W., Vodermaier, A., MacKenzie, R., & Greig, D. (2012). Anxiety and depression after cancer diagnosis: Prevalence rates by cancer type, gender, and age. *Journal of Affective Disorders, 141*(2–3), 343–351. https://doi.org/10.1016/j.jad.2012.03.025

Maass, S. W., Roorda, C., Berendsen, A. J., Verhaak, P. F., & de Bock, G. H. (2015). The prevalence of long-term symptoms of depression and anxiety after breast cancer treatment: A systematic review. *Maturitas, 82*(1), 100–108. https://doi.org/10.1016/j.maturitas.2015.04.010

Malibiran, R., Tariman, J. D., & Amer, K. (2018). Bibliotherapy: Appraisal of evidence for patients diagnosed with cancer. *Clinical Journal of Oncology Nursing, 22*(4), 377–380. https://doi.org/10.1188/18.Cjon.377-380

Mao, L., Li, P., Wu, Y., Luo, L., & Hu, M. (2023). The effectiveness of mindfulness-based interventions for ruminative thinking: A systematic review and meta-analysis of randomized controlled trials. *Journal of Affective Disorders, 321*, 83–95. https://doi.org/10.1016/j.jad.2022.10.022

Massie, M. J. (2004). Prevalence of depression in patients with cancer. *Journal of the National Cancer Institute Monographs, 2004*(32), 57–71. https://doi.org/10.1093/jncimonographs/lgh014

Mendelson, W. B. (2005). A review of the evidence for the efficacy and safety of trazodone in insomnia. *The Journal of Clinical Psychiatry, 66*(4), 469–476. https://doi.org/10.4088/jcp.v66n0409

Miller, A. H., Ancoli-Israel, S., Bower, J. E., Capuron, L., & Irwin, M. R. (2008). Neuroendocrine-immune mechanisms of behavioral comorbidities in patients with cancer. *Journal of Clinical Oncology, 26*(6), 971–982. https://doi.org/10.1200/jco.2007.10.7805

Mitchell, A. J. (2008). Are one or two simple questions sufficient to detect depression in cancer and palliative care? A Bayesian meta-analysis. *British Journal of Cancer, 98*(12), 1934–1943. https://doi.org/10.1038/sj.bjc.6604396

Nelson, C. J., Balk, E. M., & Roth, A. J. (2010). Distress, anxiety, depression, and emotional well-being in African-American men with prostate cancer. *Psycho-oncology, 19*(10), 1052–1060. https://doi.org/10.1002/pon.1659

Parpa, E., Tsilika, E., Gennimata, V., & Mystakidou, K. (2015). Elderly cancer patients' psychopathology: A systematic review: Aging and mental health. *Archives of Gerontology and Geriatrics, 60*(1), 9–15. https://doi.org/10.1016/j.archger.2014.09.008

Peng, Y. N., Huang, M. L., & Kao, C. H. (2019). Prevalence of depression and anxiety in colorectal cancer patients: A literature review. *International Journal of Environmental Research and Public Health, 16*(3), 411. https://doi.org/10.3390/ijerph16030411

Raison, C. L., & Miller, A. H. (2003). Depression in cancer: New developments regarding diagnosis and treatment. *Biological Psychiatry, 54*(3), 283–294. https://doi.org/10.1016/s0006-3223(03)00413-x

Sheppard, V. B., Llanos, A. A., Hurtado-de-Mendoza, A., Taylor, T. R., & Adams-Campbell, L. L. (2013). Correlates of depressive symptomatology in African-American breast cancer patients. *Journal of Cancer Survivorship, 7*(3), 292–299. https://doi.org/10.1007/s11764-013-0273-y

Singh, B., Spence, R. R., Steele, M. L., Sandler, C. X., Peake, J. M., & Hayes, S. C. (2018). A systematic review and meta-analysis of the safety, feasibility, and effect of exercise in women with stage II+ breast cancer. *Archives of Physical Medicine and Rehabilitation, 99*(12), 2621–2636. https://doi.org/10.1016/j.apmr.2018.03.026

Smarr, K. L., & Keefer, A. L. (2011). Measures of depression and depressive symptoms: Beck depression inventory-II (BDI-II), Center for Epidemiologic Studies Depression Scale (CES-D), Geriatric Depression Scale (GDS), Hospital Anxiety and Depression Scale (HADS), and Patient Health Questionnaire-9 (PHQ-9). *Arthritis Care & Research, 63*(S11), HQ–9. https://doi.org/10.1002/acr.20556

Smith, H. R. (2015). Depression in cancer patients: Pathogenesis, implications and treatment. *Oncology Letters*, *9*(4), 1509–1514.

Thekkumpurath, P., Walker, J., Butcher, I., Hodges, L., Kleiboer, A., O'Connor, M., Wall, L., Murray, G., Kroenke, K., & Sharpe, M. (2011). Screening for major depression in cancer outpatients: The diagnostic accuracy of the 9-item patient health questionnaire. *Cancer*, *117*(1), 218–227. https://doi.org/10.1002/cncr.25514

Torres, M. A., Pace, T. W., Liu, T., Felger, J. C., Mister, D., Doho, G. H., Kohn, J. N., Barsevick, A. M., Long, Q., & Miller, A. H. (2013). Predictors of depression in breast cancer patients treated with radiation: Role of prior chemotherapy and nuclear factor kappa B. *Cancer*, *119*(11), 1951–1959. https://doi.org/10.1002/cncr.28003

Wang, X., Wang, N., Zhong, L., Wang, S., Zheng, Y., Yang, B., Zhang, J., Lin, Y., & Wang, Z. (2020). Prognostic value of depression and anxiety on breast cancer recurrence and mortality: A systematic review and meta-analysis of 282,203 patients. *Molecular Psychiatry*, *25*(12), 3186–3197. https://doi.org/10.1038/s41380-020-00865-6

Watts, S., Leydon, G., Eyles, C., Moore, C. M., Richardson, A., Birch, B., Prescott, P., Powell, C., & Lewith, G. (2015). A quantitative analysis of the prevalence of clinical depression and anxiety in patients with prostate cancer undergoing active surveillance. *BMJ Open*, *5*(5), e006674. https://doi.org/10.1136/bmjopen-2014-006674

Watts, S., Prescott, P., Mason, J., McLeod, N., & Lewith, G. (2015). Depression and anxiety in ovarian cancer: A systematic review and meta-analysis of prevalence rates. *BMJ Open*, *5*(11), e007618. https://doi.org/10.1136/bmjopen-2015-007618

Xing, L., Guo, X., Bai, L., Qian, J., & Chen, J. (2018). Are spiritual interventions beneficial to patients with cancer? A meta-analysis of randomized controlled trials following PRISMA. *Medicine (Baltimore)*, *97*(35), e11948. https://doi.org/10.1097/md.0000000000011948

Yang, M., Liu, L., Gan, C. E., Qiu, L. H., Jiang, X. J., He, X. T., & Zhang, J. E. (2020). Effects of home-based exercise on exercise capacity, symptoms, and quality of life in patients with lung cancer: A meta-analysis. *European Journal of Oncology Nursing*, *49*, 101836. https://doi.org/10.1016/j.ejon.2020.101836

Zhang, Q., Zhao, H., & Zheng, Y. (2019). Effectiveness of mindfulness-based stress reduction (MBSR) on symptom variables and health-related quality of life in breast cancer patients-a systematic review and meta-analysis. *Supportive Care in Cancer*, *27*(3), 771–781. https://doi.org/10.1007/s00520-018-4570-x

Zhao, L., Li, X., Zhang, Z., Song, C., Guo, C., Zhang, Y., Zhang, Y., Li, L., Lu, G., Zheng, G., Wang, K., Pei, W., & Han, L. (2014). Prevalence, correlates and recognition of depression in Chinese inpatients with cancer. *General Hospital Psychiatry*, *36*(5), 477–482. https://doi.org/10.1016/j.genhosppsych.2014.05.005

CHAPTER 27

DISTRESS

INTRODUCTION

Distress is a multifactorial unpleasant experience of cognitive, behavioral, emotional, social, spiritual, and/or physical nature that interferes with the ability to cope effectively with cancer symptoms and treatment (https://www.nccn.org/professionals/physician_gls/pdf/distress.pdf). It is regarded as the sixth vital sign in oncology (Ownby, 2019). Distress encompasses a spectrum from normal feelings about cancer (e.g., sadness and fear) to more disabling symptoms such as anxiety and depression, which are presented in Chapters 25 and 26. Distress impacts on the adjustment to the disease for both the patient and their partner (Kayser et al., 2018) and contributes to avoidance behaviors (Morris et al., 2018). The experience of uncertainty is inherent in the cancer experience and is a source of distress for many (Ghodraty Jabloo et al., 2017). High distress may contribute to mortality, particularly for those with colorectal, prostate, pancreatic, and esophageal cancer, as well as leukemia (Batty et al., 2017).

PREVALENCE

Distress is common among cancer survivors; the prevalence in different types of cancer is presented in Figure 27.1.

Those with a history of more than one primary cancer have a significantly increased risk of distress and so asking about history of other cancers is important (Belcher et al., 2017).

CONTRIBUTING FACTORS

Multiple contributing factors predispose cancer survivors to cancer-related distress (Emidio et al., 2022; Silva et al., 2022). These include the following:

- history of psychiatric disorder or substance abuse
- history of trauma or abuse

SECTION VIII • PSYCHOSOCIAL SYMPTOMS

- cognitive impairment
- communication barriers (poor health literacy or language barriers)
- younger age
- belonging to a sexual minority group
- race
- ongoing physical changes
- sexual problems
- fertility concerns
- persistent health concerns
- financial concerns
- low social support
- lower education attainment (Figure 27.2)

Type of Cancer	Percentage of Prevalence	Reference
Hematologic cancer	43%	Rusiewicz et al., (2008); Syrjala et al., 2004
Lung cancer	43%	Zabora et al., (2001)
Breast cancer	36%	Ploos van Amstel et al., (2013)
Head and neck	35%	Epstein et al., (2002)
Colorectal	31%	Zabora et al., (2001)
Gynecologic	29%	Zabora et al., (2001)

Figure 27.1 Prevalence of distress.

- From suspicion of cancer to diagnosis
- While waiting for treatment to start and during the treatment trajectory including changes in treatment and treatment failure
- At the end of active treatment including moving into survivorship or transitioning to end-of-life care

Figure 27.2 Distress is experienced across the disease spectrum.

ASSESSMENT

Screening for distress should occur on an ongoing basis, from diagnosis to end of life, by a member of the oncology team. Scores on screening tools should be reviewed in a timely manner and referrals made to appropriate services (Smith, Loscalzo et al., 2018). The two most commonly used measures of distress are the National Comprehensive Cancer Network (NCCN) Distress Thermometer (Cutillo et al., 2017;

Ownby, 2019) and the Symptom Distress Scale (SDS; McCorkle & Young, 1978).

- The NCCN Distress Thermometer is a single-item visual Likert scale that goes from 0 (no distress) to 10 (extreme distress). It is accompanied by a 39-item problem list that allows the patient to identify common problems in five domains (physical, emotional, social, practical, and spirit/religious concerns). A cutoff score of 3 on the Distress Thermometer indicates clinically elevated distress (Cutillo et al., 2017).

- The SDS is a 13-item measure of 11 common symptoms that people with advanced cancer experience. These include fatigue, appetite, pain frequency and intensity, appearance, insomnia, cough, outlook, concentration, breathing, bowel pattern, and nausea intensity and frequency; gender comprises the last two items. The higher the score, the greater the distress experienced.

- The Hospital Anxiety and Depression Scale (Zigmond & Snaith, 1983) can also be used to identify distress (Granek et al., 2019).

CASE STUDY

Your patient is a 27-year-old woman who has recently been diagnosed with acute myeloid leukemia. She scores a 5 on the Distress Thermometer.

1. What should you do next?

She responds negatively to your suggestions and states that she is "fine" and will cope as soon as her stem cell transplant is over.

2. What can you offer her based on her response?

She accepts the handout you offer her but you remain concerned.

3. What are your next steps?

The *State of Spirituality Scale* is suggested as a tool to measure spiritual distress (Stephenson et al., 2022). Using a visual analog scale, the tool measures five dimensions of spirituality (meaning, beliefs, relationships, acceptance, and value) from well-being to distress.

MANAGEMENT

Management of distress requires screening with a validated tool, such as those presented in the previous section, with subsequent patient and caregiver education, appropriate referral, and follow-up (Smith, Kuhn et al., 2018; Figure 27.3).

Patients should be screened for supportive care needs and provided with education and support.	20% will ONLY require this level of support.
Many will need additional education and support, as well as encouragement to seek additional help.	30% will ALSO require this level of support.
Some will require specialized intervention for distress.	35%–40% will ALSO require special intervention.
A few will require more complex care.	10%–15% will ALSO require more complex care.

Figure 27.3 Fitch's model of a supportive care framework.

Source: From Fitch, M. I. (2008). Supportive care framework. *Canadian Oncology Nursing Journal, 18*(1), 6–24. https://doi.org/10.5737/1181912x181614.

A *step-care model* for intervention involves providing education on signs and symptoms of depression and instruction on obtaining additional support; this should be provided to all patients. Patients should also be provided with information about support groups and self-management tools such as exercise, mindfulness, and nutrition. Patients with elevated distress should be offered referral to a psychosocial specialist (Smith, Kuhn et al., 2018).

A mobile app—the *Cancer Distress Coach* (CaDC)—provides assessment, education, resources, and cognitive behavioral therapy-based activities for posttraumatic stress disorder (PTSD) symptoms that are experienced by one in three cancer survivors (Smith, Loscalzo et al., 2018).

GUIDELINES

- **American Society of Clinical Oncology (ASCO)**

  Screening, Assessment, and Care of Anxiety and Depressive Symptoms in Adults With Cancer: An American Society of Clinical Oncology Guideline Adaptation (adaptation of the CAPO guideline; Andersen et al., 2014)

- **Canadian Association of Psychosocial Oncology (CAPO)**

  A Pan Canadian Practice Guideline: Screening, Assessment and Care of Psychosocial Distress, Depression, and Anxiety in Adults With Cancer (Howell et al., 2015)

- **National Comprehensive Cancer Network (NCCN)**

  NCCN Guidelines Version 2.2023 Distress Management

  https://www.nccn.org/docs/default-source/patient-resources/nccn_distress_thermometer.pdf

SUMMARY

Distress is regarded as the sixth vital sign and can lead to significant depression and anxiety. It is experienced all along the disease trajectory from diagnosis to end of life. Screening for distress using validated tools such as the Distress Thermometer and acting on the score is key to providing comprehensive psychosocial care.

A robust set of instructor resources designed to supplement this text is located at http://connect.springerpub.com/content/reference-book/978-0-8261-8524-2.
Qualifying Instructors may request access by emailing textbook@springerpub.com.

REFERENCES

Andersen, B., DeRubeis, R., Berman, B., Gruman, J., Champion, V., Massie, M., Holland, J. C., Partridge, A. H., Bak, K., Somerfield, M. R., & Rowland, J. (2014). Screening, assessment, and care of anxiety and depressive symptoms in adults with cancer: An America n Society of Clinical Oncology guideline adaptation. *Journal of Clinical Oncology*, 32(15), 1605–1619. https://doi.org/10.1200/JCO.2013.52.4611

Batty, G. D., Russ, T. C., Stamatakis, E., & Kivimäki, M. (2017). Psychological distress in relation to site specific cancer mortality: Pooling of unpublished data from 16 prospective cohort studies. *BMJ*, 356, j108. https://doi.org/10.1136/bmj.j108

Belcher, S. M., Hausmann, E. A., Cohen, S. M., Donovan, H. S., & Schlenk, E. A. (2017). Examining the relationship between multiple primary cancers and psychological distress: A review of current literature. *Psychooncology*, 26(12), 2030–2039. https://doi.org/10.1002/pon.4299

Cutillo, A., O'Hea, E., Person, S., Lessard, D., Harralson, T., & Boudreaux, E. (2017). The distress thermometer: Cutoff points and clinical use. *Oncology Nursing Forum*, 44(3), 329–336. https://doi.org/10.1188/17.Onf.329-336

Emidio, O. M., Cutrona, S. L., Person, S. D., Mazor, K. M., Frisard, C., & Lemon, S. C. (2022). Association of neighborhood-level social determinants of health with psychosocial distress in patients newly diagnosed with lung cancer. *Cancer Reports (Hoboken)*, 5(11), e1734. https://doi.org/10.1002/cnr2.1734

Epstein, J. B., Phillips, N., Parry, J., Epstein, M. S., Nevill, T., & Stevenson-Moore, P. (2002). Quality of life, taste, olfactory and oral function following high-dose chemotherapy and allogeneic hematopoietic cell transplantation. *Bone Marrow Transplant*, 30(11), 785–792. https://doi.org/10.1038/sj.bmt.1703716

Fitch, M. I. (2008). Supportive care framework. *Canadian Oncology Nursing Journal*, 18(1), 6–24. https://doi.org/10.5737/1181912x181614

Ghodraty Jabloo, V., Alibhai, S. M. H., Fitch, M., Tourangeau, A. E., Ayala, A. P., & Puts, M. T. E. (2017). Antecedents and outcomes of uncertainty in older adults with cancer: A scoping review of the literature. *Oncology Nursing Forum, 44*(4), E152–E167. https://doi.org/10.1188/17.Onf.E152-e167

Granek, L., Nakash, O., Ariad, S., Shapira, S., & Ben-David, M. (2019). Mental health distress: Oncology nurses' strategies and barriers in identifying distress in patients with cancer. *Clinical Journal of Oncology Nursing, 23*(1), 43–51. https://doi.org/10.1188/19.Cjon.43-51

Howell, D., Keshavarz, H., Esplen, M.J. Hack, T., Hamel, M., Howes, J., Li, M., Manii, D., McLeod, D., Mayer, C., Sellick, S., Riahizadeh, S., Noroozi, H., & Ali, M. (2015, July 30). *Pan-Canadian Practice Guideline: Screening, Assessment and Management of Psychosocial Distress, Depression and Anxiety in Adults with Cancer.* https://www.capo.ca/resources/Documents/Guidelines/3APAN-~1.PDF

Kayser, K., Acquati, C., Reese, J. B., Mark, K., Wittmann, D., & Karam, E. (2018). A systematic review of dyadic studies examining relationship quality in couples facing colorectal cancer together. *Psychooncology, 27*(1), 13–21. https://doi.org/10.1002/pon.4339

McCorkle, R., & Young, K. (1978). Development of a symptom distress scale. *Cancer Nursing, 1*(5), 373–378. https://doi.org/10.1097/00002820-197810000-00003

Morris, N., Moghaddam, N., Tickle, A., & Biswas, S. (2018). The relationship between coping style and psychological distress in people with head and neck cancer: A systematic review. *Psychooncology, 27*(3), 734–747. https://doi.org/10.1002/pon.4509

Ownby, K. K. (2019). Use of the distress thermometer in clinical practice. *Journal of the Advanced Practitioner in Oncology, 10*(2), 175–179. https://doi.org/10.6004/jadpro.2019.10.2.7

Ploos van Amstel, F. K., van den Berg, S. W., van Laarhoven, H. W., Gielissen, M. F., Prins, J. B., & Ottevanger, P. B. (2013). Distress screening remains important during follow-up after primary breast cancer treatment. *Supportive Care in Cancer, 21*(8), 2107–2115. https://doi.org/10.1007/s00520-013-1764-0

Rusiewicz, A., DuHamel, K. N., Burkhalter, J., Ostroff, J., Winkel, G., Scigliano, E., Papadopoulos, E., Moskowitz, C., & Redd, W. (2008). Psychological distress in long-term survivors of hematopoietic stem cell transplantation. *Psychooncology, 17*(4), 329–337. https://doi.org/10.1002/pon.1221

Silva, S., Bártolo, A., Santos, I. M., Pereira, A., & Monteiro, S. (2022). Towards a better understanding of the factors associated with distress in elderly cancer patients: A systematic review. *International Journal of Environmental Research and Public Health, 19*(6), 3424. https://doi.org/10.3390/ijerph19063424

Smith, S. K., Kuhn, E., O'Donnell, J., Koontz, B. F., Nelson, N., Molloy, K., Chang, J., & Hoffman, J. (2018). Cancer distress coach: Pilot study of a mobile app for managing posttraumatic stress. *Psycho-oncology, 27*(1), 350–353. https://doi.org/10.1002/pon.4363

Smith, S. K., Loscalzo, M., Mayer, C., & Rosenstein, D. (2018). Best practices in oncology distress management: Beyond the screen. *American Society of Clinical Oncology Educational Book, 38*, 813–821. https://doi.org/10.1200/EDBK_201307

Stephenson, P., Sheehan, D., & Hansen, D. (2022). The state of spirituality scale as a screening tool for spiritual distress. *Clinical Journal of Oncology Nursing, 26*(6), 593–596. https://doi.org/10.1188/22.Cjon.593-596

Syrjala, K. L., Langer, S. L., Abrams, J. R., Storer, B., Sanders, J. E., Flowers, M. E., & Martin, P. J. (2004). Recovery and long-term function after hematopoietic cell transplantation for leukemia or lymphoma. *JAMA, 291*(19), 2335–2343. https://doi.org/10.1001/jama.291.19.2335

Zabora, J., BrintzenhofeSzoc, K., Curbow, B., Hooker, C., & Piantadosi, S. (2001). The prevalence of psychological distress by cancer site. *Psychooncology, 10*(1), 19–28. https://doi.org/10.1002/1099-1611(200101/02)10:1<19::aid-pon501>3.0.co;2-6

Zigmond, A. S., & Snaith, R. P. (1983). The hospital anxiety and depression scale. *Acta Psychiatrica Scandinavica, 67*, 361–370. https://doi.org/10.1111/j.1600-0447.1983.tb09716.x

CHAPTER 28

ANSWERS TO CASE STUDIES

CHAPTER 3

1. Assess for fatigue, depression, and sleep deprivation.

2. The National Comprehensive Cancer Network (NCCN) Fatigue Screening Question or the Edmonton Symptom Assessment Scale Revised (ESAS-r) for a more nuanced assessment.

3. Focus on energy preservation to allow for participation in priority activities.

4. Exercise has the most support in the literature.

5. There are no medications with good evidence to support use for this woman. Medications have side effects that impact on quality of life.

CHAPTER 4

1. The patient is requesting a highly addictive medication that has a high risk of misuse.

2. A comprehensive assessment of the patient's pain (e.g., location, intensity) is necessary, as is a physical examination. It is also important to ask about other methods of pain relief that he is using.

3. He may be using illicit drugs or is overdosing on his opioids and this may be causing his somnolence.

4. Asking him about the psychosocial challenges he is facing may result in clues as to why he is fatigued. There may be other reasons for this, including problems with shelter, alcohol use, and so on.

CHAPTER 5

1. A full assessment of her sleep patterns will reveal what problems she is having. She should be asked about her shift schedule as this is likely to be an important contributor to her sleep problems.

Keeping a sleep diary will provide you with additional information about activities that might be impacting on her sleep.

2. She should be told that there is limited evidence on the effectiveness of naturopathic interventions for sleep disturbance.

3. Hypnotics are not recommended for sleep disturbance. They are addictive and often abused and many people become tolerant to them. Getting regular exercise and practicing common sense sleep hygiene are likely to be more effective without the risk of harm.

CHAPTER 6

1. Her sister's experience is not predictive of her recovery or her risk of developing lymphedema.

2. If her insurance covers this, she should see a lymphedema specialist who will assess both arms and provide her with information about prevention of lymphedema and other strategies to maintain the health of her arm after surgery.

3. She should be vigilant in keeping the arm on the affected side clean and avoiding any trauma to that arm. If she has seen a lymphedema specialist who has recommended compression garments to prevent the development of lymphedema, she should follow the instructions exactly as given.

4. Maintaining a healthy weight and doing progressive resistance exercises under supervision can also help prevent lymphedema.

CHAPTER 7

1. He may be depressed due to his condition (advanced prostate cancer on chemotherapy), but hiding his body may suggest that he is ashamed of the changes in his body, especially the loss of body hair that is symbolic of masculinity for some men.

2. Despite the thinking that men are not affected by alterations to their body and a negative impact on body image, men are indeed conscious of how they look and the physical changes from treatment for advanced prostate cancer, including androgen deprivation and second-line chemotherapy for castrate-resistant disease.

3. Validating his experience and allowing his spouse to hear what is bothering him may normalize the situation. A referral for counseling may also be offered.

4. There are limited options for treating alopecia generally and nothing specifically for loss of body hair.

CHAPTER 8

1. A lubricant or saliva substitute may be helpful.

2. Sucking candies or eating fruits/vegetables that are acidic may help promote saliva production.

CHAPTER 9

1. Assume that she has febrile neutropenia based on her history. Treatment with a broad-spectrum antimicrobial should begin within 1 hour of presentation to the ED.

2. Complete blood cell (CBC) and platelet count, creatinine, bilirubin and creatine, hepatic transaminase enzymes, and electrolytes should be ordered, as well as two blood cultures from separate venipunctures.

3. If she is at low risk or has poor outcomes after considering contributing factors, she may be discharged on oral antimicrobials but needs to report if her fever continues for more than 2 days.

CHAPTER 10

1. Keeping a diary describing the intensity and frequency of the hot flashes and identifying any triggers may help address any behaviors that can be modified. Asking her to complete the Hot Flash Related Daily Interference Scale on a regular basis may help monitor any improvement or lack thereof.

2. Hypnosis or acupuncture may provide some relief. Assessing for signs of depression and/or anxiety may provide evidence to start an antidepressant at this time.

3. While effective in treating hot flashes, most of the selective serotonin reuptake inhibitors have sexual side effects that may cause additional impact on her quality of life. These should be discussed with her in detail before initiating treatment.

CHAPTER 11

1. A brief assessment of bowel function can allow you to make an appropriate referral, whether that is to a nutritionist or other allied health clinician.

2. Involving the patient in the conversation and asking about his bowel movements can be helpful in identifying the cause of his weight loss. For example, he may have lost interest in eating if he is constipated with a feeling of fullness.

3. Increasing his fluid intake and eating high-fiber foods are the first steps in providing some relief. If these are not helpful, laxatives such as stool softeners and/or senna tablets may help. A staged

278 SECTION VIII • PSYCHOSOCIAL SYMPTOMS

approach to managing this symptom is necessary before considering alternative analgesia.

CHAPTER 12

1. The perianal irritation may be caused by loose stools and you should ask about this even if the patient does not mention it.

2. If the plant-based diet contains a lot of fiber, this may contribute to the development of loose stools. A description of what she is eating or a food diary may help identify any foods that may be contributing to this.

3. If she does not want to alter her diet, an offer of a prescription for loperamide may be made. She should also be advised to avoid alcohol and caffeine.

CHAPTER 13

1. You can ask him about his past use of cannabis, what form it takes, and what he is afraid of. It is also important to ask him where he intends going to meet his friends and what they are going to do. Any activities that expose him to health risks should be discussed with him.

2. It is important to tell him that medication will be prescribed both before his initial dose of chemotherapy as well as on the following days and also if he experiences breakthrough nausea and vomiting. You are not likely to be able to persuade him that smoking marijuana is not good for his respiratory tract and trying to do this may make him defensive. A harm reduction approach may be more effective.

3. Leaving the hospital poses a risk to his survival; taking a harm reduction approach and involving a pharmacist and the oncologist in this situation may be necessary. His oncologist may be willing to prescribe an approved cannabinoid in addition to the antiemetic regimen, and the pharmacist should be able to provide additional advice.

CHAPTER 14

1. He appears very thin and there is obvious muscle wasting of his upper arms and shoulders.

2. The Fearon criteria provides greater detail than physical examination.

   - Precachexia reflects weight loss of ≤5%.

   - Cachexia reflects weight loss of >5% or body mass index (BMI) of <20; or sarcopenia with >2% weight loss.

   - Refractory cachexia reflects a variable degree of cachexia with disease not responsive to cancer treatment.

The Weight Loss Grading System (WLGS) includes BMI in the classification of cachexia, and the Karnofsky score will also provide additional information in the assessment of his condition.

3. The development of cachexia causes distress in family members, who may feel guilty that they are not providing good care to the patient. It is also distressing to see someone losing weight as this indicates that treatment is not working or has not worked and that the end of life is near. Their concerns should be validated and the process of cachexia explained to them, with the assurance that this is not their fault.

4. A discussion about potential treatments should be conducted with the patient, his wife, and his sister present. Treatment options for grade 2 according to the WLGS are somewhat limited, but *progesterone analogs* (megestrol acetate) or *short-term corticosteroids* may be prescribed for a limited time but only if the patient agrees. Acupuncture may also help if he is not interested in taking medication. The assessment of competence can only be made by the appropriate healthcare clinician, and a declaration of incompetence will not change the outcome.

CHAPTER 15

1. Despite his apparent health and his history of being a nonsmoker and nondrinker, his diagnosis is likely caused by the human papillomavirus (HPV) and not by anything that he has done.

2. His body mass index (BMI) is at the low end of normal and he is likely to experience dysphagia as well as significant pain as a result of the treatment. You should advise him of the importance of maintaining his nutritional status. He should also be given anticipatory guidance that his training regimen may not be possible during his treatment. This is going to be upsetting to him and it is important to allow him to express his concerns and possible anger with the situation.

3. He would benefit from a referral to a registered nutritionist who will work with him on optimizing his diet. Consulting a kinesiologist who can work with him on balancing his desire to continue a modified training regimen would also be helpful.

CHAPTER 16

1. It is important to know how many pads he is using and how often he needs to change them or how wet they are.

2. A bladder diary may be helpful in identifying any activities that increase the leakage or any dietary or liquid intake that may worsen the incontinence. While there are formal questionnaires to assess incontinence, many are lengthy and not useful in clinical practice.

280 SECTION VIII • PSYCHOSOCIAL SYMPTOMS

3. Men tend to be more distressed by climacturia (urinary leakage during arousal or orgasm) when it occurs with a partner present. However, leakage during masturbation may cause anticipatory distress for a man who intends to be sexual with a partner in the future. Using a condom (if a rigid erection is possible) or a silicone tension loop (known colloquially as a *cock ring*) may help. Pelvic floor muscle exercises/training is effective for both daily incontinence as well as climacturia.

4. There is no evidence that supplements are helpful. The most effective intervention is pelvic floor muscle exercises/training.

CHAPTER 17

1. You should ask her what changes have occurred in her relationship. You should also ask how she feels about her body and the lack of breast. Ask how this has impacted on her relationship and sexual functioning.

2. Sertraline is a selective serotonin reuptake inhibitor (SSRI) and this class of drugs has multiple side effects, including fatigue, headache, insomnia, and importantly loss of libido and absent orgasm.

3. Tell her that the issue with orgasms is likely related to the SSRI she is taking but also to other issues in her life. Encourage her to share with her partner how she is feeling. They may benefit from talking to a counselor, and ask if you can refer them to someone.

CHAPTER 18

1. Ask him what his erections were like before treatment and normalize that erections change with age. Also ask about his relationship (length of relationship, age of partner) and if he has talked to his partner and what her response to his disclosure about his difficulties has been. It is also important to assess if he is taking the medication correctly.

2. Advise him that there are other similar medications that might work better and also that there are other interventions that might work (penile pump, intracavernosal injections).

3. It is important to assess for depression and suicidal ideation in anyone who says "I don't know what I am going to do."

4. It is important to involve his partner in any discussion about his sexual function. He may have not talked to her and may be assuming that she will leave him, and this could not be accurate at all. If he hears from her that she is not going to leave and that they can work through this, he may be satisfied with her response.

CHAPTER 19

1. Ask the patient to describe what he is feeling. Using a formal assessment tool may provide additional information. A chest x-ray and/or a CT scan will help identify the extent of the metastases and if there is a treatable cause of his dyspnea.

2. If he is hypoxic, oxygen by mask or nasal prongs may help alleviate his discomfort. A stepwise approach, starting with non-pharmacologic measures, should be initiated.

3. Consultation with the palliative care team or specialist is warranted. A review of any medications he is taking will help guide what other treatments may be helpful.

4. Helping his daughter understand what palliative sedation is and what it is not is the first step in managing the situation. Palliative sedation should only occur after a comprehensive discussion and with the consent of the patient if possible and with the involvement of the family.

CHAPTER 20

1. A review of the history of his cancer is warranted, including which treatments he has had. Brachytherapy and bevacizumab should suggest potential cavitation of the tumor.

2. Hemoglobin, hematocrit, and a chest x-ray should be ordered. A CT scan with intravenous (IV) contrast may be considered.

3. Reassure the patient that the bleeding is usually self-limiting, but also warn him about the risk of life-threatening bleeding (roughly a half cup of blood in 24 hours).

CHAPTER 21

1. He may have preexisting hearing impairment.

2. Poor health literacy and anxiety may also be impacting on his ability to comprehend or actively listen due to what you are telling him.

3. Family involvement may be of benefit, but he may become defensive if he is pressured to undergo testing.

4. Educate family members that the chemotherapy may further impact his hearing so that they are aware and can report further deterioration in his hearing, at which point he may be willing to undergo auditory testing and potential intervention, such as an assisted hearing device.

CHAPTER 22

1. She is at risk of developing chemotherapy-induced peripheral neuropathy (CIPN) due to the chemotherapy she is prescribed; it contains a taxane. You can encourage her to talk to her oncologist about alternative regimens, but you can also reassure her that most women do not experience long-term symptoms.

2. In order to best advise her, you need to know exactly what difficulties she is having. Is it cold intolerance or motor difficulties?

3. If she replies that she has cold intolerance, she can be advised to wear gloves and warm socks when going outside in the winter. She can also use gloves when taking cold items out of the fridge or freezer. If she is having problems with her balance or gait, she can be advised to ask for help, or to use an assistive device such as a cane. Advice must be tailored to her specific challenges.

CHAPTER 23

1. Explain that changes in memory are among the more common cognitive changes seen in women with breast cancer who have had chemotherapy.

2. Formal questionnaires have limited sensitivity, and self-reports of cognitive changes should be taken seriously. The following questions will add details about the symptoms she is experiencing:

   - Are you having difficulty paying attention? Multitasking?
   - Do you frequently leave tasks incomplete?
   - Are you having difficulty finding words?
   - Do you have difficulty remembering things?
   - Are you finding that prompts like notes or reminders need to be used more frequently?
   - Does it take you longer to think through problems and does your thinking seem slower?
   - Have you noticed an impact on functional performance or job performance?

3. Cognitive training, psychoeducation, mindfulness-based stress reduction, as well as exercise may be helpful in mitigating or improving cognitive dysfunction.

CHAPTER 24

1. Assess the affected nail for pain, bleeding, signs of infection, and a history of trauma.

CHAPTER 28 • ANSWERS TO CASE STUDIES **283**

2. Reassure her that this is a common side effect of certain chemotherapy agents, including the docetaxel that she received.

3. The pathology result confirms that this is melanosis (black or brown discoloration of the nail plate) and no further treatment is necessary. You can reassure her that with time and growth of the affected nail, the dark color should disappear.

CHAPTER 25

1. Assess for anxiety and depression. Ask about her precancer mental status and any history of anxiety or depression. Review her medication history and ask about her coping behaviors. If she admits to moderate to severe anxiety, assess for self-harm or harm to others and refer for urgent mental health specialist assessment.

2. Exercise is helpful in relieving both anxiety and depression. There are a range of psychosocial interventions that are effective, for example, yoga, mindfulness-based interventions, and cognitive behavioral therapy. She may be willing to explore pharmaceutical interventions if these are not effective.

CHAPTER 26

1. The spouse's description of how many hours of sleep he is getting is suggestive of depression. There are other considerations: Is he severely fatigued? What medications is he taking? Is he using alcohol or drugs to avoid being awake? You need to speak to the patient to assess more fully and to hopefully elicit answers from him.

2. The Patient Health Questionnaire (PHQ)-2 is a brief assessment for depression. If he reports that he is experiencing little interest or pleasure in doing things, or if he is feeling down, depressed, or hopeless, you may want to assess him more fully with the PHQ-9. The patient should be told that he appears depressed and should be offered intervention to help with this.

3. If the patient is not willing to use medication to treat his depression, the first step is to offer supportive care, such as a referral to a therapist who can provide cognitive behavioral therapy. He should also be encouraged to get some physical activity every day. Other supportive care interventions can also be offered, such as mindfulness meditation (many mobile phone apps are available to download). You can also suggest that he speak with his urologist if he has anxiety about the upcoming surgery or the need for more information that may help him worry or ruminate less.

CHAPTER 27

1. A score of 5 on the Distress Thermometer suggests moderate distress and requires interventions such as referral to a psychosocial specialist (social worker or psychologist). You should also offer screening for depression using one or more of the depression screening tools presented in Chapter 26.

2. At a minimum, you can offer education and support, as well as validation that what she is experiencing is normal after a diagnosis of a life-threatening cancer. Anticipatory guidance about what she may also experience during and after a stem cell transplant may result in her agreeing to specialized psychosocial support.

3. You cannot force her to accept a referral for further support, but you should make a note in her chart that your offer of additional support was refused. She should also continue to be screened for distress and/or depression at future visits and during preparation for the transplant, as well as during all treatments and follow-up.

Index

abdomen, physical examination of, 101–102
abiraterone, 187
absolute neutrophil count (ANC), 86
absorbent pad, 147
ACCP. *See* American College of Chest Physicians
acneiform rash, 237
ACS. *See* American Cancer Society
A/CS. *See* Anorexia/Cachexia Subscale
activities of daily living (ADL), 243
acupuncture, 60, 76, 92, 93, 130, 151, 199
  with electrostimulation, 103
acute and chronic pain, 25
ADL. *See* activities of daily living
ADT. *See* androgen deprivation therapy
alopecia, 67–71
  agents causing, 68
  assessment, 68–69
  botanical and herbal supplements, 70
  pharmaceutical agents, 71
  scalp cooling devices, 69–70
alpha-adrenergic agonists, 91
American Academy of Audiology, 217
American Academy of Sleep Medicine, 48
American Board of Physical Therapy Specialties, 166
American Cancer Society (ACS), 110
American College of Chest Physicians (ACCP), 32, 208
American College of Obstetricians and Gynecologists, 172
American College of Physicians, 48–49
American Society of Clinical Oncology (ASCO), 29, 33, 61, 76–77, 86, 110, 120, 129, 171, 188, 200, 222, 253, 260, 262
American Society of Colon and Rectal Surgeons, 151

American Society of Pain and Neuroscience (ASPN), 33
American Speech-Language-Hearing Association, 217
American Thoracic Society, 200
American Urological Association (AUA), 188
Analgesic Ladder, 28
analgesics, 34
anamorelin, 129
ANC. *See* absolute neutrophil count
androgen deprivation therapy (ADT), 92, 93, 186–187
anorexia, 125–132
Anorexia/Cachexia Subscale (A/CS), 127
anticipatory nausea, 115, 118
anticonvulsants, 28, 91
antidepressants, 28, 90, 261
antiemetic-induced constipation, 103
antimuscarinics, 147, 150
anxiety, 44, 149, 249–253, 257
APRN, 3
aquatic exercises, 60
artificial urinary sphincters, 147
ASCO. *See* American Society of Clinical Oncology
ASPN. *See* American Society of Pain and Neuroscience
AUA. *See* American Urological Association
audiologist/auditory clinic, 217
auricular acupressure, 104
automated symptom monitoring system, 221
avanafil, 185
axillary lymph node dissection, 55
axillary radiation therapy, 55

Baseline Dyspnea Index (BDI), 198
BDI. *See* Baseline Dyspnea Index
Beau's lines, 240
benzodiazepines, 199
benzydamine mouthwash, 79
beta-3 agonists, 147, 150
bethanechol, 76
BETTER model, 162
bevacizumab, 207
BFI. *See* Bowel Function Index
bibliotherapy, 261
bimatoprost, 70
BMI. *See* body mass index
Bodily Sensations of Orgasm questionnaire, 169
body mass index (BMI), 128
body-worn sensors, 221
botanical and herbal supplements, 70
Bowel Function Index (BFI), 102
brachytherapy, 183, 207
brain fog, 227
brain tumors, radiation therapy for, 228
breast cancer, 56, 227
    survivors, 56–57, 148
breast sensuality, 170
    loss of, 170–171
Bristol Stool Chart, 102
Bristol Stool Scale, 109
British Society of Gastroenterology, 110
bronchodilators, 199
bronchoscopy, 208
bupropion, 90

cachexia, 125–132
CaDC. *See* Cancer Distress Coach
CADS. *See* Chemotherapy-Induced Alopecia Distress Scale
CALM. *See* Cancer and Living Meaningfully
Canadian Association of Psychosocial Oncology (CAPO), 270
Canadian Urological Association, 152
Cancer and Living Meaningfully (CALM), 230
cancer cachexia, 125
cancer care, 3
Cancer Distress Coach (CaDC), 270
cancer pain, 25–34
    assessment, 26–27
    barriers to pain management, 29

contributing factors, 25–26
    guidelines, 32–34
    management, 28–32
    nonpharmaceutical management, 29
    prevalence, 25
    self-management, 32
cancer-related fatigue (CRF), 15–19
    assessment, 16–17
    contributing factors, 15–16
    guidelines, 19
    management, 17–19
    nonpharmaceutical interventions, 18
    pharmaceutical interventions, 18
    prevalence, 15
    psychosocial interventions, 18–19
    self-management, 19
Cancer Worry Scale, 252
cannabinoids (dronabinol), 118, 119, 130
    types of, 31
cannabis, 29–31, 119
capecitabine, 237
capecitabine plus irinotecan, 107
CAPO. *See* Canadian Association of Psychosocial Oncology
CARD model, 162
CARE. *See* Consultation and Relational Empathy
case studies, 275–284
CBT. *See* cognitive behavioral therapy
CCIS. *See* Cleveland Clinic Fecal Incontinence Severity Scoring System
CDT. *See* complex lymphatic therapy
cervical cancer, 56, 169
chemo brain, 227
chemotherapy, 15, 67, 70, 85
chemotherapy agents, 115, 116, 238
chemotherapy-associated nail changes, 242, 243
Chemotherapy-Induced Alopecia Distress Scale (CADS), 68–69
chemotherapy-induced diarrhea (CID), 108
chemotherapy-induced menopause, 162
chemotherapy-induced nausea and vomiting (CINV), 115–118
    complementary therapies for, 119
chemotherapy-induced peripheral neuropathy (CIPN), 219, 220, 222
cholinergic agents, 76
Choosing Wisely initiative, 47
chronic obstructive pulmonary disease (COPD), 197

CID. *See* chemotherapy-induced diarrhea
CINV. *See* chemotherapy-induced nausea and vomiting
CIPN. *See* chemotherapy-induced peripheral neuropathy
Cleveland Clinic Fecal Incontinence Severity Scoring System (CCIS), 151
climacturia, 146
clinical assessment, 5
clonidine, 91
Cochrane review, 130
cognitive behavioral interventions, 46
cognitive behavioral therapy (CBT), 18, 92, 260
cognitive changes, 227
cognitive dysfunction, 227–230
cognitive rehabilitation, 229
CO$_2$ laser treatment, 149
Common Terminology Criteria for Adverse Events (CTCAE), 68, 108, 138, 139, 215
National Cancer Institute, 221
complementary therapies, 118, 119
complex lymphatic therapy (CDT), 59
computer-based cognitive training, 230
condom catheter, 147
conserving energy, 19
constipation, 101–104
antiemetic-induced, 103
first-line agents for, 102
nonpharmaceutical management, 103
pharmaceutical management, 103
Consultation and Relational Empathy (CARE), 8
Continence Product Advisor, 149
cooling system, 70
COPD. *See* chronic obstructive pulmonary disease
corticosteroids, 129
CRF. *See* cancer-related fatigue
cryotherapy, 79
CTCAE. *See* Common Terminology Criteria for Adverse Events
cyproterone acetate, 93
cystoscopy, 146
cytokines, 125

DADDS. *See* Death and Dying Distress Scale
DAQ. *See* Death Anxiety Questionnaire

Dean Scale, 68, 69
Death and Dying Distress Scale (DADDS), 252
death anxiety, 252
Death Anxiety Questionnaire (DAQ), 252
decongestive lymphatic therapy (DLT), 59
dehydroepiandrosterone (DHEA), 165, 168
depression, 44, 149, 257–262
assessment, 258–259
contributing factors, 257–258
management, 260
prevalence, 258
symptoms, 258
dexamethasone, 18
DHEA. *See* dehydroepiandrosterone
diarrhea, 107–110
diet, 18
dietary intake, 127
DigniCap, 70
dilators, 166–167
distress, 26, 162, 267–271
DLT. *See* decongestive lymphatic therapy
docetaxel, 239
drug–drug interactions, 31
dry mouth, 76
Dysfunctional Beliefs and Attitudes About Sleep Scale for Cancer Patients (C-DBAS-14), 45
dyspareunia, 164–168
dilators, 166–167
lasers and energy-based devices, 167
lubricants, 165–166
management, 165
mindfulness meditation, 167
moisturizers, 165
dysphagia, 137–140
assessment, 138–139
assessment tools, 139
contributing factors, 137–138
management, 139
dyspnea, 197–200

early palliative care, 27
ED. *See* erectile dysfunction
Edmonton Symptom Assessment Scale Revised (ESAS-r), 16–17, 45
electroacupuncture, 93, 149
electronic patient-reported outcome measures (ePROMs), 5, 7
emesis, risk categories for, 116

288 INDEX

emetogenic agents, 117
emotional health, 6
environmental factors, 219
enzalutamide, 187
ePROMs. *See* electronic patient-reported outcome measures
erectile dysfunction (ED), 183–186
ESAS-r. *See* Edmonton Symptom Assessment Scale Revised
ESMO. *See* European Society for Medical Oncology
European Association of Urology (EAU), 152
European Society for Medical Oncology (ESMO), 28, 33, 110, 120, 129, 244
evidence-based interventions, 3
exercise, 18, 46, 59–60, 130, 251
external lymphedema, 58

FAACT. *See* Functional Assessment of Anorexia/Cachexia Therapy
Faces Pain Rating Scale, 27
FACIT-Fatigue. *See* Functional Assessment of Chronic Illness Therapy-Fatigue Scale
FACT-C. *See* Functional Assessment of Cancer Therapy-Colorectal
family caregivers, 32
fatigue, 44
fear of cancer recurrence, 251–252
febrile neutropenia, 85–87
fecal incontinence, 145, 150–151
Fecal Incontinence Quality of Life Scale, 151
Female Sexual Function Index (FSFI), 164
fever, 85–87
Fitch's model, 270
5 A's model, 162
fixed-dose oxycodone/naloxone prolonged-release tablets (OXN PR), 103
fluoxetine, 90
Food and Drug Administration (FDA), 70, 169
formal pad testing, 146
FSFI. *See* Female Sexual Function Index
Functional Assessment of Anorexia/Cachexia Therapy (FAACT), 127

Functional Assessment of Cancer Therapy (FACT-G), 116
Functional Assessment of Cancer Therapy-Colorectal (FACT-C), 151
Functional Assessment of Chronic Illness Therapy-Fatigue Scale (FACIT-Fatigue), 17

gabapentin, 28, 91, 93
GAD-7. *See* seven-item Generalized Anxiety Disorder
gaming systems, 221
Gastrointestinal Quality of Life Index, 150
gastrointestinal symptoms, 3
G-CSF. *See* granulocyte-colony stimulating factor
gemcitabine, 239
general symptoms, 3
genitourinary symptoms, 3
grading systems, 126–127
granulocyte-colony stimulating factor (G-CSF), 86
gut microbiome, 107
gynecologic cancer, 56, 149, 167, 168

HADS. *See* Hospital Anxiety and Depression Scale
hair loss, 67
hand–foot skin reaction (HFSR), 237, 239
head and neck cancer, 58, 78, 137
healthy diet, 59
hearing loss, 213–217
hemoptysis, 207–208
HFSR. *See* hand–foot skin reaction
high body mass, 56
high-fiber diet, 110
hormonal therapies, 93
Hospital Anxiety and Depression Scale (HADS), 259, 269
hot flashes, 89–94
Hot Flash Related Daily Interference Scale, 89, 90
human papillomavirus (HPV), 137
hyaluronic gel, 239
hybrid lubricants, 166
hyperbaric oxygen treatment, 76
hypnosis, 91, 251

IMRT. *See* intensity modulated radiation therapy
incontinence, 145–152
  fecal, 145, 150–151
  measures, 147
  in men, 145–148
  urinary, 145
  in women, 148–150
inflammation, 125, 128
Insomnia Severity Index (ISI), 45
inspiratory muscle training, 199
integrative therapies, for pain, 30
intensity modulated radiation therapy (IMRT), 75
intermittent therapy, 187
International Cognition and Cancer Task Force, 230
International Society of Oral Oncology (ISOO), 76–77, 79, 80
intravaginal testosterone, 169
ISI. *See* Insomnia Severity Index
ISOO. *See* International Society of Oral Oncology

Jenkins Sleep Scale (JSS), 45
JSS. *See* Jenkins Sleep Scale

ketamine, 28
kinesio taping, 60

laparoscopic nerve-sparing radical hysterectomy, 148
LARS. *See* low anterior resection syndrome
lasers and energy-based devices, 167
lidocaine, 167
Li-ESWT. *See* low-intensity extracorporeal shockwave therapy
life-threatening hemoptysis, 207
Likert scale, 101, 116, 151, 252, 269
local low-dose estrogen, 168
loperamide, 110, 151
loss of breast sensuality, 170–171
loss of libido, 162–163, 186–187
low anterior resection syndrome (LARS), 150
low-dose intravaginal estriol, 150
lower limb lymphedema, 57, 60
low-income ethnic minority, 257

low-intensity extracorporeal shockwave therapy (Li-ESWT), 186
lubricants, 165–166
lung cancer, 197
lymphatic therapy, 59
lymphedema, 55–62
  assessment, 56–58
  contributing factor, 55–56
  guidelines, 61
  lymphatic therapy, 59
  patient-reported outcome measures for, 57
  prevalence, 55
  prevention, 59
  stages, 58

Manchester Health Questionnaire, 151
manual lymphatic drainage (MLD), 59
manual lymph drainage, 60
MASCC. *See* Multinational Association of Supportive Care in Cancer
MASCC Antiemesis Tool (MAT), 116
MAT. *See* MASCC Antiemesis Tool
MBSR. *See* mindfulness-based stress reduction
MD Anderson Symptom Inventory (MDASI), 17
MDASI. *See* MD Anderson Symptom Inventory
Mees' lines, 240, 241
megestrol acetate, 129
Memorial Symptom Assessment Scale, 116
men
  incontinence in, 145–148
  sexual dysfunction in, 183–188
menopause
  genitourinary syndrome, 164
  surgical, 162
metastatic bone pain, 29
methylphenidate, 18
mHealth. *See* mobile health
mild hot flashes, 91
mind–body interventions, 30, 46, 47
mindfulness-based sex therapy, 163
mindfulness-based stress, 230
mindfulness-based stress reduction (MBSR), 250
mindfulness meditation, 167, 185
Mini-Mental State Examination (MMSE), 228
minoxidil, 70

MLD. *See* manual lymphatic drainage
MMSE. *See* Mini-Mental State Examination
mobile app, 270
mobile health (mHealth), 19
MOCA. *See* Montreal Cognitive Assessment
modafinil, 18
moderate neutropenia, 86
moisturizers, 165
monitoring program, 215
Montreal Cognitive Assessment (MOCA), 228
Muehrcke lines, 240, 241
Multinational Association of Supportive Care in Cancer (MASCC), 76–77, 79, 80, 120
  Risk Index for Febrile Neutropenia, 86

nail bed, 240
nail changes, 240–244
nail matrix, 240
nail plate, 240
NAMS. *See* North American Menopause Society
National Cancer Institute (NCI), 33, 120
National Comprehensive Cancer Network (NCCN), 28, 33, 49, 57, 61, 94, 120, 171, 188, 230, 253, 262, 270
  screening question, 17, 46
National Lymphedema Network, 61
nausea and vomiting, 115–121
NCCN. *See* National Comprehensive Cancer Network
NCCN Distress Thermometer, 269
NCI. *See* National Cancer Institute
nebulized opioids, 199
nerve stimulation, 151
neurologic symptoms, 4, 219–223
neuropathic pain, 26, 29, 30
nociceptive pain, 26
nonhormonal therapies, 93
nonlife-threatening hemoptysis, 207
nontargeted chemotherapy agents, 238
North American Menopause Society (NAMS), 171
Numeric Rating Scale (NRS), 26–27

OIBD. *See* opioid-induced bowel dysfunction
olanzapine, 118, 129

OMAS. *See* Oral Mucositis Assessment Scale
oncology nurse, 3
Oncology Nursing Society (ONS), 33, 94, 120, 172, 188, 222, 244, 262
ONS. *See* Oncology Nursing Society
opioid-induced bowel dysfunction (OIBD), 101
opioid-induced constipation, 101
opioids, 29, 199
oral mucositis, 77–80
Oral Mucositis Assessment Scale (OMAS), 78
oromucosal spray (Sativex), 31
ospemifene, 168
ototoxicity, 217
oxaliplatin, 219
OXN PR. *See* fixed-dose oxycodone/ naloxone prolonged-release tablets

paclitaxel, 219
PAC Symptoms Questionnaire. *See* Patient Assessment of Constipation Symptoms Questionnaire
pain, 25
  additional questions related to, 26
  cancer. *See* cancer pain
  cannabis for, 30
  and distress, 26
  and fatigue, 44
  integrative therapies for, 30
  management, 26, 28
  measures, 27
  metastatic bone, 29
  with penetration (dyspareunia), 162
  treatment-related, 26
pain–fatigue–sleep disturbance cluster, 19
palliative care, 27
palliative sedation, 199–200
palmar-plantar erythrodysesthesia, 237
PAMORAs. *See* peripherally acting mu-opioid receptor antagonists
papulopustular rash, 237
parenteral nutrition, 130
paronychia, 242
paroxetine, 90, 93
Patient Assessment of Constipation (PAC) Symptoms Questionnaire, 101–102
patient education, 59, 80, 109, 151
Patient Health Questionnaire-2 (PHQ-2), 258, 259

INDEX **291**

patient-reported outcome measures (PROMs), 5–8
  barriers to use, 7
  electronic, 7
  for lower extremity lymphedema, 58
  for lymphedema, 57
patient-reported outcomes (PROs), 5
  domain framework and outcome measures, 6
Patient-Reported Outcomes (PRO)-CTCAE scale, 68
Patient-Reported Outcomes Measurement Information System (PROMIS), 17, 165
  Sleep Disturbance Short Form, 45
patient-reported experience measures (PREMs), 5, 7–8, 26
Paxman system, 70
pelvic floor dysfunction, 169
pelvic floor muscle exercises/training, 146–147, 149, 151
pelvic floor muscle therapy, 186
pelvic floor physiotherapy, 166
penile clamp, 147
penile implant, 185
penile pump, 185
penile rehabilitation, 185
peripherally acting mu-opioid receptor antagonists (PAMORAs), 103
peripheral neuropathy, 18, 220
periungual pyogenic granuloma, 242
perometry, 58
Peyronie disease, 188
pharmaceutical agents, 71
pharmaceutical sleep agents, 47
photobiomodulation therapy, 60
PHQ-2. *See* Patient Health Questionnaire-2
physical examination, 127
physical exercise, 260
physical health, 6
Pittsburgh Sleep Quality Index (PSQI), 44–45
placebo effect, 92
platinum-based chemotherapy, 213
platinum-based therapy, 217
PLISSIT model, 162
postmenopausal women, 164
pregabalin, 28, 91
PREMs. *See* patient-reported experience measures
preoperative pelvic muscle training, 147

prescription strength laxatives, 103
probiotics, 80, 110
progesterone analogs, 129
progressive resistance exercise, 130
PROMIS. *See* Patient-Reported Outcomes Measurement Information System
PROMs. *See* patient-reported outcome measures
PROs. *See* patient-reported outcomes
prostate cancer, 145, 227
PSQI. *See* Pittsburgh Sleep Quality Index
psychoeducation, 261
psychoeducation methods, 230
psychosocial interventions, 18–19
psychosocial symptoms, 4
psychostimulants, 262
pulmonary cancer, 207
pulmonary symptoms, 4

radiation-induced oral mucositis grading scale, 78
radiation therapy, 15, 29, 183, 213
  agents, 117
  for brain tumors, 228
  head or neck cancer, 75
radiation therapy-induced nausea and vomiting (RINV), 115, 117
Radiation Therapy Oncology Group (RTOG) Dysphagia Grading Scale, 138
radical prostatectomy, 145
RDAS. *See* Revised Death Anxiety Scale
rectal or anal cancer, 169
resistance exercise, 59
Revised Death Anxiety Scale (RDAS), 252
Revised Hearing Handicap Inventory (RHHI), 214
RHHI. *See* Revised Hearing Handicap Inventory
RINV. *See* radiation therapy-induced nausea and vomiting
RTOG Dysphagia Grading Scale. *See* Radiation Therapy Oncology Group Dysphagia Grading Scale

sacral nerve stimulation, 151
saliva, 76
sarcopenia, 15
SBRT. *See* stereotactic body radiation

292 INDEX

scalp cooling devices, 69–70
scanxiety, 249
selective estrogen receptor modulator (SERM), 168
selective serotonin reuptake inhibitors, 90, 261
self-management, 19
SERM. *See* selective estrogen receptor modulator
serotonin–norepinephrine reuptake inhibitors, 261
seven-item Generalized Anxiety Disorder (GAD-7), 250
sex therapy, 163
sexual dysfunction
  in men, 183–188
  side effects, 187–188
  in women, 161–172
    alterations in orgasms, 169
    assessment, 161–162
    body image changes, 169–170
    dyspareunia, 164–168
    loss of breast sensuality, 170–171
    loss of libido, 162–163
sexuality, assessment models, 162
short-term corticosteroids, 129
short-term systemic corticosteroids, 199
silicone lubricants, 166–167
skin, 237–239
sleep disturbances, 17, 43, 93
  assessment, 44–46
  cognitive behavioral interventions, 46
  contributing factors, 43–44
  exercise, 46
  guidelines, 48–49
  nonpharmaceutical interventions, 46
  objective measures, 45
  prevalence, 43
  sleep hygiene, 46, 47
sleep hygiene, 46, 47
smoking cannabis, 31
social health, 6
Society for Integrative Oncology, 33
sorafenib, 126
squamous cell lung cancer, 207
State of Spirituality Scale, 269
stenosis, 166
step-care model, 270
stepped-care approach, 261
stereotactic body radiation (SBRT), 183

STIDAT. *See* Systemic Therapy-Induced Assessment Tool
stress urinary incontinence (SUI), 145, 146
SUI. *See* stress urinary incontinence
surgical menopause, 162
swallowing, 138
swimming exercises, 60
"symptom management," 27
systematic pain assessment, 29
Systemic Therapy-Induced Assessment Tool (STIDAT), 109

targeted chemotherapy agents, 238
T-DAS. *See* Templer's Death Anxiety Scale
TEC. *See* toxic erythema of chemotherapy
Templer's Death Anxiety Scale (T-DAS), 252
tetrahydrocannabinol (THC), 30
THC. *See* tetrahydrocannabinol
therapeutic exercise, 30
tinnitus, 213
  grading, 215
Tinnitus Primary Function Questionnaire (TPFQ), 215–216
toxic erythema of chemotherapy (TEC), 237–239
TPFQ. *See* Tinnitus Primary Function Questionnaire
transcutaneous electrostimulation, 76
trazadone, 261
treatment-related diarrhea, 108
treatment-related pain, 26
tricyclic antidepressants, 261
Trimix, 185
tube feeding, 130
tyrosine kinase inhibitors, 107

unrelieved severe pain, 25
urethral bulking agents, 148
urge urinary incontinence (UUI), 145, 146
urinary incontinence, 145, 148. *See also* incontinence
urodynamics, 146
UUI. *See* urge urinary incontinence

vacuum device. *See* penile pump
Vaginal Assessment Scale (VAS), 164
vaginal mesh surgery, 150

INDEX **293**

vaginal moisturizers, 165
VAS. *See* Visual Analog Scale
visceral pain, 26
Visual Analog Scale (VAS), 27, 127
vitamins, 18
VuAS. *See* Vulvar Assessment Scale
Vulvar Assessment Scale (VuAS), 164
vulvovaginal atrophy (VVA), 164
VVA. *See* vulvovaginal atrophy

water-based lubricants, 166
water displacement, 58
weight loss, 126
  anorexia and, 128

Weight Loss Grading System (WLGS),
  127, 128
Wexner Score, 151
WHO. *See* World Health Organization
WLGS. *See* Weight Loss Grading System
women
  incontinence in, 148–150
  sexual dysfunction in, 161–172
World Health Organization (WHO), 34

xerostomia, 75–77

yoga, 18, 91

www.ingramcontent.com/pod-product-compliance
Lightning Source LLC
LaVergne TN
LVHW061727060925
820435LV00019B/168